# Modern Approaches for Evaluation and Treatment of GI Motility Disorders

*Editor*

HENRY P. PARKMAN

## GASTROENTEROLOGY CLINICS OF NORTH AMERICA

www.gastro.theclinics.com

*Consulting Editor*
ALAN L. BUCHMAN

September 2020 • Volume 49 • Number 3

**ELSEVIER**

1600 John F. Kennedy Boulevard • Suite 1800 • Philadelphia, Pennsylvania, 19103-2899
http://www.theclinics.com

**GASTROENTEROLOGY CLINICS OF NORTH AMERICA Volume 49, Number 3
September 2020 ISSN 0889-8553, ISBN-13: 978-0-323-71299-6**

Editor: Kerry Holland
Developmental Editor: Julia McKenzie

*Gastroenterology Clinics of North America* (ISSN 0889-8553) is published quarterly by Elsevier Inc., 360 Park Avenue South, New York, NY 10010-1710. Months of issue are March, June, September, and December. Business and Editorial Offices: 1600 John F. Kennedy Blvd., Suite 1800, Philadelphia, PA 19103-2899. Customer Service Office: 6277 Sea Harbor Drive, Orlando, FL 32887-4800. Periodicals postage paid at New York, NY and additional mailing offices. Subscription prices are $365.00 per year (US individuals), $100.00 per year (US students), $730.00 per year (US institutions), $387.00 per year (Canadian individuals), $100.00 per year (Canadian students), $896.00 per year (Canadian institutions), $463.00 per year (international individuals), $220.00 per year (international students), and $896.00 per year (international institutions). Foreign air speed delivery is included in all *Clinics* subscription prices. All prices are subject to change without notice. **POSTMASTER:** Send address changes to *Gastroenterology Clinics of North America*, Elsevier Health Sciences Division, Subscription Customer Service, 3251 Riverport Lane, Maryland Heights, MO 63043. **Telephone: 1-800-654-2452 (U.S. and Canada); 314-447-8871 (outside U.S. and Canada). Fax: 314-447-8029. E-mail: journalscustomerservice-usa@elsevier.com (for print support); journalsonlinesupport-usa@elsevier.com (for online support).**

*Reprints.* For copies of 100 or more, of articles in this publication, please contact the Commercial Reprints Department, Elsevier Inc., 360 Part Avenue South, New York, New York 10010-1710. Tel. 212-633-3874, Fax: 212-633-3820, E-mail: reprints@elsevier.com.

*Gastroenterology Clinics of North America* is also published in Italian by Il Pensiero Scientifico Editore, Rome, Italy; and in Portuguese by Interlivros Edicoes Ltda., Rua Commandante Coelho 1085, 21250 Cordovil, Rio de Janeiro, Brazil.

*Gastroenterology Clinics of North America* is covered in *MEDLINE/PubMed (Index Medicus), Excerpta Medica, Current Contents/Clinical Medicine, Science Citation Index, ISI/BIOMED,* and *BIOSIS.*

# Contributors

## CONSULTING EDITOR

**ALAN L. BUCHMAN, MD, MSPH, FACP, FACN, FACG, AGAF**
Professor of Clinical Surgery, Medical Director, Intestinal Rehabilitation and Transplant Center, The University of Illinois at Chicago/UI Health, Chicago, Illinois

## EDITOR

**HENRY P. PARKMAN, MD**
Professor of Medicine, GI Section, Stanley Lorber Chair of Gastroenterology, Director of GI Motility Laboratory, Vice Chair of Research, Department of Medicine, Lewis Katz School of Medicine, Temple University and Temple University Hospital, Philadelphia, Pennsylvania

## AUTHORS

**ABBAS E. ABBAS, MD, MS, FACS**
Professor and Surgeon-in-Chief, Department of Thoracic Medicine and Surgery, Temple University Hospital, Lewis Katz School of Medicine, Temple University, Philadelphia, Pennsylvania

**CHARLES T. BAKHOS, MD, MS, FACS**
Associate Professor, Department of Thoracic Medicine and Surgery, Temple University Hospital, Lewis Katz School of Medicine, Temple University, Philadelphia, Pennsylvania

**JUSTIN BRANDLER, MD**
Division of Gastroenterology and Hepatology, Mayo Clinic, Rochester, Minnesota

**MICHAEL CAMILLERI, MD**
Professor of Medicine, Pharmacology, and Physiology, Mayo Clinic College of Medicine and Science, Consultant, Division of Gastroenterology and Hepatology, Mayo Clinic, Rochester, Minnesota

**WILLIAM D. CHEY, MD, AGAF, FACG, FACP**
University of Michigan – Michigan Medicine, Ann Arbor, Michigan

**LAKSHMIKANTH L. CHIKKAMENAHALLI, PhD**
Research Fellow, Enteric NeuroScience Program, Divisions of Gastroenterology and Hepatology, and Physiology and Biomedical Engineering, Mayo Clinic, Rochester, Minnesota

**ERICA N. DONNAN, MD**
Instructor of Medicine, Division of Gastroenterology and Hepatology, Department of Medicine, Feinberg School of Medicine, Northwestern University, NMH/Arkes Family Pavilion, Chicago, Illinois

**ROMULO A. FAJARDO, MD**
Resident, Department of General Surgery, Temple University Hospital, Philadelphia, Pennsylvania

**GIANRICO FARRUGIA, MD**
Professor of Medicine, Professor of Physiology and Biomedical Engineering, Enteric NeuroScience Program, Divisions of Gastroenterology and Hepatology, and Physiology and Biomedical Engineering, Mayo Clinic, Rochester, Minnesota

**BRIAN GINNEBAUGH, MD, MS**
Gastroenterology Fellow, Internal Medicine, University of Michigan, Ann Arbor, Michigan

**MADHUSUDAN GROVER, MBBS**
Assistant Professor of Medicine, Assistant Professor of Physiology and Biomedical Engineering, Enteric NeuroScience Program, Divisions of Gastroenterology and Hepatology, and Physiology and Biomedical Engineering, Mayo Clinic, Rochester, Minnesota

**C. PRAKASH GYAWALI, MD, MRCP**
Professor of Medicine, Division of Gastroenterology, Washington University School of Medicine, St Louis, Missouri

**WILLIAM L. HASLER, MD**
Professor, Division of Gastroenterology and Hepatology, University of Michigan Health System, Ann Arbor, Michigan

**ALICE C. JIANG, MD**
Division of Gastroenterology, Department of Internal Medicine, Rush University Medical Center, Chicago, Illinois

**ZUBAIR MALIK, MD**
Assistant Professor of Medicine, Lewis Katz School of Medicine, Temple University, Director, Esophageal Program, GI Section, Temple University Hospital, Philadelphia, Pennsylvania

**ALAN H. MAURER, MD**
Department of Radiology, Nuclear Medicine Section, Department of Medicine, Gastroenterology Section, Lewis Katz School of Medicine, Temple University, Temple University Hospital, Philadelphia, Pennsylvania

**AMI PANARA, MD**
Division of Gastroenterology, Department of Internal Medicine, University of Miami Leonard M. Miller School of Medicine, Miami, Florida

**JOHN E. PANDOLFINO, MD, MSCI**
Chief of Gastroenterology and Hepatology, Professor of Medicine, Division of Gastroenterology and Hepatology, Department of Medicine, Feinberg School of Medicine, Northwestern University, NMH/Arkes Family Pavilion, Chicago, Illinois

**HENRY P. PARKMAN, MD**
Professor of Medicine, GI Section, Stanley Lorber Chair of Gastroenterology, Director of GI Motility Laboratory, Vice Chair of Research, Department of Medicine, Lewis Katz School of Medicine, Temple University and Temple University Hospital, Philadelphia, Pennsylvania

**PANKAJ J. PASRICHA, MBBS, MD**
Professor of Medicine, Professor of Neurosciences, Division of Gastroenterology and Hepatology, Center for Neurogastroenterology, Johns Hopkins School of Medicine, Baltimore, Maryland

**ROMAN V. PETROV, MD, PhD, FACS**
Associate Professor, Department of Thoracic Medicine and Surgery, Temple University Hospital, Lewis Katz School of Medicine, Temple University, Philadelphia, Pennsylvania

**SATISH S.C. RAO, MD, PhD**
Professor of Medicine, Division of Gastroenterology and Hepatology, Augusta University Medical Center, Augusta, Georgia

**BENJAMIN D. ROGERS, MD**
Division of Gastroenterology, Washington University School of Medicine, St Louis, Missouri

**RICHARD SAAD, MD, MS, FACG**
University of Michigan – Michigan Medicine, Ann Arbor, Michigan

**RON SCHEY, MD, FACG**
Director Neurogastroenterology and Esophageal Program, Division of Gastroenterology/Hepatology, Department of Internal Medicine, University of Florida College of Medicine, Jacksonville, Florida

**KARTIK SHENOY, MD**
Associate Professor, Thoracic Medicine and Surgery, Lewis Katz School of Medicine, Temple University, Director, Lung Volume Reduction Surgery Program, Temple University Hospital, Philadelphia, Pennsylvania

**STUART JON SPECHLER, MD**
Division of Gastroenterology, Center for Esophageal Diseases, Baylor University Medical Center, Center for Esophageal Research, Baylor Scott & White Research Institute, Dallas, Texas

**LAUREN STEMBOROSKI, DO**
Division of Gastroenterology/Hepatology, Department of Internal Medicine, University of Florida College of Medicine, Jacksonville, Florida

**YUN YAN, MD**
Division of Gastroenterology and Hepatology, Department of Internal Medicine, Augusta University, Augusta, Georgia

# Contents

High-resolution manometry evaluates esophageal motor function using 10 supine water swallows. Superimposing impedance over high-resolution manometry pressure topography assesses the relationship between contraction and bolus propulsion and identifies inadequate clearance. Ancillary techniques and maneuvers augment the standard supine high-resolution manometry evaluation by challenging peristaltic function. Increasing bolus volume (rapid drink challenge) and altering bolus consistency (standardized test meal, solid swallows) enhance identification of esophageal outflow obstruction syndromes. Physiologic maneuvers (multiple rapid swallows, abdominal compression) address the ability of the esophageal smooth muscle to augment contraction vigor. Pharmacologic challenge is less commonly used clinically, and elucidates pathophysiology of esophageal motor disorders.

The functional luminal imaging probe (FLIP) uses high-resolution planimetry to provide a three-dimensional image of the esophageal lumen by measuring diameter, volume, and pressure changes. Literature surrounding use of FLIP has demonstrated its clinical utility as a diagnostic tool and as a device to guide and measure response to therapy. FLIP can assess and guide treatments for esophageal disease states including gastroesophageal reflux disease, achalasia, and eosinophilic esophagitis. FLIP may become the initial test for patients with undifferentiated dysphagia at their index endoscopy. This article summarizes use of FLIP in assessing sphincter function, wall stiffness, and motility to guide treatments.

Despite the exceptional efficacy of proton pump inhibitors (PPIs) in healing reflux esophagitis complicating gastroesophageal reflux disease (GERD), up to 40% of patients who take PPIs for GERD complain of persistent GERD symptoms. There is no clear consensus on the type, dosing, and duration of PPI therapy required to establish a diagnosis of PPI-refractory GERD symptoms, but most authorities do not consider patients "PPI-refractory" unless they have been on double-dose PPIs. This article discusses the mechanisms that might underlie heartburn that does not respond PPIs and an approach to the management of patients with PPI-refractory GERD symptoms.

Lung transplantation is a high-risk, but lifesaving, procedure for patients with end-stage lung disease. Although 1-year survival is high, long-term survival is not nearly as high, due mainly to acute and chronic rejection. Bronchiolitis obliterans syndrome is the most common type of chronic rejection and often leads to poor outcomes. For this reason, esophageal testing in the lung transplant population has become a major issue, and this article discusses the evidence behind esophageal testing, the importance of esophageal dysmotility gastroesophageal reflux disease, both acidic and nonacidic reflux, and aspiration and the treatment of these findings.

The incidence of gastroesophageal reflux disease (GERD) remains on the rise. Pathophysiology of GERD is multifactorial, revolving around an incompetent esophagogastric junction as an antireflux barrier, with other comorbid conditions contributing to the disease. Proton pump inhibitors remain the most common treatment of GERD. Endoscopic therapy has gained popularity as a less invasive option. The presence of esophageal dysmotility complicates the choice of surgical fundoplication. Most literature demonstrates that fundoplication is safe in the setting of ineffective or weak peristalsis and that postoperative dysphagia cannot be predicted by preoperative manometry parameters. More data are needed on the merits of endoluminal approaches to GERD.

Achalasia is a progressive neurodegenerative disorder characterized by failure of relaxation of the lower esophageal sphincter (LES) and altered motility of the esophagus. The traditional, highly effective, surgical approach to relieve obstruction at the LES includes cardiomyotomy. Fundoplication is added to decrease risk of postoperative reflux. Per oral endoscopic myotomy is a new endoscopic procedure that allows division of the LES via transoral route. It has several advantages including less invasiveness, cosmesis, and tailored approach to the length on the myotomy. However, it is associated with increased rate of post-procedural reflux. Various endoscopic interventions are used to address this problem.

## Gastric

This article reviews the latest enhancements in standards and technology for performing gastric emptying and associated small bowel and colon transit scintigraphic studies. It discusses how developments in appropriate use criteria, American Medical Association Current Procedural Terminology coding, and advanced commercial software permit clinicians to obtain more comprehensive physiologic studies of gastric, small bowel, and colon gastrointestinal motility disorders. It shows how gastrointestinal scintigraphy has expanded to permit assessments of global and regional (fundic and antral) gastric motility and how it permits a single study (whole-gut transit scintigraphy), including measurement of solid and liquid gastric emptying and small bowel and colon transit.

Gastroparesis presents with nausea, vomiting, and other upper gut symptoms, and is diagnosed by confirming delayed gastric emptying. A related condition, chronic unexplained nausea and vomiting, has similar symptoms but with normal emptying. Both conditions are managed using therapies with diverse mechanisms of action. Even though prokinetic treatments are proposed to improve gastroparesis by accelerating gastric emptying, there is limited evidence that they provide benefit by virtue of transit stimulating effects. Other tests can delineate alterations in other gut sensorimotor parameters in patients with suspected gastroparesis, but their relation to symptoms and their capability to guide treatment are largely unproved.

Gastroparesis is a complex chronic debilitating condition of gastric motility resulting in the delayed gastric emptying and multiple severe symptoms, which may lead to malnutrition and dehydration. Initial management of patients with gastroparesis focuses on the diet, lifestyle modification and medical therapy. Various endoscopic and surgical interventions are reserved for refractory cases of gastroparesis, not responding to conservative therapy. Pyloric interventions, enteral access tubes, gastric electrical stimulator and gastrectomy have been described in the care of patients with gastroparesis. In this article, the authors review current management, indications, and contraindications to these procedures.

The cellular and molecular understanding of human gastroparesis has markedly improved due to studies on full-thickness gastric biopsies. A decrease in the number of interstitial cells of Cajal (ICC) and functional changes in ICC constitutes the hallmark cellular feature of gastroparesis. More recently, in animal models, macrophages have also been identified to play a central role in development of delayed gastric emptying. Activation of macrophages leads to loss of ICC. In human gastroparesis, loss of anti-inflammatory macrophages in gastric muscle has been shown. Deeper molecular characterization using transcriptomics and proteomics has identified macrophage-based immune dysregulation in human gastroparesis.

Small intestinal bacterial overgrowth (SIBO) is a condition with presentation that can vary from asymptomatic to steatorrhea and malnutrition. Small bowel aspiration and culture is the current gold standard of diagnosis; however, this is invasive and is not without risk to the patient. Breath testing is a noninvasive and less expensive alternative method; however, it lacks diagnostic sensitivity and specificity. Novel diagnostic methods being studied include gas-sensing capsules. The mainstay of treatment is antibiotics; alternative therapies include herbal medications, dietary modifications, and prokinetic agents. Further investigation into less invasive and less harmful diagnostic methods and treatment options is warranted.

Constipation and fecal incontinence are commonly encountered complaints in the gastrointestinal clinic. Assessment of anorectal function includes comprehensive history, rectal examination, and prospective stool diary or electronic App diary that accurately captures bowel symptoms, evaluation of severity, and quality of life of measure. Evaluation of a suspected patient with dyssynergic constipation includes anorectal manometry, balloon expulsion test, and defecography. Investigation of a suspected patient with fecal incontinence includes high-resolution anorectal manometry; anal ultrasound or MRI; and neurophysiology tests, such as translumbosacral anorectal magnetic stimulation or pudendal nerve latency. This article provides an approach to the assessment of anorectal function.

Irritable bowel syndrome (IBS) is probably the most common diagnosis in gastroenterology involving the brain-gut axis. By definition, pain is the most frequent symptom experienced by patients. It is important to understand the biopsychosocial and physiologic aspects of the disease when discussing treatment of IBS. Such therapies as lifestyle modifications, changes in diet, and cognitive behavioral therapy should be used in conjunction with pharmacotherapy rather than pharmacotherapy alone. The pathophysiologic mechanisms are reviewed in this article along with the current treatments available, in the era of growing demand for more effective treatments for the pain component of IBS.

Patients are often referred for treatment of refractory constipation that may result from uncontrolled underlying disease or ineffective treatment. This article reviews clinical testing in patients with refractory constipation, differentiating subtypes of primary chronic idiopathic constipation, and common pitfalls in assessment of refractory chronic constipation. The constipation may also be refractory because of significant associated diseases affecting the colon and resulting in slow transit constipation. The choice of therapy is best guided by the subtype. Management of refractory constipation requires correct diagnosis and individualized treatment, which may rarely include conservative surgery (loop ileostomy).

# GASTROENTEROLOGY
# CLINICS OF NORTH AMERICA

**SERIES OF RELATED INTEREST**

*Gastrointestinal Endoscopy Clinics of North America*
(Available at: https://www.giendo.theclinics.com)
*Clinics in Liver Disease*
(Available at: https://www.liver.theclinics.com)

**THE CLINICS ARE AVAILABLE ONLINE!**
Access your subscription at:
www.theclinics.com

# Foreword

# New Advances in Motility of the Digestive Tract

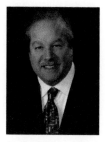

Alan L. Buchman, MD, MSPH
*Consulting Editor*

Dr Parkman has assembled a world-renowned group of experts to provide clinical review articles on motility of the digestive tract. Gastrointestinal absorption affects multiple aspects of life: it affects food intake, digestion, absorption, vitamin synthesis, and also clinical symptoms of bloating, pain, diarrhea, and constipation. The intestinal microbiome is also affected. New diagnostic techniques are allowing for greater insight into these problems, although our medical and surgical therapeutic regimen has yet to catch up to these advances. This issue of *Gastroenterology Clinics of North America*, edited by Dr Parkman, focuses on patient diagnosis and management, the proper use of available clinical testing, the appropriate use of therapies currently available as well as those coming down the pipe, albeit it ever so slowly. The discussions of dyspepsia in patients who fail to respond to management of GERD, gastroparesis, constipation, and small bowel bacterial overgrowth are particularly relevant.

Alan L. Buchman, MD, MSPH
Intestinal Rehabilitation and Transplant Center
Department of Surgery/UI Health
University of Illinois at Chicago
840 South Wood Street
Suite 402 (MC958)
Chicago, IL 60612, USA

*E-mail address:*
buchman@uic.edu

Gastroenterol Clin N Am 49 (2020) xiii
https://doi.org/10.1016/j.gtc.2020.06.002
0889-8553/20/© 2020 Published by Elsevier Inc.

# Preface

# Modern Approaches for Evaluation and Treatment of Gastrointestinal Motility Disorders

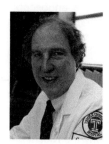

Henry P. Parkman, MD
*Editor*

The time is ripe for this issue of *Gastroenterology Clinics of North America* on the modern approaches for the evaluation and treatment of gastrointestinal (GI) motility disorders. New developments have taken place in the evaluation of patients with symptoms of GI motility disorders: new equipment and new protocols for their use. How to place these new developments into context in the evaluation and management of patients needs clarification. There are also new pharmacologic and surgical treatments currently available. When to use these novel treatments, often endosurgical treatments, is not clear. These tests and treatments are now available not only at academic medical centers but also throughout GI practices, both at academic medical centers and in private practice. The topics chosen for this issue frequently come up in patient management and will be of interest to many others; they are both timely and relevant.

The esophageal section starts out with high-resolution esophageal manometry, discussing how to enhance the study using provocative maneuvers during the testing protocol. The use of endoscopic functional luminal imaging probe (EndoFLIP) is discussed using this technology to assess the lower esophageal sphincter in gastroesophageal reflux disease (GERD) and achalasia, the esophageal lumen in eosinophilic esophagitis, as well as for esophageal manometry during an endoscopic procedure. Gastroenterologists continue to see GERD patients, now often seeing patients with persistent reflux symptoms despite proton-pump inhibitor treatment; evaluation and treatment of these patients are covered. Tailoring endoscopic and surgical treatments for the patient with either GERD or achalasia is discussed. Finally, many academic centers are performing lung transplantation for end-stage lung disease; the esophageal

Gastroenterol Clin N Am 49 (2020) xv–xvi
https://doi.org/10.1016/j.gtc.2020.06.001

evaluation and management of esophageal dysfunction, particularly GERD, which is often led by the gastroenterologist, are covered.

The gastric section starts out with an article on scintigraphy, first discussing gastric emptying and how to enhance the study to better delineate pathophysiology and better correlate symptoms to gastric motility disturbances. Scintigraphy can also assess small bowel transit and colonic transit. The whole-gut transit scintigraphic test can provide valuable information to the clinician to help care for the patient. Does the patient with constipation really have delayed colonic transit, or is it part of a diffuse GI motility disturbance? Knowing this may impact patient management, especially if surgery is being contemplated. Gastroparesis is discussed in several articles, covering the use of clinical tests to guide diagnosis of patients with gastroparesis and treatments for gastroparesis, including medical treatments as well as the endoscopic and surgical treatments for gastroparesis. Finally, full-thickness gastric biopsies can be obtained in patients with gastroparesis; the authors discuss how these full-thickness gastric biopsies provide insights into gastric neuromuscular disorders to help with treatment.

The controversial entity of small intestinal bacterial overgrowth (SIBO) is presented, covering how to diagnose SIBO and then how to treat this disorder initially as well as in case of relapse, which so often happens. Assessing anorectal function with a number of different tests in patients with constipation and fecal incontinence is covered. Importantly, treating chronic abdominal pain is discussed, particularly the recent additions to medical therapy that may help avoid narcotic analgesics. Finally, evaluation and treatment of patients with refractory chronic constipation, a commonly seen entity by gastroenterologists, are discussed.

Reading these articles will provide updates in many areas on modern approaches for the evaluation and treatment of patients with suspected GI motility disorders. I certainly learned a tremendous amount in reading each article. I hope you do also. I would like to thank the many authors contributing to this issue: Thank you, and I hope you like your free copy!

Finally, I am writing this preface to this issue at the height of the COVID-19 pandemic in Philadelphia. I, like most physicians, have spent the last month not performing procedures and seeing patients using telemedicine. I am looking forward to restarting our GI motility laboratory. Another reason this issue will be timely!

Henry P. Parkman, MD
Department of Medicine
GI Motility Laboratory
Lewis Katz School of Medicine
Temple University
Philadelphia, PA, USA

*E-mail address:*
henry.parkman@temple.edu

# ESOPHAGUS

ESOPHAGUS

# Enhancing High-Resolution Esophageal Manometry
## Use of Ancillary Techniques and Maneuvers

Benjamin D. Rogers, MD, C. Prakash Gyawali, MD, MRCP*

### KEYWORDS

- High-resolution impedance manometry • Multiple rapid swallows
- Rapid drink challenge • Standardized test meal
- Postprandial high-resolution manometry

### KEY POINTS

- Impedance topographs can be superimposed on high-resolution manometry Clouse plots, with novel metrics to quantify bolus retention and transit.
- Two simple ancillary high-resolution manometry maneuvers—multiple rapid swallows and rapid drink challenge—identify smooth muscle contraction reserve and unveil obstructive motor physiology, respectively.
- Several other novel mechanical and pharmacologic provocative measures are being evaluated and show promise, but there is insufficient evidence to recommend routine use.

## INTRODUCTION

Conventional manometry, introduced in the 1970s, relied on widely spaced, water-perfused channels to generate linear representations of esophageal pressure changes with water swallows, typically displayed in stacked line tracing format.[1] High-resolution manometry (HRM) was conceived in the 1990s, with significantly higher pressure recording sites in the esophagus and spatiotemporal display of pressure data.[2] This concept changed not just the manometry protocol, but also uncovered novel insights into the mechanics of peristalsis itself. For the first time, esophageal peristalsis was recognized as a synchronized and coordinated chain of contracting muscle segments, anchored by sphincters at either end.[3] The introduction of solid state circumferential pressure sensors further enhanced the technology and allowed visualization of pressure events from the entire esophageal in colorful topographic plots, termed Clouse plots in honor of Ray Clouse who conceived and pioneered HRM.[2] Because pressure data are acquired and assimilated digitally, software tools

Division of Gastroenterology, 660 S. Euclid Ave, Campus Box 8124, St. Louis, MO 63110, USA
* Corresponding author.
E-mail address: cprakash@wustl.edu

Gastroenterol Clin N Am 49 (2020) 411–426
https://doi.org/10.1016/j.gtc.2020.04.001
0889-8553/20/© 2020 Elsevier Inc. All rights reserved.

can be used to interrogate motor function and define physiologic parameters. Shortly after its development, it became apparent that a standardized HRM classification scheme would be required for the characterization of these newly defined physiologic parameters.

The Chicago Classification, soon to be in its fourth iteration, has become the internationally accepted paradigm for describing motor patterns.[4] Within the context of expanding HRM use for the diagnosis of esophageal symptoms, the Chicago Classification has provided a framework for the standardized description of motor patterns in the context of dysphagia and chest pain and has led to improved outcomes from tailored treatment of especially achalasia subtypes.[5]

Standardizing manometry has not been without consequences that have rendered the procedure unphysiologic and not representative of normal swallowing. To evaluate the contribution of esophageal peristalsis in stripping the esophagus of luminal content, gravitational effect is negated by performing the procedure in the supine position.[6] Additionally, to decrease the effects temperature and volume on peristalsis, 5 mL of ambient temperature water are used for each swallow.[4,7] Because these standardized maneuvers do not fully represent normal physiology, provocative measures are often used to enhance the workload of the esophageal smooth muscle, using increased bolus volume,[8] solid swallows,[9] and repetitive swallowing,[10,11] particularly when the standard protocol does not demonstrate motor abnormalities to explain symptoms (**Table 1**).

This review discusses the enhancements that can be made to the 10 water swallow protocol of standard HRM in the evaluation of symptomatic esophageal disorders, using physiologic and pharmacologic provocation maneuvers.

## HIGH-RESOLUTION IMPEDANCE MANOMETRY

By incorporating pairs of electrodes along the length of HRM catheters, stationary impedance can be generated and overlaid into the topographic plot[12] (**Fig. 1**). Impedance decreases when a liquid bolus is present adjacent to an electrode pair in the esophagus, and returns to baseline once the bolus moves beyond the electrodes. Conversely, impedance is high when air is present. Impedance recordings from multiple pairs of electrodes can be assimilated using dedicated software and superimposed on pressure topography to allow visualization of a bolus as it is propelled distally through the esophagus.

The ability to monitor the passage of both liquid and air along the length of the esophagus allows for characterization of bolus movement through the esophageal lumen in both the anterograde and retrograde directions.[13,14] This added dimension assesses and localizes bolus escape in direct correlation with peristalsis.[7,12] (**Table 1**) Although the relationship between bolus transit and esophageal pressurization is imperfect, bolus clearance from combined high-resolution impedance manometry (HRIM) and video fluoroscopy are concordant with that obtained from barium studies, both in healthy individuals and patients with dysphagia.[15] Thus, HRIM could potentially serve as a surrogate for barium studies under certain circumstances,[15] particularly where frequent testing is expected, because this strategy can decrease the amount of radiation a patient receives.

Beyond visualization of bolus movement, HRIM has been shown to correlate with symptoms. The perception of dysphagia associates with time from the nadir impedance, representing intrabolus pressure[16] to peak pressure in the ensuing contraction.[17] Automated analyses of such metrics (automated impedance manometry) applied to HRIM studies demonstrate that nadir impedance and impedance at peak

**Table 1**
Common ancillary maneuvers during clinical esophageal HRM

| | Indications | Methodology | Expected Findings | Abnormal Findings |
|---|---|---|---|---|
| HRIM | As part of routine HRM<br>Regurgitation and belching syndromes<br>Assessment of bolus transit | Use of 5 mL electrolyte solution, for example, saline rather than water during HRM test swallows | Normal bolus transit without bolus escape or bolus retention<br>Normal esophageal impedance integral<br>Normal bolus flow time | Bolus retention<br>Abnormal esophageal impedance integral<br>Abnormal bolus flow time |
| Upright swallows | When EGJ outflow obstruction is seen on supine swallows | Administration of 5 mL swallows in the seated position | Integrated relaxation pressure of <12 mm Hg<br>Normal bolus transit on HRIM | Elevated integrated relaxation pressure<br>Bolus retention |
| Changing bolus volume (rapid drink challenge) | As part of routine HRM<br>Dysphagia<br>Achalasia after therapy | 100–200 mL water through a straw as fast as possible while upright during HRM or HRIM | Inhibition of contraction during swallows, low EGJ gradient<br>Contraction sequence may or may not be present after swallows | Esophageal pressurization and/or high EGJ gradient, indicating obstructive process at EGJ<br>Bolus retention measured as impedance bolus height in cm |
| Changing bolus consistency | Esophageal transit symptoms (dysphagia) not explained on standard HRM with liquid swallows | Viscous swallows[a]<br>Bread swallows[a]<br>Marshmallow swallows[a]<br>Standardized test meal | Normal bolus transit<br>Augmented contraction vigor | Bolus retention<br>Integrated relaxation pressure of >25 mm Hg on standardized test meal<br>Obstructive motor pattern<br>Development of dysphagia |
| Physiologic challenge (multiple rapid swallows) | As part of routine HRM<br>Hypomotility disorders<br>Symptomatic patients with normal motility<br>Before antireflux surgery | Five 2-mL water swallows <3 s apart while supine | Inhibition of contraction during swallows<br>Augmented contraction following swallows (contraction reserve) | Contraction during swallows (abnormal inhibition)<br>No augmentation of contraction following swallows (lack of contraction reserve) |
| Postprandial monitoring | Regurgitation<br>Belching syndromes<br>Postprandial PPI-refractory esophageal symptoms | Variable test meal followed by monitoring for 30–60 min (HRIM can be useful) | Normal motor pattern<br>Infrequent TLESRs | Rumination episodes<br>Supragastric belching episodes<br>Frequent TLESRs |

*Abbreviations:* HRIM, high-resolution impedance manometry; HRM, high-resolution manometry; IRP, integrated relaxation pressure; PPI, proton pump inhibitor; TLESR, transient lower esophageal sphincter relaxation.
[a] Data are limited regarding interpretation of findings.

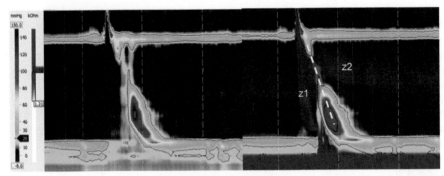

**Fig. 1.** High-resolution impedance manometry (HRIM). Superimposed topographic plots of bolus presence (*violet*) depict bolus presence during esophageal HRIM. Bolus presence is expected before the contraction sequence (z1). Identification of bolus presence following the contraction sequence (z2) constitutes bolus escape or bolus retention. The ratio between z2 and z1 provides the esophageal impedance integral for quantification of bolus escape.

pressures can distinguish normal patients from those with dysphagia. Symptomatic individuals with dysphagia had higher intrabolus pressures and nadir impedance pressures, as well as shorter interval times between nadir and peak pressures. Further, an impedance threshold of 2400 Ω at peak pressure predicted dysphagia with a sensitivity of 0.83, specificity of 0.93, and kappa of 0.77.[17] Thus, these findings suggest that automated impedance manometry can distinguish even subtle abnormalities,[18] paving the way for new insight into bolus transit and symptom generation, and opening new analysis paradigms that are potentially more sensitive that existing ones.[18]

Conversely, where peristaltic breaks are present or when peristalsis fails entirely, both ingested boluses and refluxate can be retained within the esophageal lumen. The likelihood of bolus retention increases significantly with 5 cm or greater breaks in peristaltic integrity (using a 20 mm Hg isobaric contour). The quantification of bolus escape has proven more difficult, but advanced analytical algorithms have been developed in this arena as well, the most intuitive being the esophageal impedance integral.[19] This involves sophisticated processing of HRIM data to measure bolus presence before (Z1) and following peristalsis (Z2) and generating a ratio Z2:Z1 (termed esophageal impedance integral ratio) (**Fig. 1**). The esophageal impedance integral ratio correlates significantly with data from video fluoroscopy (r = 0.96),[19] and allows quantification of bolus transit, not just when breaks are present, but also in normal peristalsis without breaks. Using HRIM with video fluoroscopy, 4 distinct phases of deglutition are identified: upper esophageal sphincter opening, upper esophageal sphincter closure to transition zone, transition zone to contractile deceleration point, and contractile deceleration point to bolus emptying completion.[16] The distinction of these phases relies on the recognition of mechanical esophageal states and intrabolus pressure classification, which may allow for identification of pathology subtypes based on discrete abnormalities.[16]

Stationary impedance facilitates direct evaluation of bolus passage across the esophagogastric junction (EGJ) using the bolus flow time.[20] The bolus flow time is measured by identifying concurrent drops in EGJ basal pressure as well as impedance values to signify bolus passage through a relaxed EGJ. The metric has been validated using concurrent fluoroscopy and shows potential in parsing out obstructive EGJ syndromes among those with dysphagia. A recent analysis has also demonstrated that there is good inter-rater agreement, which would allow for its broader adaptation, should it prove useful as an outcome predictive metric.[21]

HRIM has particular value in the evaluation of aerophagia and belching syndromes. The presence of air in the esophagus creates a characteristic impedance pattern that is easily recognized. Correlating antegrade and/or retrograde air movement with esophageal physiologic phenomena allows segregation of supragastric belching from physiologic gastric air eructation in patients with belching syndromes. Three patterns of supragastric belching have been described: primary supragastric belching, where air is injected into the esophagus by pharyngeal contraction or sucked into the esophagus by diaphragmatic crural contraction, followed by eructation through an open upper esophageal sphincter; secondary supragastric belching, which is associated with a transient lower esophageal sphincter (LES) relaxation, and secondary supragastric belching associated with rumination. Postprandial monitoring (discussed elsewhere in this article) may have added value in identification of these belching syndromes.

Although the combination of HRM and stationary impedance has enhanced the value of HRM by allowing bolus quantification, the lack of a reproducible metric has handicapped the interpretation of HRIM thus far. Incorporation of intuitive metrics such as the esophageal impedance integral and bolus flow time will further enhance documentation of bolus transit, whereas automated impedance manometry analysis has potential for improving understanding of bolus transit and symptom generation in esophageal disorders.

## UPRIGHT SWALLOWS DURING HIGH-RESOLUTION MANOMETRY AND HIGH-RESOLUTION IMPEDANCE MANOMETRY

The manometry catheter is placed with the patient in the upright seated position, which is most conducive to normal swallowing.[7] If there is difficulty in negotiating the catheter through the EGJ or if the catheter curls up in the esophageal lumen, standing the patient up and having the patient raise their arms above their head can straighten the esophagus and facilitate catheter placement.[22] Separation between the LES and the crural diaphragm becomes less profound in the upright position, and small hiatus hernias may not be appreciated anymore. Consequently, the catheter can be negotiated past a hiatus hernia better in the standing position. Beyond favorable positioning for catheter placement, changing positions can be beneficial in the elucidation of hiatus hernias. Having patients stand has been shown to be significantly more sensitive for their detection than either endoscopy or supine manometry and provided new diagnostic information in a substantial proportion of patients.[23]

In the upright position, bolus transit is assisted by gravity. Consequently, obstructive motor findings, esophageal pressurization, or compartmentalization that persists in the upright position has particular significance. To this point, recent investigations have demonstrated that an integrated relaxation pressure (IRP) of greater than 12 mm Hg in the upright position correlates with esophageal outflow obstruction on fluoroscopic investigations.[24] Values of less than 12 mm Hg, even in those with elevated IRP in the supine position, would therefore stand as an argument against surgically corrective measures for EGJ outflow obstruction. Performing upright swallows during an HRM protocol may therefore be of value in better defining EGJ outflow obstruction, especially when the IRP is high in asymptomatic individuals in supine swallows (**Table 1**).

## BOLUS VOLUME AND CONSISTENCY

The standard HRM protocol consists of supine water swallows, which is not how most patients experience esophageal symptoms. Therefore, studies have evaluated the effects of altering bolus volume and consistency to replicate normal swallowing, with the purpose of replicating symptoms to evaluate motor patterns in relationship to symptoms (**Table 1**).

The rapid drink challenge (RDC) consists of a large fluid bolus administered in the seated position. The patient is asked to drink 100 to 200 mL of fluid as fast as they can through a straw. The duration of time taken by the patient to complete the maneuver is recorded. In healthy normal volunteers, repetitive swallowing results in inhibition of esophageal peristalsis and profound relaxation of the LES, converting the tubular esophagus into a passive conduit for flow of liquid to the stomach without resistance (**Fig. 2**).[25] After the drink challenge, an exaggerated contraction sequence is identified in approximately one-quarter of healthy volunteers as well as controls.[25] The primary value of the RDC is in demonstrating a latent outflow obstruction pattern, especially when this is not evident in standard supine water swallows. Obstruction can manifest as panesophageal compartmentalization of pressure, a pressure gradient between the esophageal and gastric lumen favoring the esophagus, or esophageal shortening and contraction (see **Fig. 2**).[26] Obstructive features identified during RDC, particularly the IRP, correlate with the severity of dysphagia evaluated using validated questionnaires.[27–29] The presence of these obstructive features warrants further evaluation for obstructive processes, both motor and mechanical, using alternate tests such as barium radiography (especially solid bolus barium swallow or timed upright barium esophagram) or functional lumen imaging probe. The RDC was recommended as a standard provocative maneuver to be incorporated into routine manometry protocols by a consensus group of esophageal experts.[30]

Among other techniques used to study the effects of increasing bolus volume, the upright impedance bolus height on HRIM 5 minutes after the administration of a 200-mL of liquid bolus is of particular value in quantifying the effect of esophageal outflow obstruction in achalasia.[31] The impedance bolus height measured in this fashion correlates well with the height of the barium column on a timed upright barium swallow, and therefore can be a surrogate for barium esophagography in assessing response to management of esophageal outflow obstruction. Although 10-mL volumes have been sporadically used as a provocative maneuver, this test is not a standard part of the HRM protocol and its clinical value is questionable.

The administration of a standardized test meal (STM) provides for varied bolus consistency that replicates normal, day-to-day eating.[32] Obstructive features can be uncovered during test meals, particularly if the patient is asked to bring a meal or a food item that typically triggers dysphagia. STMs increase the diagnostic yield of the identification of major motor disorders and of contraction reserve. However, the variability in esophageal peristalsis seen during the ingestion of a meal also adds to the difficulty in interpretation of motor findings during STM. Although normative values have been developed and published,[9] the adoption of an STM as a standard part of the HRM protocol is not widespread.[33] The STM is likely to remain a niche procedure, used under special circumstances where routine esophageal testing, including standard HRM or HRIM, does not uncover the mechanism for solid food dysphagia.

There is increased esophageal body contraction vigor with single solid boluses of bread or marshmallows in healthy individuals as well as patients with evidence of reflux.[34] Further, solid boluses can obstruct in the esophagus, and can generate obstructive motor physiology, even when liquid swallows do not. However, viscous and solid boluses are not often used during HRM and HRIM, mainly because objective outcomes data from findings related to these boluses are lacking and because more useful clinical information can be obtained from RDC and STM.

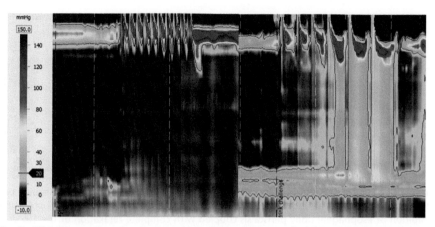

**Fig. 2.** RDC. The patient is asked to drink 100 to 200 mL of ambient temperature water through a straw as fast as possible in the seated position. As with multiple rapid swallows, profound inhibition of esophageal body contraction and of LES tone are expected during repetitive swallowing (*left*). However, a contraction sequence is not always seen following the last swallow of the sequence, even in healthy volunteers. In the presence of esophago-gastric junction obstructive syndromes, there is pressure compartmentalization during RDC that can be visually evident (*right*).

## PHYSIOLOGIC PROVOCATIVE MANEUVERS

Deglutitive inhibition and augmentation of contraction after repetitive swallowing are esophageal physiologic phenomena that are essential for normal swallowing. During repetitive swallowing of small boluses during normal eating and drinking, esophageal body peristalsis and LES tone are inhibited as part of deglutitive inhibition.[10] This phenomenon is essential for normal drinking, because each successive bolus would obstruct if each swallow resulted in esophageal smooth muscle contraction and lumen closure. Consequently, initiation of a second swallow within 2 to 3 seconds of an initial swallow results in inhibition of peristalsis of the first swallow. Each successive swallow continues to inhibit progression of the previous swallow, until the last swallow of the sequence, which is followed by an augmented contraction wave. The ability of esophageal smooth muscle to augment contraction vigor is important for the clearance of retained content in the esophagus,[6] and for bolus transit in the setting of a distal obstructive process[35] (**Fig. 3**).

Multiple rapid swallows (MRS) is the most commonly used physiologic maneuver during HRM,[33] and consists of five 2-mL swallows administered in rapid succession.[36] (**Table 1**) This maneuver evaluates both the integrity of esophageal neural innervation and the ability of esophageal smooth muscle to contract. When esophageal inhibitory innervation is intact, there is inhibition of smooth muscle contraction and profound LES relaxation during swallows (see **Fig. 2**). When esophageal excitation is intact and esophageal smooth muscle has normal contractile function, the vigor of contraction after the final swallow of the sequence surpasses that seen with single water swallows, termed contraction reserve.[10,36] Augmentation of contraction is evaluated using the MRS distal contractile integral to mean single swallow distal contractile integra ratio, and is greater than 1 in the presence of contraction reserve.[36] There can be variability in response between consecutive MRS maneuvers, and a recent report suggests that a minimum of 3 MRS maneuvers are needed for demonstration of a consistent pattern.[37]

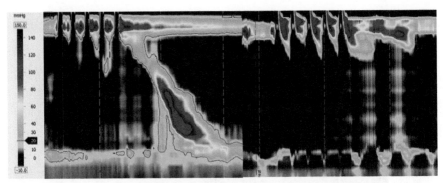

**Fig. 3.** MRS. Five 2-mL water boluses are administered in rapid succession in the supine position, with less than 3 seconds between swallows. A normal response consists of profound inhibition of esophageal body peristalsis coupled with complete relaxation of the LES during repetitive swallowing, followed by an augmented contraction response and reestablishment of LES tone after the final swallow of the sequence (*left*). Augmentation of contraction is termed presence of contraction reserve. Absence of contraction following the final swallow (*right*) is an abnormal finding that can predict persistence or progression of hypomotility states like ineffective esophageal motility, and can indicate a higher likelihood of postfundoplication dysphagia after antireflux surgery.

Evaluation for abnormal inhibition during MRS can be used as a confirmatory marker for inhibitory dysfunction in spastic disorders and achalasia spectrum disorders[38] (see **Fig. 3**). This evaluation can also be used as a physiologic tool to study the pathophysiology spastic disorders.[39] For instance, hypercontractile disorders have been found to demonstrate abnormal inhibition similar to that seen with type 3 achalasia,[40] suggesting that these 2 types of disorders may share a common pathophysiology. Further, a hypercontractile esophageal body pattern can be associated with EGJ outflow obstruction from abnormal LES relaxation, which can also demonstrate a similar pattern of abnormal inhibition.[40]

Within the spectrum of hypomotility disorders, lack of contraction reserve has been associated with a higher likelihood of late postfundoplication dysphagia after antireflux surgery, especially in the setting of ineffective esophageal motility.[36,41] When esophageal motor function is assessed in patients with gastroesophageal reflux disease, the lack of contraction reserve may be a marker for new development of ineffective esophageal motility and/or progression of ineffective esophageal motility over time.[42] Insufficient augmentation has been linked to increased pathologic bolus exposure, suggesting abnormal acid exposure may result in part from loss of reserve in peristalsis and subsequent inability to clear refluxate.[43]

LES competence is necessary for the prevention of reflux of gastric content into the esophagus, especially during times when the pressure gradient across the EGJ favors retrograde movement of gastric content. Maneuvers aimed at increasing abdominal pressure and thus assessing competency of the LES barrier are being evaluated (**Table 2**). Studies in children using abdominal binders that can gradually increase intra-abdominal pressure have demonstrated that an intact LES plays a major role in preventing reflux.[44] Similar studies using abdominal binders in adults can evaluate esophageal peristaltic performance against resistance of increased intra-abdominal pressure. A straight leg raise maneuver during manometry also increases intra-abdominal pressure and can provide similar information on the integrity of the EGJ barrier, including presence of hiatus hernia.[45] As the prevalence of obesity increases, the relationship between intra-abdominal pressure and acid reflux will need further investigation.

## PHARMACOLOGIC PROVOCATIVE MANEUVERS

Eliciting symptoms during manometry can have clinical value, because it allows for direct correlation of physiologic changes with subjective sensation. Pharmacologic provocation involves the administration of medications by inhalation or parenterally during esophageal HRM. Edrophonium, an acetylcholinesterase inhibitor, was shown in early studies to significantly increase LES pressures in patients with achalasia, but not in healthy individuals.[46] (**Table 2**) Edrophonium administration induces chest pain in nearly one-third of patients with known noncardiac chest pain by increasing the duration of distal esophageal contractions, without significant effects on coronary arteries.[47] The test is hampered by a lack of clear pressure thresholds or distinguishing characteristics between normal and abnormal patients.[48] Further, the potential for cardiorespiratory adverse effects has effectively limited the use of this agent.

**Table 2**
**Investigation of esophageal physiology and pathophysiology using HRM**

|  | Methodology | Expected Findings | Potential Clinical Value |
|---|---|---|---|
| Physiologic challenge | Abdominal compression | Increased reflux as intra-abdominal pressures are increased when LES tone is diminished, augmented esophageal body contractile vigor and intrabolus pressure | Evaluation of symptomatic patients at risk for reflux when intra-abdominal pressures are elevated |
|  | Straight leg raise | Same as abdominal compression | Same as abdominal compression but less invasive |
| Pharmacologic challenge | Amyl nitrite | Inhibition of LES tone | Identification of patients that might respond to LES disruption |
|  | Cholecystokinin | Phasic esophageal body contraction, esophageal body shortening, reduction of LES tone, induction of TLESR | Stratification of achalasia subtypes and EGJ outflow obstruction |
|  | Atropine | Reduction of LES pressures and esophageal body contraction vigor | Identification of intact cholinergic innervation |
| Ambulatory manometry | Ambulatory recording of motor patterns using a catheter and recording system | Normal motor patterns | Correlation of unexplained esophageal symptoms with abnormal motor patterns |

Amyl nitrite is a potent nitric oxide donor that is inhaled and then rapidly distributed throughout the body thereby inhibiting LES contraction.[49,50] Therefore, in EGJ outflow obstruction, a lack of inhibition of LES tone or pressure after amyl nitrite inhalation may signify a structural or mechanical cause, whereas the inhibition of LES contraction may indicate an achalasia-like disorder. In unselected patients with EGJ outflow obstruction, roughly one-half will respond in this fashion.[51] Although the addition of this pharmacologic challenge is posited as an adjunct to standard testing to ascertain which patients might respond to LES therapies, its availability and potential side effects from vasodilation limit routine use.

Cholecystokinin is a pharmacologic provocative agent that attenuates LES contraction in the postprandial period[52] and induces transient LES relaxation.[53] A biphasic response can be seen where LES relaxation is followed by phasic esophageal smooth muscle contraction as well as longitudinal esophageal muscle contraction in healthy individuals.[54] This response may be attenuated when inhibitory function is impaired; therefore, cholecystokinin is postulated to potentially stratify achalasia subtypes and EGJ outflow obstruction, but this requires further study.

Cholinergic contribution to esophageal contraction has been studied for decades, and the administration of anticholinergic agents (eg, atropine) decreases LES pressures in both normal controls and patients with achalasia by 30% to 60%.[50] Cholinergic postganglionic transmission at the LES serves as the basis for the use of botulinum toxin in achalasia. Heterogeneity in symptom response has been explained as demonstrative, in some cases, of the variable amount of cholinergic preservation. Alternatively, excessive cholinergic drive has been associated with hypercontractility and asynchrony between circular and longitudinal muscle contractions that has been abolished in studies using atropine.[55] Although not widely used during manometric testing, atropine may provide insights into its pathogenesis and may identify intact cholinergic transmission in subsets of patients.

Less frequent reports exist of other types of chemical provocation during standard manometry. In animal studies, nitro-L-argine methyl ester, a selective nitric oxide inhibitor, has been shown to eradicate LES relaxation[56] and recombinant hemoglobin designed to inactive nitric oxide was shown to induce esophageal contraction and prevent LES relaxation.[57] However, neither of these agents have undergone rigorous analysis nor are they used routinely.

## POSTPRANDIAL MONITORING

For the 40% of symptomatic patients with persistent reflux symptoms who report an incomplete response to proton pump inhinitors,[58] HRIM can evaluate for pathophysiologic mechanisms supporting or refuting reflux, and alternative explanations for regurgitation such as rumination (**Table 1**). One promising methodology for this consists of extending HRIM beyond the standard liquid supine protocol to include a refluxogenic meal and prolonged monitoring (**Figs. 4** and **5**). Postprandial HRIM was able to identify a behavioral explanation for symptoms in 62% of 94 symptomatic proton pump inhibitor nonresponders in a recent study, 42% of whom were diagnosed with rumination syndrome (see **Fig. 4**) and 20% with supragastric belching (see **Fig. 5**).[59]

Transient lower esophageal sphincter relaxations (TLESR) are common physiologic events both in health and reflux disease[60,61] and HRM is the current gold standard for their identification.[62] Recent work has sought to characterize these events and consensus definition relies on crural diaphragm inhibition, absence of swallowing within 4 seconds before event onset, and LES relaxation lasting more than 10

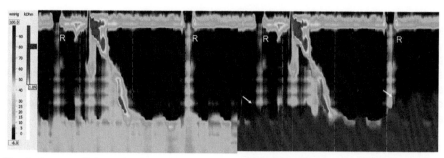

**Fig. 4.** Postprandial monitoring using HRIM demonstrates episodes of rumination (R) in a patient with postprandial regurgitation. There is simultaneous increase in both the intra-abdominal and intraesophageal pressure, with open lower and upper esophageal sphincters, which constitutes the 'r' wave of rumination. The impedance plots on the left image demonstrate retrograde movement of gastric content into the esophagus during the 'r' wave (*arrows*).

seconds.[63] The proportion of TLESR associated with reflux of gastric content is significantly increased in the postprandial period both in normal subjects and those with evidence of reflux.[64] Postprandial HRM or HRIM, however, have a greater value in the identification of supragastric belching and rumination syndrome rather than TLESR.

## AMBULATORY MANOMETRY

Recent reports have demonstrated that prolonged HRM monitoring is feasible, with the potential for TLESR identification as well as understanding relationships between longitudinal muscle physiology and symptoms.[65] (**Table 2**) Despite the potential for accurate TLESR evaluation, this evaluation is typically not part of stationary or ambulatory monitoring in clinical practice, mainly because esophageal reflux burden, a surrogate metric relating to TLESRs, is easier to acquire using reflux monitoring. However, the evaluation of motor patterns on ambulatory HRM could provide

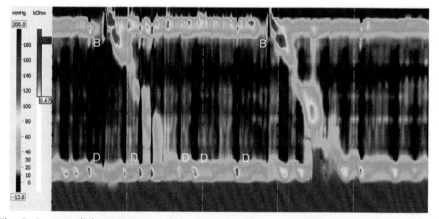

**Fig. 5.** Postprandial monitoring using HRIM identifies supragastric belching in a patient with excessive air eructation. Air is either sucked into the esophagus during forceful diaphragmatic crural contraction (D), or injected into the esophagus by pharyngeal contraction. The patient then expels the air out through an open upper esophageal sphincter (B).

explanations for refractory esophageal symptoms. Literature exists suggesting that longitudinal esophageal muscle contraction plays a role in esophageal peristalsis as well as LES relaxation[66] and therefore may play a role in symptoms when that contraction is sustained, specifically in esophageal chest pain.[67] HRM is unable to conclusively detect vertical esophageal shift in correlation with longitudinal muscle activation, but so-called LES lift is felt to represent a potential surrogate.[68] The field of ambulatory manometry needs further research before this technique can become a routine diagnostic tool.

## FUTURE RESEARCH

Manometry-based research is an expanding field with the promise of continued growth in the coming years. It is anticipated that impedance-centered analyses will provide new insights into the physiology of bolus propulsion and how aberrancy relates to symptoms. Future research will help to evaluate the precise role of level, degree, and frequency of bolus escape in leading to both symptoms and outcomes. Changes in bolus consistency and volume, evaluation during STMs, and prolonged monitoring through the postprandial period will help to better appreciate peristaltic changes associated with real world scenarios and offer new insights into symptomatic deglutitive disorders. The standardization of TLESR and provocative testing metrics are, therefore, timely and are anticipated to contribute to our understanding of the processes that affect reflux, its clearance, and the factors that put patients at risk for disease states pertaining to abnormal motor function and abnormal bolus transit.

New clinical testing methods are anticipated to better personalize esophageal physiologic testing to each individual's precise presentation. The potential mechanisms for this range from physiologic and potentially pharmacologic challenge in outflow obstruction syndromes to ambulatory monitoring in unexplained chest pain to measures to increase intra-abdominal pressure to better evaluate the consequences of compromised LES barrier function. Importantly, these tools will also allow us to determine, with increasing accuracy, where interventions are likely to be successful and where the field needs further improvement.

Finally, the time is right for advanced analytics using data from an increasingly collaborative multicenter approach, where major themes and patterns can be better identified and pathophysiologic paradigms can be tested.

## SUMMARY

Used judicially, ancillary techniques and measures can enhance HRM findings and can aid in a more informed management approach in symptomatic individuals. These maneuvers, properly applied, serve the crucial function of clarifying physiologic responses to stressing the esophagus by creating conditions that more closely resemble normal swallowing. In particular, 2 simple measures—MRS and RDC—can evaluate for contraction reserve signifying esophageal resilience, or reveal a latent obstructive pattern, respectively. Although the existing body of evidence is sufficient to warrant the routine use of MRS and RDC in standard manometric evaluation, more research is needed to understand the precise niche of these maneuvers in clinical esophagology.

## DISCLOSURE

C.P. Gyawali has received honoraria for consulting from Medtronic, Diversatek, Torax, Ironwood, and Quintiles, and is on the speaker's bureau for Medtronic and Diversatek. B.D. Rogers has no conflicts of interest to disclose. No conflicts of interest exist.

## REFERENCES

1. Murray JA, Clouse RE, Conklin JL. Components of the standard oesophageal manometry. Neurogastroenterol Motil 2003;15:591–606.
2. Gyawali CP. High resolution manometry: the Ray Clouse legacy. Neurogastroenterol Motil 2012;24(Suppl 1):2–4.
3. Clouse RE, Staiano A. Topography of the esophageal peristaltic pressure wave. Am J Physiol 1991;261:G677–84.
4. Kahrilas PJ, Bredenoord AJ, Fox M, et al. The Chicago Classification of esophageal motility disorders, v3.0. Neurogastroenterol Motil 2015;27:160–74.
5. Rohof WO, Salvador R, Annese V, et al. Outcomes of treatment for achalasia depend on manometric subtype. Gastroenterology 2013;144:718–25 [quiz: e13-4].
6. Sweis R, Anggiansah A, Wong T, et al. Normative values and inter-observer agreement for liquid and solid bolus swallows in upright and supine positions as assessed by esophageal high-resolution manometry. Neurogastroenterol Motil 2011;23:509.e198.
7. Gyawali CP, Patel A. Esophageal motor function: technical aspects of manometry. Gastrointest Endosc Clin N Am 2014;24:527–43.
8. Osmanoglou E, Van Der Voort IR, Fach K, et al. Oesophageal transport of solid dosage forms depends on body position, swallowing volume and pharyngeal propulsion velocity. Neurogastroenterol Motil 2004;16:547–56.
9. Sweis R, Anggiansah A, Wong T, et al. Assessment of esophageal dysfunction and symptoms during and after a standardized test meal: development and clinical validation of a new methodology utilizing high-resolution manometry. Neurogastroenterol Motil 2014;26:215–28.
10. Fornari F, Bravi I, Penagini R, et al. Multiple rapid swallowing: a complementary test during standard oesophageal manometry. Neurogastroenterol Motil 2009; 21:718.e41.
11. Elvevi A, Mauro A, Pugliese D, et al. Usefulness of low- and high-volume multiple rapid swallowing during high-resolution manometry. Dig Liver Dis 2015;47:103–7.
12. Holloway RH. Combined impedance-manometry for the evaluation of esophageal disorders. Curr Opin Gastroenterol 2014;30:422–7.
13. Zerbib F, des Varannes SB, Roman S, et al. Normal values and day-to-day variability of 24-h ambulatory oesophageal impedance-pH monitoring in a Belgian-French cohort of healthy subjects. Aliment Pharmacol Ther 2005;22:1011–21.
14. Zerbib F, Roman S, Ropert A, et al. Esophageal pH-impedance monitoring and symptom analysis in GERD: a study in patients off and on therapy. Am J Gastroenterol 2006;101:1956–63.
15. Bogte A, Bredenoord AJ, Oors J, et al. Assessment of bolus transit with intraluminal impedance measurement in patients with esophageal motility disorders. Neurogastroenterol Motil 2015;27:1446–52.
16. Lin Z, Yim B, Gawron A, et al. The four phases of esophageal bolus transit defined by high-resolution impedance manometry and fluoroscopy. Am J Physiol Gastrointest Liver Physiol 2014;307:G437–44.
17. Rommel N, Van Oudenhove L, Tack J, et al. Automated impedance manometry analysis as a method to assess esophageal function. Neurogastroenterol Motil 2014;26:636–45.
18. Nguyen NQ, Holloway RH, Smout AJ, et al. Automated impedance-manometry analysis detects esophageal motor dysfunction in patients who have non-

obstructive dysphagia with normal manometry. Neurogastroenterol Motil 2013;25: 238–45, e164.

19. Lin Z, Nicodeme F, Lin CY, et al. Parameters for quantifying bolus retention with high-resolution impedance manometry. Neurogastroenterol Motil 2014;26: 929–36.

20. Lin Z, Imam H, Nicodeme F, et al. Flow time through esophagogastric junction derived during high-resolution impedance-manometry studies: a novel parameter for assessing esophageal bolus transit. Am J Physiol Gastrointest Liver Physiol 2014;307:G158–63.

21. Carlson DA, Lin Z, Kou W, et al. Inter-rater agreement of novel high-resolution impedance manometry metrics: bolus flow time and esophageal impedance integral ratio. Neurogastroenterol Motil 2018;30:e13289.

22. Gyawali CP. Making the most of imperfect high-resolution manometry studies. Clin Gastroenterol Hepatol 2011;9:1015–6.

23. Hashmi S, Rao SS, Summers RW, et al. Esophageal pressure topography, body position, and hiatal hernia. J Clin Gastroenterol 2014;48:224–30.

24. Triggs JR, Carlson DA, Beveridge C, et al. Upright integrated relaxation pressure facilitates characterization of esophagogastric junction outflow obstruction. Clin Gastroenterol Hepatol 2019;17(11):2218–26.e2.

25. Marin I, Cisternas D, Abrao L, et al. Normal values of esophageal pressure responses to a rapid drink challenge test in healthy subjects: results of a multicenter study. Neurogastroenterol Motil 2017;29(6):e13021.

26. Marin I, Serra J. Patterns of esophageal pressure responses to a rapid drink challenge test in patients with esophageal motility disorders. Neurogastroenterol Motil 2016;28:543–53.

27. Ang D, Hollenstein M, Misselwitz B, et al. Rapid drink challenge in high-resolution manometry: an adjunctive test for detection of esophageal motility disorders. Neurogastroenterol Motil 2017;29(1):e12902.

28. Biasutto D, Mion F, Garros A, et al. Rapid drink challenge test during esophageal high resolution manometry in patients with esophago-gastric junction outflow obstruction. Neurogastroenterol Motil 2018;30:e13293.

29. Woodland P, Gabieta-Sonmez S, Arguero J, et al. 200 mL rapid drink challenge during high-resolution manometry best predicts objective esophagogastric junction obstruction and correlates with symptom severity. J Neurogastroenterol Motil 2018;24:410–4.

30. Gyawali CP, Roman S, Bredenoord AJ, et al. Classification of esophageal motor findings in gastro-esophageal reflux disease: conclusions from an international consensus group. Neurogastroenterol Motil 2017;29.

31. Cho YK, Lipowska AM, Nicodeme F, et al. Assessing bolus retention in achalasia using high-resolution manometry with impedance: a comparator study with timed barium esophagram. Am J Gastroenterol 2014;109(6):829–35.

32. Ang D, Misselwitz B, Hollenstein M, et al. Diagnostic yield of high-resolution manometry with a solid test meal for clinically relevant, symptomatic oesophageal motility disorders: serial diagnostic study. Lancet Gastroenterol Hepatol 2017;2: 654–61.

33. Sweis R, Heinrich H, Fox M, et al. Variation in esophageal physiology testing in clinical practice: results from an international survey. Neurogastroenterol Motil 2018;30(3):e13215.

34. Daum C, Sweis R, Kaufman E, et al. Failure to respond to physiologic challenge characterizes esophageal motility in erosive gastro-esophageal reflux disease. Neurogastroenterol Motil 2011;23:517.e200.

35. Gyawali CP, Kushnir VM. High-resolution manometric characteristics help differentiate types of distal esophageal obstruction in patients with peristalsis. Neurogastroenterol Motil 2011;23:502.e197.
36. Shaker A, Stoikes N, Drapekin J, et al. Multiple rapid swallow responses during esophageal high-resolution manometry reflect esophageal body peristaltic reserve. Am J Gastroenterol 2013;108:1706–12.
37. Mauro A, Savarino E, De Bortoli N, et al. Optimal number of multiple rapid swallows needed during high-resolution esophageal manometry for accurate prediction of contraction reserve. Neurogastroenterol Motil 2018;30:e13253.
38. Kushnir V, Sayuk GS, Gyawali CP. Multiple rapid swallow responses segregate achalasia subtypes on high-resolution manometry. Neurogastroenterol Motil 2012;24:1069.e561.
39. Mauro A, Quader F, Tolone S, et al. Provocative testing in patients with jackhammer esophagus: evidence for altered neural control. Am J Physiol Gastrointest Liver Physiol 2019;316(3):G397–403.
40. Quader F, Mauro A, Savarino E, et al. Jackhammer esophagus with and without esophagogastric junction outflow obstruction demonstrates altered neural control resembling type 3 achalasia. Neurogastroenterol Motil 2019;31(9):e13678.
41. Hasak S, Brunt LM, Wang D, et al. Clinical characteristics and outcomes of patients with postfundoplication dysphagia. Clin Gastroenterol Hepatol 2019; 17(10):1982–90.
42. Mello MD, Shriver AR, Li Y, et al. Ineffective esophageal motility phenotypes following fundoplication in gastroesophageal reflux disease. Neurogastroenterol Motil 2016;28:292–8.
43. Min YW, Shin I, Son HJ, et al. Multiple rapid swallow maneuver enhances the clinical utility of high-resolution manometry in patients showing ineffective esophageal motility. Medicine (Baltimore) 2015;94:e1669.
44. Goldani HA, Fernandes MI, Vicente YA, et al. Lower esophageal sphincter reacts against intraabdominal pressure in children with symptoms of gastroesophageal reflux. Dig Dis Sci 2002;47:2544–8.
45. Bitnar P, Stovicek J, Andel R, et al. Leg raise increases pressure in lower and upper esophageal sphincter among patients with gastroesophageal reflux disease. J Bodyw Mov Ther 2016;20:518–24.
46. Cohen S, Fisher R, Tuch A. The site of denervation in achalasia. Gut 1972;13:556–8.
47. Dalton CB, Hewson EG, Castell DO, et al. Edrophonium provocative test in noncardiac chest pain. Evaluation of testing techniques. Dig Dis Sci 1990;35:1445–51.
48. Richter JE, Hackshaw BT, Wu WC, et al. Edrophonium: a useful provocative test for esophageal chest pain. Ann Intern Med 1985;103:14–21.
49. Dodds WJ, Stewart ET, Kishk SM, et al. Radiologic amyl nitrite test for distinguishing pseudoachalasia from idiopathic achalasia. AJR Am J Roentgenol 1986;146:21–3.
50. Holloway RH, Dodds WJ, Helm JF, et al. Integrity of cholinergic innervation to the lower esophageal sphincter in achalasia. Gastroenterology 1986;90:924–9.
51. Babaei A, Shad S, Szabo A, et al. Pharmacologic interrogation of patients with esophagogastric junction outflow obstruction using amyl nitrite. Neurogastroenterol Motil 2019;31:e13668.
52. Liu JF, Zhang J, Liu XB, et al. Investigation of cholecystokinin receptors in the human lower esophageal sphincter. World J Gastroenterol 2014;20:6554–9.
53. Hirsch DP, Mathus-Vliegen EM, Holloway RH, et al. Role of CCK(A) receptors in postprandial lower esophageal sphincter function in morbidly obese subjects. Dig Dis Sci 2002;47:2531–7.

54. Babaei A, Mittal R. Cholecystokinin induces esophageal longitudinal muscle contraction and transient lower esophageal sphincter relaxation in healthy humans. Am J Physiol Gastrointest Liver Physiol 2018;315:G734–42.
55. Korsapati H, Bhargava V, Mittal RK. Reversal of asynchrony between circular and longitudinal muscle contraction in nutcracker esophagus by atropine. Gastroenterology 2008;135:796–802.
56. Yamato S, Saha JK, Goyal RK. Role of nitric oxide in lower esophageal sphincter relaxation to swallowing. Life Sci 1992;50:1263–72.
57. Murray JA, Ledlow A, Launspach J, et al. The effects of recombinant human hemoglobin on esophageal motor functions in humans. Gastroenterology 1995;109:1241–8.
58. Cicala M, Emerenziani S, Guarino MP, et al. Proton pump inhibitor resistance, the real challenge in gastro-esophageal reflux disease. World J Gastroenterol 2013; 19:6529–35.
59. Yadlapati R, Tye M, Roman S, et al. Postprandial high-resolution impedance manometry identifies mechanisms of nonresponse to proton pump inhibitors. Clin Gastroenterol Hepatol 2018;16:211–8.e1.
60. He S, Jell A, Huser N, et al. 24-hour monitoring of transient lower esophageal sphincter relaxation events by long-term high-resolution impedance manometry in normal volunteers: the "mirror phenomenon". Neurogastroenterol Motil 2019; 31:e13530.
61. Sifrim D, Holloway R, Silny J, et al. Composition of the postprandial refluxate in patients with gastroesophageal reflux disease. Am J Gastroenterol 2001;96:647–55.
62. Roman S, Zerbib F, Belhocine K, et al. High resolution manometry to detect transient lower oesophageal sphincter relaxations: diagnostic accuracy compared with perfused-sleeve manometry, and the definition of new detection criteria. Aliment Pharmacol Ther 2011;34:384–93.
63. Roman S, Holloway R, Keller J, et al. Validation of criteria for the definition of transient lower esophageal sphincter relaxations using high-resolution manometry. Neurogastroenterol Motil 2017;29(2):e12920.
64. Cucchiara S, Bortolotti M, Minella R, et al. Fasting and postprandial mechanisms of gastroesophageal reflux in children with gastroesophageal reflux disease. Dig Dis Sci 1993;38:86–92.
65. Mittal RK, Karstens A, Leslie E, et al. Ambulatory high-resolution manometry, lower esophageal sphincter lift and transient lower esophageal sphincter relaxation. Neurogastroenterol Motil 2012;24:40–6.e2.
66. Dogan I, Bhargava V, Liu J, et al. Axial stretch: a novel mechanism of the lower esophageal sphincter relaxation. Am J Physiol Gastrointest Liver Physiol 2007; 292:G329–34.
67. Balaban DH, Yamamoto Y, Liu J, et al. Sustained esophageal contraction: a marker of esophageal chest pain identified by intraluminal ultrasonography. Gastroenterology 1999;116:29–37.
68. Pandolfino JE, Kwiatek MA, Nealis T, et al. Achalasia: a new clinically relevant classification by high-resolution manometry. Gastroenterology 2008;135: 1526–33.

# EndoFLIP in the Esophagus
## Assessing Sphincter Function, Wall Stiffness, and Motility to Guide Treatment

Erica N. Donnan, MD[a,b,*], John E. Pandolfino, MD, MSCI[a,b]

### KEYWORDS

- Impedance • Achalasia • Dysphagia • FLIP • EndoFLIP • Gastroesophageal reflux

### KEY POINTS

- The FLIP has demonstrated its clinical utility as a diagnostic tool and as a device that is used to guide and measure response to therapy.
- The FLIP can assess and guide treatments for esophageal disease states including gastroesophageal reflux disease, achalasia, and eosinophilic esophagitis.
- The FLIP can assess the sphincter function through the Esophagogastric Junction-Distensibility Index.
- The wall stiffness is measured by the FLIP by measuring esophageal narrowing and the mechanical characteristics of the esophageal body.
- Motility is classified by FLIP panometry, a combination of Esophagogastric Junction-Distensibility Index and contraction pattern at the time of upper endoscopy.

## INTRODUCTION

The techniques used to measure esophageal and sphincter physiology have evolved over time with high-resolution manometry and the functional luminal imaging probe (FLIP) taking center stage over the past 10 years. Currently high-resolution manometry in combination with the Chicago Classification v3.0 is the gold standard for the clinical assessment of esophageal motility disorders.[1] However, a growing body of literature surrounding the use of the FLIP has demonstrated its clinical utility as a diagnostic tool and as a device that is used to guide and measure response to therapy.

The FLIP provides a three-dimensional image of the esophageal lumen through use of high-resolution impedance planimetry to measure pressure changes, diameter, and volume. By measuring distensibility, the FLIP can measure esophageal wall stiffness

<sup>a</sup> Division of Gastroenterology and Hepatology, Department of Medicine, Feinberg School of Medicine, Northwestern University, Chicago, IL, USA; <sup>b</sup> NMH/Arkes Family Pavilion, Suite 1400, 676 North Saint Clair, Chicago, IL 60611, USA
* Corresponding author. NMH/Arkes Family Pavilion, Suite 1400, 676 North Saint Clair, Chicago, IL 60611.
E-mail address: erica.donnan@northwestern.edu

Gastroenterol Clin N Am 49 (2020) 427–435
https://doi.org/10.1016/j.gtc.2020.04.002
0889-8553/20/© 2020 Elsevier Inc. All rights reserved.

and the dynamics of esophagogastric junction (EGJ) opening.[2] The Esophagogastric Junction-Distensibility Index (EGJ-DI) is the measure of sphincter distensibility and is derived by dividing the median narrowest cross-sectional area by the median intraballoon pressure over a set timeframe. The use of the EGJ-DI combined with contraction patterns, known as FLIP panometry, allows for the classification of esophageal motility.[3]

There are now published normative data from healthy control patients that allow the FLIP to be applied to clinical practice.[4] In 2017 the American Gastroenterological Association Institute's Clinical Practice Updates Committee published an Expert Review of FLIP. The paper summarized the best practice advice recommending that although the FLIP should not be used in isolation to make diagnostic or treatment decisions, it is a complementary tool to assess EGJ opening dynamics and stiffness of the esophageal wall.[5] The purpose of this review article is to summarize the use of the FLIP in assessing motility, the sphincter function, and wall stiffness to guide treatments.

## THE FUNCTIONAL LUMINAL IMAGING PROBE CATHETER, STUDY PROTOCOL, AND DATA ANALYSIS

The FLIP is comprised of a catheter with a distal overlying balloon. Within the balloon there are 16 paired impedance planimetry electrodes and a solid-state pressure transducer located distally. There is a continuous low electric current that is emitted by excitation electrodes located on both ends of the balloon. The balloon is inflated with saline enabling the measurement of voltage across the impedance planimetry electrodes. This allows for the measurement of the luminal cross-sectional area.

The FLIP is typically placed in a sedated patient at the time of endoscopy and can be placed and performed in less than 5 minutes.[6] The FLIP is placed transorally and is positioned within the esophagus through the identification of the waist on a display figure with 20 mL of saline in the balloon. The catheter often moves during the study as the esophagus contracts; using the waist on the display figure allows for readjustment of the balloon during the study. Once the catheter is at the correct position, the balloon is distended typically stepwise in 10-mL increments up to 70 mL.

There was previously a delay between the upper endoscopy and the interpretation of FLIP panometry because the FLIP required the use of a customized analysis program before interpretation. However, the manufacturer (Medtronic Inc, Shoreview, MN) has created FLIP 2.0 with a screen that displays 40 seconds of continuous FLIP topography during the time of the endoscopy so that now the operator can interpret the measurements in real time using FLIP panometry (**Fig. 1**). Carlson and colleagues[7] recently demonstrated this in a prospective multicentered study with excellent agreement between real-time and post hoc FLIP panometry interpretation of abnormal motility.

## ASSESSING MOTILITY
### Repetitive Antegrade Contractions, Repetitive Retrograde Contractions, Disordered Contractility

When the esophagus is distended by the FLIP, contractions are induced that are currently subdivided into three categories: (1) repetitive antegrade contractions (RACs), (2) repetitive retrograde contractions, and (3) diminished-disordered contractile response (**Fig. 2**).[3,8,9] FLIP panometry combines the EGJ-DI along with the contractility pattern to categorize the esophageal motility. The classification scheme has been previously published and is initially designated by the presence or absence of EGJ outflow obstruction defined by an abnormal EGJ-DI and then the

FLIP 2.0: Catheter    FLIP 2.0: Real-time FLIP-panometry

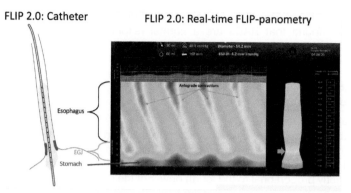

**Fig. 1.** Diagram of catheter and placement through the EGJ. The FLIP 2.0 display provides real-time measurement of the EGJ-DI, which is measured as the narrowest CSA (*green arrow*) divided by the simultaneous pressure. The pattern represents a normal response to volumetric distention and is defined as repetitive antegrade contractions. CSA, cross-sectional area. (*Courtesy of* the Esophageal Center at Northwestern, Chicago, IL.)

# FLIP topography: Contractile patterns

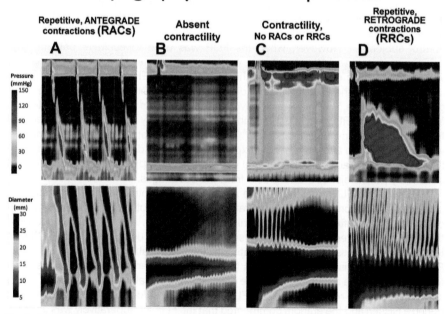

**Fig. 2.** Motility patterns in response to volumetric distention. The *top panels* are the high-resolution manometry image and the *bottom panels* are the FLIP topography image of the representative patient. (*A*) Normal subject with an RAC pattern. (*B*) Patient with type I achalasia. The FLIP depicts an absent contractile response and a poorly relaxing sphincter. (*C*) Type II achalasia. The FLIP suggests that there are disordered nonoccluding contractions in the body of the esophagus and the sphincter does not open. (*D*) Patient with type III achalasia. The FLIP topography reveals an abnormal pattern where the contractions are retrograde and rapid in terms of the rate of contractions. (*Courtesy of* the Esophageal Center at Northwestern, Chicago, IL.)

contractility pattern.[3] Recently published data from 20 asymptomatic healthy control patients found that RACs are a normal response to sustained esophageal distention.[4]

## ASSESSING THE SPHINCTER FUNCTION
### *Lower Esophageal Sphincter*

#### *Gastroesophageal reflux disease*

It is hypothesized that increased EGJ distensibility and dimension should increase the volume of reflux in patients with gastroesophageal reflux disease (GERD). This is based on Poiseuille's law of flow, which states that flow rate of a liquid through a tube is directly proportional to the fourth power of the radius of the tube and inversely related to the length and viscosity of the tube. The EGJ of patients with GERD with a hiatal hernia was found to be shorter and more distensible than normal subjects in a study that combined concurrent esophageal manometry, fluoroscopy, and stepwise controlled barostatic distention of the EGJ.[10] Most research involving GERD and the FLIP has focused on the EGJ-DI; however, the results have shown conflicting data. The best practice statement from the American Gastroenterological Association Institute's Clinical Practice Updates Committee Expert Review recommends against using the FLIP for routine GERD management.[5]

In a study using the FLIP to evaluate patients with hiatal hernia and Barrett esophagus compared with control subjects, the lower esophageal sphincter in patients with a hiatal hernia had a lower pressure and was more distensible than the EGJ in control subjects.[11] In a different study the EGJ is more distensible in reflux patients than in control subjects.[12] However, when the FLIP was used to evaluate patients with GERD symptoms in addition to 48-hour wireless esophageal pH monitoring compared with asymptomatic control subjects, the patients with GERD were found to have a lower EGJ-DI and the EGJ-DI was not different between normal or abnormal esophageal acid exposure.[13] Another study evaluated 25 patients undergoing reflux testing for suspected GERD with the FLIP and with ambulatory wireless esophageal pH testing off of proton-pump inhibitors.[14] The EGJ-DI did not differ between abnormal acid exposure time and normal acid exposure time. They did, however, find that patients with RACs had a lower total acid exposure time, supporting the importance of secondary peristalsis for clearing acid from the esophagus.[14]

The use of the FLIP for preoperative assessment and intraoperative use has been studied for GERD procedures. Preoperative EGJ-DI was not found to be predictive of clinical outcomes after transoral incisionless fundoplication.[15] In one study fundoplication did reduce distensibility to normal levels.[16] The goal of using intraoperative FLIP is to tailor the tightness of the fundoplication to the individual. Intraoperative use of the FLIP to measure distensibility during a laparoscopic Nissen fundoplication has been found to be feasible and in one instance changed intraoperative management.[17] There is a published case report of using the FLIP to replace the rigid bougie commonly used during a Nissen and the authors commented that the FLIP intraoperatively was useful to evaluate the orientation and the position of the Nissen.[18] It has not been studied if intraoperative use of FLIP for Nissen fundoplication can change outcomes.

The conflicting data about GERD and the EGJ-DI may reflect that the EGJ-DI is not the most important measurement in assessing reflux because the opening dimensions and pressure gradient for reflux are much lower than those produced during swallowing. Future studies in GERD should assess the rate of opening and the yield pressure for opening because the dynamic relationship between opening at lower pressures may be more relevant.

### Achalasia

The hallmark feature of achalasia is the failure of the lower esophageal sphincter to relax. The FLIP is ideally suited to assess the lower esophageal sphincter and has thus proven to be a useful tool in the diagnosis and management of achalasia. FLIP topography is a sensitive marker of achalasia; it has been found to identify abnormalities in esophageal motility including 100% of patients with achalasia in several studies.[3,7]

Focusing on assessment of the lower esophageal sphincter through the EGJ-DI and the EGJ cross-sectional area, the FLIP can be used during the treatment of achalasia. Intraoperative FLIP has been studied during per-oral endoscopic myotomy for achalasia with the findings that EGJ cross-sectional area correlates with clinical response in addition to post-procedure reflux.[19] Intraoperative FLIP has been used for patients undergoing surgical myotomy to evaluate the EGJ cross-sectional area, with the finding that surgical myotomy significantly decreases contractile vigor.[20]

The EGJ-DI has been found to be predictive of immediate clinical response to pneumatic dilation in achalasia. A prospective study measured the EGJ-DI immediately before and after pneumatic dilation in patients with idiopathic achalasia and found that an incremental increase of the EGJ distensibility index of greater than 1.8 mm$^2$/mm Hg after the pneumatic dilation was able to accurately predict clinical response.[21] With this information physicians can provide appropriate follow-up and schedule anticipated needed procedures at the time of the initial pneumatic dilation. When the DI was prospectively evaluated in patients with achalasia post-treatment, it was found to be the single most useful measure of EGJ opening.[22]

The FLIP is helpful clinically to diagnose achalasia in patients with features of achalasia that do not meet the manometric criteria for achalasia. One study evaluated a subgroup of patients with clinical and radiologic features of achalasia but did not have an integrated relaxation pressure (IRP) greater than 15 as required by the Chicago Classification for diagnosis. These patients were found to have decreased EGJ distensibility and they symptomatically improved after treatment of achalasia.[23]

### Esophagogastric junction outflow obstruction

EGJ outflow obstruction as a diagnosis under the Chicago Classification of esophageal motility disorders on high-resolution manometry is a challenging category to diagnose and treat because it represents a heterogeneous group of diseases including mechanical obstruction, evolving achalasia, or an artifact of the manometry catheter.[24] The FLIP can help confirm a true obstruction. We recommend using the FLIP for the investigation of nonobstructive dysphagia (**Fig. 3**).[3]

### Upper Esophageal Sphincter

The upper esophageal sphincter (UES) is essential for oropharyngeal swallowing and is comprised of the cricopharyngeus muscle, the proximal cervical esophagus, and the inferior pharyngeal constrictor muscle. The UES is an interesting area of potential future FLIP application. The current methods to assess the UES include video fluoroscopy, direct visualization with a nasopharyngeal scope, and pharyngeal manometry. The FLIP has been shown to be feasible and safe to evaluate the distensibility of the UES in postlaryngectomy patients.[25] Additionally, the FLIP has been used to measure upper sphincter distensibility and opening patterns during swallowing in healthy control subjects.[23] More studies are required for potential clinical application of the FLIP in the evaluation of the UES.

# FUNCTIONAL LUMINAL IMAGING PROBE PANOMETRY: A METHOD TO DISTINGUISH TRUE EGJOO

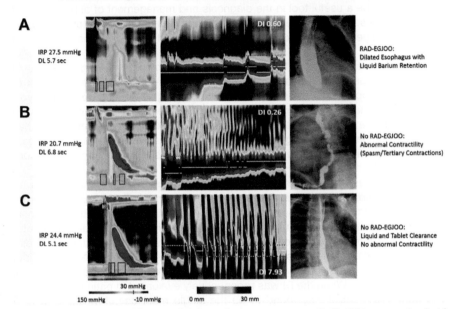

**Fig. 3.** Representative swallows on high-resolution manometry (*left*), FLIP panometry (*middle*), and esophagram (*right*) for three patients diagnosed with esophagogastric junction outflow obstruction (EGJOO) based on IRP >15 mm Hg. (*A*) True-EGJOO (achalasia) with a FLIP DI <2 mm²/mm Hg. (*B*) Borderline abnormal manometry with some early compartmentalized pressurization during the swallow. However, the FLIP topography suggests a true EG-JOO with FLIP DI <2 mm²/mm Hg and erratic contractions that are disordered and retrograde. This is more consistent with what is seen on the esophagram (*rosary beads and corkscrew*). (*C*) False-positive EGJOO on high-resolution manometry as the FLIP reveals a normal RAC pattern and a normal EGJ-DI. The esophagram supports normal emptying. IRP, integrated relaxation pressure; DL, distal latency; RAD, radiographic. (*Courtesy of* the Esophageal Center at Northwestern, Chicago, IL.)

## ASSESSING WALL STIFFNESS
### Eosinophilic Esophagitis

Eosinophilic esophagitis (EoE) is a chronic immune-mediated disease of the esophagus with chronic inflammation that leads to fibrosis of the esophageal lumen resulting in esophageal narrowing. Esophageal symptoms of EoE include dysphagia, regurgitation, chest pain, and food impactions. Esophageal biopsies are histologically characterized by increased eosinophils.[26] The FLIP is used in EoE to assess esophageal narrowing and the mechanical characteristics of the esophageal body. This includes measuring esophageal remodeling from fibrosis. The distensibility plateau is identified through measuring the narrowest esophageal body cross-sectional area and the corresponding intraballoon pressure during volume distention (**Fig. 4**). Compared with control patients, EoE patients have decreased compliance of the esophageal body.[27] Decreased distensibility using the FLIP has been shown in adults with EoE and is a risk factor for severity of rings and strictures seen endoscopically, need for dilation, and food impaction.[28] The

Distal distensibility plateau: 10.1 mm; proximal distensibility plateau: 12 mm

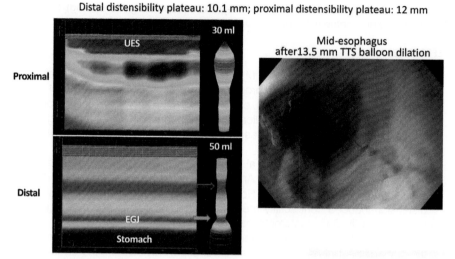

**Fig. 4.** Two representative FLIP 2.0 images of the distal and proximal esophagus. Note the sphincter landmark in each. They had a narrow-caliber esophagus with a dominant EGJ stricture around 10 mm (*green arrow*) and another distal body stricture (*purple arrow*) around 12 mm. Note the tear in the esophagus after a balloon dilation to 13.5 mm. TTS, through the scope. (*Courtesy of* the Esophageal Center at Northwestern, Chicago, IL.)

FLIP may be superior to current practices of monitoring disease activity through upper endoscopy with biopsies because sampling may be inconsistent. Esophageal fibrosis measured endoscopically has been found to be inaccurate compared with fluoroscopy.[29]

The FLIP was recently studied in a pediatric population by Menard-Katcher and colleagues[30] and they found that esophageal distensibility is decreased in children with EoE compared with control subjects and this corresponded to a 2-mm difference in esophageal caliber. Distensibility in patients with EoE was negatively correlated with eosinophil density and children without EoE had increasing distensibility with age, which was not found in the children with EoE. This points to esophageal remodeling results in decreased distensibility in children with EoE.

## SUMMARY

The FLIP has demonstrated its clinical utility as a diagnostic tool and a tool to guide and measure treatment response. With published normative data from healthy control patients and real-time interpretation of FLIP panometry during the endoscopy now available, FLIP is poised to become the initial test for the evaluation of dysphagia.

## DISCLOSURE

J.E. Pandolfino holds shared intellectual property rights and ownership surrounding FLIP panometry systems, methods, and apparatus with Medtronic Inc. J.E. Pandolfino discloses Crospon, Inc (stock options), Given Imaging (Consultant, Grant, Speaking), Sandhill Scientific (Consulting, Speaking), Takeda (Speaking), Astra Zeneca

(Speaking), Medtronic (Speaking, Consulting), Torax (Speaking, Consulting), Ironwood (Consulting), and Impleo (Grant). E.N. Donnan has nothing to disclose.

## REFERENCES

1. Kahrilas PJ, Bredenoord AJ, Fox M, et al. The Chicago Classification of esophageal motility disorders, v3.0. Neurogastroenterol Motil 2015;27(2):160–74.
2. McMahon BP, Frokjaer JB, Liao D, et al. A new technique for evaluating sphincter function in visceral organs: application of the functional lumen imaging probe (FLIP) for the evaluation of the oesophago-gastric junction. Physiol Meas 2005; 26(5):823–36.
3. Carlson DA, Kahrilas PJ, Lin Z, et al. Evaluation of esophageal motility utilizing the functional lumen imaging probe. Am J Gastroenterol 2016;111(12):1726–35.
4. Carlson DA, Kou W, Lin Z, et al. Normal values of esophageal distensibility and distension-induced contractility measured by functional luminal imaging probe panometry. Clin Gastroenterol Hepatol 2019;17(4):674–81.e1.
5. Hirano I, Pandolfino JE, Boeckxstaens GE. Functional lumen imaging probe for the management of esophageal disorders: expert review from the clinical practice updates committee of the AGA institute. Clin Gastroenterol Hepatol 2017; 15(3):325–34.
6. Ahuja NK, Agnihotri A, Lynch KL, et al. Esophageal distensibility measurement: impact on clinical management and procedure length. Dis Esophagus 2017; 30(8):1–8.
7. Carlson DA, Gyawali CP, Kahrilas PJ, et al. Esophageal motility classification can be established at the time of endoscopy: a study evaluating real-time functional luminal imaging probe panometry. Gastrointest Endosc 2019;90(6):915–23.e1.
8. Carlson DA, Lin Z, Kahrilas PJ, et al. The functional lumen imaging probe detects esophageal contractility not observed with manometry in patients with achalasia. Gastroenterology 2015;149(7):1742–51.
9. Carlson DA, Lin Z, Rogers MC, et al. Utilizing functional lumen imaging probe topography to evaluate esophageal contractility during volumetric distention: a pilot study. Neurogastroenterol Motil 2015;27(7):981–9.
10. Pandolfino JE, Shi G, Curry J, et al. Esophagogastric junction distensibility: a factor contributing to sphincter incompetence. Am J Physiol Gastrointest Liver Physiol 2002;282(6):G1052–8.
11. Lottrup C, McMahon BP, Ejstrud P, et al. Esophagogastric junction distensibility in hiatus hernia. Dis Esophagus 2016;29(5):463–71.
12. Kwiatek MA, Pandolfino JE, Hirano I, et al. Esophagogastric junction distensibility assessed with an endoscopic functional luminal imaging probe (EndoFLIP). Gastrointest Endosc 2010;72(2):272–8.
13. Tucker E, Sweis R, Anggiansah A, et al. Measurement of esophago-gastric junction cross-sectional area and distensibility by an endolumenal functional lumen imaging probe for the diagnosis of gastro-esophageal reflux disease. Neurogastroenterol Motil 2013;25(11):904–10.
14. Carlson DA, Kathpalia P, Craft J, et al. The relationship between esophageal acid exposure and the esophageal response to volumetric distention. Neurogastroenterol Motil 2018;30(3).
15. Smeets FG, Keszthelyi D, Bouvy ND, et al. Does measurement of esophagogastric junction distensibility by EndoFLIP predict therapy- responsiveness to endoluminal fundoplication in patients with gastroesophageal reflux disease? J Neurogastroenterol Motil 2015;21(2):255–64.

16. Kwiatek MA, Kahrilas K, Soper NJ, et al. Esophagogastric junction distensibility after fundoplication assessed with a novel functional luminal imaging probe. J Gastrointest Surg 2010;14(2):268–76.
17. Ilczyszyn A, Botha AJ. Feasibility of esophagogastric junction distensibility measurement during Nissen fundoplication. Dis Esophagus 2014;27(7):637–44.
18. Perretta S, Dallemagne B, McMahon B, et al. Video. Improving functional esophageal surgery with a "smart" bougie: Endoflip. Surg Endosc 2011;25(9):3109.
19. Ngamruengphong S, von Rahden BH, Filser J, et al. Intraoperative measurement of esophagogastric junction cross-sectional area by impedance planimetry correlates with clinical outcomes of peroral endoscopic myotomy for achalasia: a multicenter study. Surg Endosc 2016;30(7):2886–94.
20. Campagna RAJ, Carlson DA, Hungness ES, et al. Intraoperative assessment of esophageal motility using FLIP during myotomy for achalasia. Surg Endosc 2020 Jun;34(6):2593–600.
21. Wu PI, Szczesniak MM, Craig PI, et al. Novel intra-procedural distensibility measurement accurately predicts immediate outcome of pneumatic dilatation for idiopathic achalasia. Am J Gastroenterol 2018;113(2):205–12.
22. Jain AS, Carlson DA, Triggs J, et al. Esophagogastric junction distensibility on functional lumen imaging probe topography predicts treatment response in achalasia-anatomy matters! Am J Gastroenterol 2019;114(9):1455–63.
23. Ponds FA, Bredenoord AJ, Kessing BF, et al. Esophagogastric junction distensibility identifies achalasia subgroup with manometrically normal esophagogastric junction relaxation. Neurogastroenterol Motil 2017;29(1).
24. Triggs JR, Carlson DA, Beveridge C, et al. Upright integrated relaxation pressure facilitates characterization of esophagogastric junction outflow obstruction. Clin Gastroenterol Hepatol 2019;17(11):2218–26.e2.
25. Regan J, Walshe M, Timon C, et al. Endoflip(R) evaluation of pharyngo-oesophageal segment tone and swallowing in a clinical population: a total laryngectomy case series. Clin Otolaryngol 2015;40(2):121–9.
26. Dellon ES, Gonsalves N, Hirano I, et al. ACG clinical guideline: evidenced based approach to the diagnosis and management of esophageal eosinophilia and eosinophilic esophagitis (EoE). Am J Gastroenterol 2013;108(5):679–92 [quiz 693].
27. Kwiatek MA, Hirano I, Kahrilas PJ, et al. Mechanical properties of the esophagus in eosinophilic esophagitis. Gastroenterology 2011;140(1):82–90.
28. Nicodeme F, Hirano I, Chen J, et al. Esophageal distensibility as a measure of disease severity in patients with eosinophilic esophagitis. Clin Gastroenterol Hepatol 2013;11(9):1101–7.e1.
29. Gentile N, Katzka D, Ravi K, et al. Oesophageal narrowing is common and frequently under-appreciated at endoscopy in patients with oesophageal eosinophilia. Aliment Pharmacol Ther 2014;40(11–12):1333–40.
30. Menard-Katcher C, Benitez AJ, Pan Z, et al. Influence of age and eosinophilic esophagitis on esophageal distensibility in a pediatric cohort. Am J Gastroenterol 2017;112(9):1466–73.

# Evaluation and Treatment of Patients with Persistent Reflux Symptoms Despite Proton Pump Inhibitor Treatment

Stuart Jon Spechler, MD

## KEYWORDS

- Gastroesophageal reflux disease • Reflux hypersensitivity • Functional heartburn
- Fundoplication

## KEY POINTS

- Up to 40% of patients who take proton pump inhibitors (PPIs) for gastroesophageal reflux disease (GERD) complain of persistent GERD symptoms.
- PPI-refractory GERD symptoms are those that do not respond to double-dose PPI therapy (first dose taken 30–60 minutes before breakfast, second dose taken 30–60 minutes before dinner).
- For PPI-refractory GERD symptoms, endoscopy can exclude eosinophilic esophagitis, and esophageal manometry can exclude major motility disorders.
- Reflux hypersensitivity is diagnosed when esophageal MII-pH monitoring reveals normal esophageal acid exposure with a positive symptom index (SI) and/or symptom association probability (SAP) for heartburn.
- Functional heartburn is diagnosed when esophageal MII-pH monitoring reveals normal esophageal acid exposure with a negative SI and/or SAP for heartburn.

The proton pump inhibitors (PPIs), which are powerful suppressors of gastric acid secretion, are among the most commonly used medications in the world.[1] It has been estimated that more than 7% of adults in the United States take prescription PPIs, with gastroesophageal reflux disease (GERD) being the most common indication.[2] The PPIs are widely regarded as the mainstay of medical therapy for GERD, and they are extremely effective for healing reflux esophagitis[3]; however, they are considerably less effective than once thought for eliminating GERD symptoms. Up to 40% of patients who take PPIs for GERD complain of persistent GERD symptoms,[4] and "PPI-refractory GERD" is the most common reason for GERD-related referrals to gastroenterologists.[5]

Division of Gastroenterology, Center for Esophageal Diseases, Baylor University Medical Center, Center for Esophageal Research, Baylor Scott & White Research Institute, 3500 Gaston Avenue, 2 Hoblitzelle, Suite 250, Dallas, TX 75246, USA
E-mail address: sjspechler@aol.com

Gastroenterol Clin N Am 49 (2020) 437–450
https://doi.org/10.1016/j.gtc.2020.04.003
0889-8553/20/© 2020 Elsevier Inc. All rights reserved.

The typical symptoms of GERD are heartburn and regurgitation, but GERD can have numerous atypical symptoms, such as chest pain, chronic cough, hoarseness, and throat clearing.[6] In general, the typical GERD symptom of heartburn is far more likely to respond to PPIs than the atypical symptoms, but a PPI response is neither a sensitive nor specific test for GERD, even for patients with heartburn.[7] In a study in which 299 primary care patients with heartburn, regurgitation, or chest pain were given a "PPI test" (esomeprazole 40 mg every day for 2 weeks), a symptomatic response was seen in 67% of those in whom objective tests (endoscopy, esophageal pH monitoring) eventually established a diagnosis of GERD; however, 60% of those with no objective evidence of GERD also had a symptomatic response to esomeprazole.[8]

All the PPIs are prodrugs that require acid for activation. Acid converts the PPI prodrug to a sulfenamide form that can bind covalently to (and thereby disable) proton pumps ($H^+$, $K^+$-ATPases) of the gastric parietal cells. As a result of their requirement for acid activation, PPIs can bind only to proton pumps that are actively secreting acid. In the fasting state, fewer than 10% of gastric proton pumps are active, whereas approximately 70% are active when stimulated by meals.[9] Consequently, PPIs are most effective when taken 30 to 60 minutes before meals. One study of 100 patients with persistent GERD symptoms despite PPI therapy found that 54 took their PPIs incorrectly (21 >60 minutes before meals, 16 after meals, 15 at bedtime, 2 as needed).[10] Thus, it is important to query patients with "PPI-refractory GERD" on how they are taking their PPIs, and to stress the importance of taking them 30 to 60 minutes before meals. Some patients will respond to this simple clinical maneuver.

## VARYING DEFINITIONS OF PROTON PUMP INHIBITOR–REFRACTORY GASTROESOPHAGEAL REFLUX DISEASE SYMPTOMS

There is no clear consensus on the type, dosing, and duration of PPI therapy required to establish a diagnosis of PPI-refractory GERD symptoms. The acid-suppression potency of available PPI preparations varies widely, although all have been shown to be effective for healing reflux esophagitis in their standard dosages. Based on the effects of different PPIs on mean 24-hour intragastric pH measurements, relative potencies of the individual agents can be standardized to omeprazole in terms of "omeprazole equivalents" (OEs, with omeprazole having an OE of 1.00).[11,12] By so doing, the relative potencies of standard-dose pantoprazole, lansoprazole, omeprazole, esomeprazole, and rabeprazole have been estimated at 0.23, 0.90, 1.00, 1.60, and 1.82 OEs, respectively[11,12]; that is, 4 pantoprazole tablets are needed to achieve the acid-suppressing capability of 1 omeprazole tablet. Furthermore, individual patients can exhibit considerable variability in their response to different PPIs.[13] These data provide conceptual support for the practice of switching patients with PPI-refractory symptoms from one PPI to another, preferably more potent one, although there are few clinical data that support the clinical efficacy of this maneuver.

The US Food and Drug Administration approves only once-daily dosing of PPIs for GERD, and limited studies suggest that there is only modest gain achieved by doubling the standard PPI dose for patients with refractory GERD symptoms.[14] Nevertheless, most authorities will not consider patients "PPI-refractory" until they have been on a double dose of PPIs. For double-dose PPI therapy, patients should take the first dose 30 to 60 minutes before breakfast, and the second dose 30 to 60 minutes before dinner. Sifrim and Zerbib[4] proposed that patients with heartburn and regurgitation not responding to 12 weeks of double-dose PPI treatment (ie, troublesome symptoms still occurring ≥3 times per week) can be considered to have PPI-refractory reflux symptoms. Yadlapati and Delay[15] have suggested that PPI-refractory GERD should be defined as persistent troublesome GERD symptoms and objective evidence of GERD after 8 weeks of double-dose PPI therapy. These definitions might be useful as criteria for clinical studies, but also might be too restrictive for strict application in clinical practice.

There is no clear consensus on the type of GERD symptoms that qualify for inclusion under the rubric of "PPI-refractory." Although many observational studies have reported beneficial effects of PPI treatment for extraesophageal GERD symptoms, such as throat clearing, hoarseness, and chronic cough, controlled trials have not regularly demonstrated a benefit of PPIs over placebo for these conditions.[16–20] It can be argued whether or not it is appropriate to use the term "PPI-refractory" for a condition that might never be PPI-responsive. Among the atypical GERD symptoms, noncardiac chest pain shows the best response to PPIs.[6] A systematic review of randomized controlled trials that explored PPI effects on chest pain found therapeutic gain for PPIs in 56% to 85% of patients with objective evidence of GERD by pH monitoring or endoscopy, but in only 0% to 17% of patients without such objective evidence.[21]

Regurgitation is widely regarded as a typical GERD symptom, but there is disagreement among physicians regarding the definition of regurgitation. As a gastrointestinal fellow, I was taught that regurgitation is the effortless appearance of gastric material in the mouth, in contrast to vomiting, which requires effort and is often associated with the symptom of nausea. Although I still feel that this is a useful definition of regurgitation, I can provide no reference for it. Experts at the Montreal consensus conference on GERD defined regurgitation as "the perception of flow of refluxed gastric content into the mouth or hypopharynx."[22] However, the Reflux Disease Questionnaire (RDQ), a validated instrument used in the evaluation of patients with GERD, has 2 items that can be considered regurgitation: (1) an acid taste in the mouth, and (2) unpleasant movement of material upward from the stomach. Studies using the RDQ have found that regurgitation is a troublesome symptom in approximately 50% of patients with GERD, and that PPIs relieve regurgitation only marginally better than placebo.[20,23] Because PPIs inhibit gastric acid production but do nothing to correct the diathesis for reflux in patients with GERD, it is not surprising that PPIs have little efficacy in relieving regurgitation.[24]

## PROTON PUMP INHIBITOR–REFRACTORY HEARTBURN

Heartburn, a burning sensation in the retrosternal area, is the cardinal and most frequent symptom of GERD, and GERD is the most frequent cause of heartburn.[22] However, heartburn is by no means specific for GERD. For example, a symptom indistinguishable from the heartburn of GERD can affect patients with eosinophilic esophagitis or esophageal motility disorders like achalasia, and balloon distention of the esophagus can elicit retrosternal burning typical of heartburn.[25] Furthermore, a patient's concept of what is meant by the word "heartburn" can differ substantially from the physician's concept, and it is important for physicians to ask patients who say that they have heartburn to describe the symptom.[26] When so asked, many patients will describe a symptom that clearly is not the typical heartburn of GERD, including the crushing, exercise-induced, left-sided chest pain (angina pectoris) of coronary artery disease.

There are 5 major mechanisms that might underlie heartburn that does not respond to PPIs:[27]

1. The PPIs have not normalized esophageal acid exposure.
2. The PPIs have normalized esophageal acid exposure, but persistent reflux events (acidic or nonacidic) nevertheless evoke heartburn. This condition is called reflux hypersensitivity.[28]

3. The sensation of heartburn is caused by an esophageal disorder other than GERD, such as eosinophilic esophagitis or achalasia.
4. The sensation of heartburn is caused by an extraesophageal disorder, such as heart disease or gallbladder disease.
5. The sensation of heartburn is not caused by GERD, reflux events, or any other identifiable histopathologic, motility, or structural abnormality. This condition is called functional heartburn.[28]

It is possible to distinguish among these mechanisms with a rigorous systematic evaluation that includes careful medical history, endoscopy with esophageal biopsy, esophageal manometry, and esophageal multichannel intraluminal impedance (MII)-pH monitoring. These mechanisms are discussed in detail as follows.

### Proton Pump Inhibitors Have not Normalized Esophageal Acid Exposure

Two studies that have analyzed esophageal pH monitoring studies in patients with PPI-refractory GERD symptoms who were on standard, once-daily PPI therapy showed that abnormal esophageal acid exposure persisted in approximately one-third of cases.[29,30] One of those studies also evaluated patients with PPI-refractory GERD symptoms on twice-daily PPI therapy.[29] Abnormal esophageal acid exposure was found in only 7% of 52 patients with typical GERD symptoms, and in only 1% of patients with extraesophageal GERD symptoms on PPIs twice a day. Thus, the likelihood that twice-daily PPIs have not normalized esophageal acid exposure is small. Stated differently, persistent abnormal acid reflux is a decidedly uncommon cause of persistent GERD symptoms in patients on twice-daily PPIs.

### Proton Pump Inhibitors Have Normalized Esophageal Acid Exposure, but Persistent Reflux Events Evoke Heartburn (Reflux Hypersensitivity)

Before the advent of esophageal impedance monitoring, acid hypersensitivity was diagnosed when pH monitoring studies identified patients with normal total esophageal acid exposure in whom "physiologic" episodes of acid reflux were associated with GERD symptoms. More recently, esophageal MII-pH monitoring studies have established that nonacidic reflux episodes (pH > 4) also can be associated with symptoms. Consequently, the term "acid hypersensitivity" has been dropped, and the condition in which patients with normal esophageal acid exposure have reflux episodes (acidic or nonacidic) associated with heartburn now is called reflux hypersensitivity. It has been estimated that 38% to 36% of patients who do not respond to twice-daily PPI therapy have reflux hypersensitivity.[6]

It has been assumed that refluxed acid causes symptoms by activating nociceptors in the esophageal epithelium that convey pain.[31] The mechanism whereby the reflux of nonacidic material causes heartburn is less clear. Although refluxed material with pH >4 by convention is considered "nonacidic," perhaps weakly acidic refluxate (pH >4 and <7) triggers pain through the same mechanisms as more strongly acidic material. Alternatively, the reflux of irritants other than acid (eg, bile salts) might trigger heartburn, or large-volume reflux might cause esophageal distention that elicits the sensation of heartburn. An association has been established between sustained contraction of esophageal longitudinal muscle and the sensations of heartburn and chest pain.[31,32]

Reflux hypersensitivity is diagnosed by esophageal pH or MII-pH monitoring studies that have used either the symptom index (SI) or the symptom association probability (SAP) to identify a significant association between episodes of reflux and episodes of symptoms. To calculate the SI, the total number of reflux episodes that are associated with symptom episodes is divided by the total number of symptom episodes recorded during the monitoring period.[33] An SI $\geq$50% is considered positive (ie, at least 50% of all symptom episodes are associated with an episode of reflux). A major problem with the SI is that it does not consider the total number of reflux events, and this can yield misleading results in certain situations. For example, suppose that a patient has 100 episodes of acid reflux during the monitoring period but only 1 symptom episode, which happens to correspond with one of the acid reflux episodes. That patient would have an SI of 100%, spuriously suggesting a very strong association between symptoms and reflux episodes.

The SAP was developed to circumvent the shortcomings of the SI.[34] To determine the SAP, the 24-hour monitoring period is divided into 720 two-minute increments, and each increment is evaluated for the occurrence of reflux and symptom episodes. A Fisher's exact test is performed to determine a P-value for the probability that the reflux and symptom events are randomly distributed. The SAP is determined by subtracting the calculated P-value from 1, and the remainder is multiplied by 100%. Thus, a positive SAP (>95%) establishes a significant association between reflux and symptom episodes (ie, the P-value is < .05). SAP and SI results do not always agree and, despite the theoretic advantages of the SAP, its clinical superiority over the SI has not been established unequivocally.

### Heartburn Is Caused by an Esophageal Disorder Other than Gastroesophageal Reflux Disease

Conceivably, any inflammatory disorder of the esophagus might cause the retrosternal burning discomfort of heartburn, but eosinophilic esophagitis (EoE) is the inflammatory disorder most likely to be confused with GERD. Dysphagia and food impaction usually are the predominant symptoms of EoE, but confusion with GERD can arise when heartburn is a major complaint.[35] Endoscopy revealing the typical findings of EoE (exudates, rings, edema, furrows, stricture) supports the diagnosis, which is established when esophageal biopsies show more than 15 eosinophils per high power field. One caveat for the clinician to bear in mind is that PPIs can eliminate the endoscopic and histologic signs of EoE, and so an endoscopy performed for a patient on PPIs cannot rule out EoE.[36] If possible, PPIs should be discontinued for 3 to 4 weeks before diagnostic endoscopy when EoE is a consideration. Achalasia, an esophageal motility disorder that typically causes dysphagia, frequently is associated with heartburn that can be confused with GERD.[37] It is not clear whether the sensation of heartburn in achalasia is caused by the abnormal esophageal muscle activity, or by acid in the esophagus. Abnormal esophageal acid exposure has been documented in patients with achalasia, although it is not clear whether this is due to refluxed gastric acid or to lactic acid produced by the fermentation of carbohydrate retained in the achalasic esophagus.[38] Confusion with PPI-refractory GERD occasionally has resulted in patients with achalasia undergoing fundoplication to treat symptoms mistakenly attributed to GERD. Fundoplication can cause debilitating dysphagia in this setting.[39] To avoid this potentially devastating mistake, esophageal manometry should be performed in all patients before fundoplication for the treatment of GERD.

### Heartburn Is Caused by an Extraesophageal Disorder

GERD is associated with obesity, which is strongly associated with coronary artery diseases (CAD).[40] Therefore, heartburn due to GERD is not uncommon in patients with CAD.[41] Although angina can be described as burning in character and angina might be incorrectly diagnosed as heartburn due to GERD,[42] there is surprisingly little published documentation of this error. As mentioned earlier, patients might use the word "heartburn" incorrectly to describe their typical anginal symptoms. If such patients tell their physicians that they been experiencing "heartburn," and the physicians take that history at face value without asking for a description of the heartburn symptom, then angina due to CAD might well be confused with GERD. It is not clear how often angina causes retrosternal burning discomfort that a careful history would not distinguish from the heartburn of GERD. Nevertheless, the consequences of misdiagnosing CAD as GERD can be catastrophic, and clinicians should consider the possibility that CAD might be causing a heartburn sensation that does not respond to PPIs, especially in older patients with other risk factors for CAD.

The pain of pancreatic or biliary tract disease can be referred to the epigastrium and lower chest, might be described as burning in character, and will not respond to PPIs. As is the case for angina due to CAD, however, it is not clear how often pancreaticobiliary diseases cause retrosternal burning discomfort that a careful history would not distinguish from the heartburn of GERD. Nevertheless, it is important to consider that pancreaticobiliary diseases might underlie PPI-refractory pain, especially in patients with other risk factors for those diseases.

### Functional Heartburn

The term "functional" has been used inconsistently in the medical literature, and experts continue to disagree on its proper usage. To classify the functional gastrointestinal disorders (ie, those not due to any named histopathologic, motility, or structural abnormality), a group of experts devised the "Rome criteria" in 1992. Since then, there have been another 3 iterations of the Rome criteria. The investigators of all these iterations have struggled with use of the term "functional," noting that it can be both nonspecific and potentially stigmatizing, and that patients with "functional" disorders can have subtle histopathologic and physiologic abnormalities that have no specific names. The most recent Rome iteration (Rome IV) contains a disclaimer discouraging use of the term "functional," and a proposal to change the name "functional gastrointestinal disorders" to "disorders of gut-brain interaction."[43] Nevertheless, the authors of the esophageal disorders portion of the Rome IV criteria continue to use the term "functional gastrointestinal disorders," retain the term "functional heartburn," and specifically deem reflux hypersensitivity a "functional gastrointestinal disorder."[28]

According to Rome IV, functional heartburn is defined as retrosternal burning discomfort or pain that is refractory to "optimal antisecretory therapy" in the absence of GERD, histopathologic mucosal abnormalities, major motor disorders, or structural explanations. Functional heartburn is distinguished from reflux hypersensitivity by esophageal pH or MII-pH monitoring studies that show no association between reflux episodes and heartburn episodes (ie, SI <50% and/or SAP ≤95%). It has been estimated that 29% to 39% of patients who do not respond to twice-daily PPI therapy have functional heartburn.[6]

### TREATMENTS OTHER THAN PROTON PUMP INHIBITORS
#### Antireflux Lifestyle Modifications

Antireflux lifestyle modifications include elevation of the head of the bed on 4-inch to 6-inch blocks; weight loss for overweight patients; avoiding recumbency for several hours after meals; avoiding bedtime snacks; and avoiding fatty foods, smoking, and alcoholic beverages. Data that support the efficacy of these lifestyle modifications in controlling GERD, especially GERD that is refractory to PPI therapy, are very limited. Nevertheless, it is reasonable to try these modifications, especially for patients in whom regurgitation is a prominent complaint, and for patients with reflux hypersensitivity.

## Baclofen

A major mechanism underlying episodes of gastroesophageal reflux is a sudden, protracted collapse of lower esophageal sphincter (LES) pressure called a transient LES relaxation (TLESR).[44] Unlike the brief, appropriate LES relaxations that accompany swallow-induced peristalsis, TLESRs are not preceded by swallowing and last more than 10 seconds. The TLESR is part of the normal belch reflex that is triggered by gaseous distention of the stomach. The nucleus tractus solitarius in the medulla is involved in the reflex, both in integrating sensory information from the stomach and in controlling the neural circuits that trigger the TLESR. Neurons with γ-aminobutyric acid B ($GABA_B$) receptors can inhibit TLESRs, and baclofen is a $GABA_B$ agonist that has been shown to decrease the frequency of TLESRs.[45] However, baclofen often causes intolerable drowsiness and other side effects, and studies on its efficacy for PPI-refractory GERD are very limited. Other $GABA_B$ agonists have been developed, including arbaclofen placarbil and lesogaberan, but have been abandoned because of poor clinical efficacy.[46,47]

## Alginates

In the presence of gastric acid, alginates precipitate into a gel that forms a "raft" that floats on top of the gastric contents, thereby creating a mechanical barrier that displaces the postprandial acid pocket distally into the stomach and out of the esophagus. A recent systematic review and meta-analysis concluded that alginates are more effective than placebo and antacids for treating GERD symptoms.[48] Limited data suggest that combining alginates with PPIs might yield better control of GERD symptoms than PPIs alone in patients with nonerosive reflux disease.[49]

## Adding a Histamine H2 Receptor Antagonist at Bedtime

Histamine H2 receptor antagonists (H2RAs) are considerably less effective at inhibiting gastric acid production and at healing erosive esophagitis than the PPIs. However, approximately 70% to 80% of individuals treated with twice-daily PPIs experience the phenomenon of nocturnal gastric acid breakthrough, defined as a fall in gastric pH below 4 for more than 1 hour at night. Nocturnal gastric acid breakthrough appears to be largely histamine-driven and, in the short-term, nocturnal gastric pH can be maintained above 4 by adding a bedtime dose of an H2-blocker. However, the clinical importance of nocturnal gastric acid breakthrough is not clear, and few data support the clinical efficacy of adding an H2RA at bedtime for patients with persistent GERD symptoms on PPI therapy.[50]

## Potassium-Competitive Acid Blockers

Like PPIs, the potassium-competitive acid blockers (P-CABs) also target the $H^+$, $K^+$-ATPase of the gastric parietal cell. Unlike PPIs, the P-CABs do not require an enteric coating that delays their absorption and do not require acid for their activation. Also unlike PPIs, the P-CABs bind ionically to both active and inactive proton pumps, and so do not have to be dosed around meals. Thus, the P-CABs a have more rapid onset of action than the PPIs, and they appear to block gastric acid secretion even more effectively than PPIs.[51] Presently P-CABs are not available for clinical use in the United States. The P-CAB vonoprazan is available in Japan, where it has demonstrated efficacy in healing erosive esophagitis not healed by conventional-dose PPI therapy.[52] Despite the theoretic advantages over PPIs, however, it is not clear that

P-CABs are any more effective than PPIs for treating GERD in Western patients. If and when P-CABs become available for use in Western countries, they might be especially useful for patients with persistently abnormal esophageal acid exposure on double-dose PPI therapy.

### Neuromodulators

Neuromodulators such as tricyclic antidepressants, trazadone, and selective seroto-nin reuptake inhibitors, used in dosages that allegedly do not alter mood, have been shown to have some efficacy in relieving noncardiac chest pain and heartburn in pa-tients with reflux hypersensitivity.[53–55] These agents are thought to dull visceral hyper-sensitivity through effects on central nervous system pain-processing pathways. Unfortunately, the neuromodulators often have intolerable and sometimes dangerous side effects, and studies on their efficacy for PPI-refractory heartburn are few and of short duration.

### Cognitive Behavioral Therapy

Cognitive behavioral therapy can be effective in patients with functional heartburn and reflux hypersensitivity, and a health psychologist with specialization in gastroenter-ology can be a valuable asset in patient management.[56] Unfortunately, the availability of such therapists is limited.

### Antireflux Procedures

Antireflux surgery (fundoplication) is widely regarded as the "gold-standard" among the antireflux procedures for its efficacy in improving the physiologic parameters of GERD, such as LES pressure and esophageal acid exposure time.[57] Fundoplication creates a barrier to the reflux of all gastric material (acidic and nonacidic), and therefore should be an effective treatment for PPI-refractory GERD symptoms that are reflux related. In practice, however, patients with "GERD symptoms" unre-sponsive to PPIs often do not respond to surgery either.[58] This might be due to pre-operative failure to exclude the non-GERD diseases and functional disorders that are frequent in this population, and to the use of fundoplication for the treatment of extraesophageal "GERD symptoms," such as cough and throat clearing that are not clearly reflux related. Modern laparoscopic antireflux surgery has a short-term complication rate (infection, bleeding, esophageal perforation) of approxi-mately 4%, a very low surgical mortality rate, and a GERD recurrence rate of approximately 18% within 5 years postoperatively.[59] Fundoplication also is frequently complicated by dysphagia and by inability to belch and vomit, and occa-sionally by other troublesome symptoms.

Magnetic sphincter augmentation (MSA) with the LINX Reflux Management System, a bracelet of magnetic beads that encircles the distal esophagus to bolster the LES and prevent reflux, was developed as a less invasive and more readily reversible GERD treatment than fundoplication. MSA has been shown to be an effective and du-rable therapy in carefully selected patients with GERD with symptoms incompletely controlled by PPIs, usually those with small hiatal hernias (<3 cm), mild or no reflux esophagitis, and documented abnormal esophageal acid exposure.[60] In addition, a recent randomized trial has established the unequivocal superiority of MSA over twice-daily PPIs for the control of regurgitation.[61]

A number of endoscopic therapies for GERD have been studied, and most of the devices have been removed from the marketplace because of concerns regarding safety and efficacy. Presently, the only endoscopic GERD treatments still widely avail-able are radiofrequency antireflux treatment (Stretta) and transoral incisionless fundoplication (TIF). Although some data support the use of Stretta in carefully selected patients with GERD who are dissatisfied with PPI therapy,[62] a recent systematic review and meta-analysis concluded that Stretta does not significantly alter physiologic parameters such as esophageal acid exposure and LES pressure, does not reliably enable patients to stop PPIs, and does not significantly improve health-related quality of life.[63] Randomized trials have shown that TIF is effective for treating troublesome regurgitation,[64,65] but the long-term benefit of TIF is not established and highly questionable.[57]

## MANAGEMENT OF PATIENTS WITH HEARTBURN REFRACTORY TO PROTON PUMP INHIBITOR THERAPY

An approach to management of patients who complain of heartburn refractory to PPI therapy is presented in **Fig. 1**. First, a careful medical history should be performed to confirm that the patient truly has heartburn, meaning retrosternal burning discomfort, and to identify warning symptoms such as dysphagia, weight loss, and gastrointestinal bleeding that might require expedited evaluation. The history might also provide clues regarding the presence of heart disease and other disorders that might be causing the patient's symptoms, and that might require urgent evaluation.

If the patient is not already on a regimen of twice-daily PPI therapy, that regimen should be implemented before proceeding with invasive tests. The importance of taking PPIs 30 to 60 minutes before breakfast and dinner should be stressed. Consideration also should be given to switching PPIs, especially for patients already on twice-daily PPI treatment, and for those taking pantoprazole, which is the least potent of the available PPIs for gastric acid suppression. If heartburn persists after 4 to 8 weeks of this PPI trial, PPIs can be stopped.

There is disagreement among experts regarding whether esophageal pH monitoring should be performed on or off PPIs for patients with PPI-refractory heartburn at this point in the workup.[66] The major argument for performing the test off PPI therapy is that a normal pH monitoring study eliminates GERD as a diagnostic concern, and thus should direct further diagnostic and therapeutic efforts at non-GERD disorders. The counterargument is that many patients will have an abnormal pH monitoring study off PPIs and, although this establishes that those patients have GERD, it does not establish that GERD is the cause of the PPI-refractory symptoms and it does not explain why the patients have not responded to PPIs. The physician's assessment of the pretest probability that the patient has GERD can be used to guide the choice of whether or not to perform esophageal pH monitoring off PPIs. If there is a high pretest probability that the patient has GERD (eg, a prior endoscopy showed long-segment Barrett esophagus or severe reflux esophagitis), then pH monitoring off PPIs is highly likely to be positive and highly unlikely to provide useful information. Conversely, if the pretest probability for GERD is low (eg, the heartburn description is questionable and there has been no response whatsoever to PPIs), then esophageal pH monitoring can be very helpful for guiding further evaluation and treatment.

When performing diagnostic endoscopy, it is important that PPIs are stopped for 3 to 4 weeks if possible when EoE is a diagnostic consideration. PPIs can eliminate the endoscopic and histologic signs of EoE, and so an endoscopy performed with a patient on PPI therapy cannot rule out EoE. Irrespective of the appearance of the esophagus, 2 to 4 biopsies should be taken from both the proximal and distal esophagus to look for EoE. Another advantage of stopping PPIs before endoscopy is that it will allow assessment of the presence and severity of reflux esophagitis. Although it is common for physicians to make a diagnosis of nonerosive reflux disease when endoscopy for

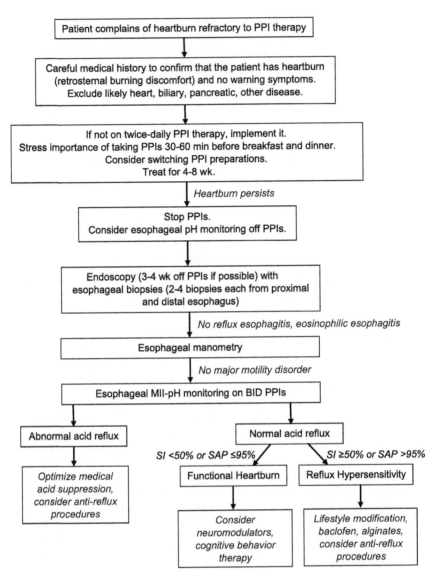

**Fig. 1.** Approach to the diagnosis and management of heartburn refractory to medical therapy. BID, twice a day.

heartburn shows no reflux esophagitis, that diagnosis is inappropriate unless PPIs were stopped because PPIs can eliminate all endoscopic signs of reflux esophagitis.

If there is no endoscopic evidence of EoE or reflux esophagitis, esophageal manometry is performed to seek major motility abnormalities like achalasia or distal esophageal spasm that can cause the symptom of heartburn. If there is no major motility disorder, then esophageal MII-pH monitoring is performed with the patient on twice-daily PPIs. If there is persistent abnormal acid reflux, then therapy can be focused on optimizing medical acid suppression or on controlling reflux with an anti-reflux procedure such as fundoplication or MSA. If there is normal acid reflux and the SI and/or SAP are negative (ie, SI <50%, SAP ≤95%), then the patient has functional heartburn, which might be treated with neuromodulators or with cognitive behavior therapy. If the SI and/or SAP are positive (ie, SI $\geq$ 50%, SAP >95%) in the patient with normal acid reflux, then reflux hypersensitivity is diagnosed. Patients with reflux hypersensitivity can be treated with antireflux lifestyle modifications, baclofen and alginates. Antireflux procedures like fundoplication and MSA can be recommended in highly selected patients.

## DISCLOSURE

S.J. Spechler has served as a consultant for Takeda Pharmaceuticals, Frazier Life Sciences, Phathom Pharmaceuticals, and Ironwood Pharmaceuticals, and receives royalties as an author for UpToDate.

## REFERENCES

1. Lanas A. We are using too many PPIs, and we need to stop: a European perspective. Am J Gastroenterol 2016;111:1085–6.
2. Kantor ED, Rehm CD, Haas JS, et al. Trends in prescription drug use among adults in the United States from 1999-2012. JAMA 2015;314:1818–31.
3. Katz PO, Gerson LB, Vela MF. Guidelines for the diagnosis and management of gastroesophageal reflux disease. Am J Gastroenterol 2013;108:308–28.
4. Sifrim D, Zerbib F. Diagnosis and management of patients with reflux symptoms refractory to proton pump inhibitors. Gut 2012;61:1340–54.
5. Fass R, Sifrim D. Management of heartburn not responding to proton pump inhibitors. Gut 2009;58:295–309.
6. Gyawali CP, Fass R. Management of gastroesophageal reflux disease. Gastroenterology 2018;154:302–18.
7. Gyawali CP, Kahrilas PJ, Savarino E, et al. Modern diagnosis of GERD: the Lyon Consensus. Gut 2018;67:1351–62.
8. Bytzer P, Jones R, Vakil N, et al. Limited ability of the proton-pump inhibitor test to identify patients with gastroesophageal reflux disease. Clin Gastroenterol Hepatol 2012;10:1360–6.
9. Shin JM, Sachs G. Pharmacology of proton pump inhibitors. Curr Gastroenterol Rep 2008;10(6):528–34.
10. Gunaratnam NT, Jessup TP, Inadomi J, et al. Sub-optimal proton pump inhibitor dosing is prevalent in patients with poorly controlled gastro-oesophageal reflux disease. Aliment Pharmacol Ther 2006;23:1473–7.
11. Kirchheiner J, Glatt S, Fuhr U, et al. Relative potency of proton-pump inhibitors-comparison of effects on intragastric pH. Eur J Clin Pharmacol 2009;65:19–31.
12. Graham DY, Tansel A. Interchangeable use of proton pump inhibitors based on relative potency. Clin Gastroenterol Hepatol 2018;16:800–8.
13. Katz PO, Koch FK, Ballard ED, et al. Comparison of the effects of immediate-release omeprazole oral suspension, delayed-release lansoprazole capsules and delayed-release esomeprazole capsules on nocturnal gastric acidity after bedtime dosing in patients with night-time GERD symptoms. Aliment Pharmacol Ther 2007;25(2):197–205.
14. Kahrilas PJ, Shaheen NJ, Vaezi MF, American Gastroenterological Association Institute, Clinical Practice and Quality Management Committee. American Gastroenterological Association Institute technical review on the management of gastroesophageal reflux disease. Gastroenterology 2008;135:1392–413.
15. Yadlapati R, DeLay K. Proton pump inhibitor-refractory gastroesophageal reflux disease. Med Clin North Am 2019;103:15–27.

16. Hom C, Vaezi MF. Extraesophageal manifestations of gastroesophageal reflux disease. Gastroenterol Clin North Am 2013;42:71–91.
17. Chang AB, Lasserson TJ, Gaffney J, et al. Gastro-oesophageal reflux treatment for prolonged non-specific cough in children and adults. Cochrane Database Syst Rev 2011;(1):CD004823.
18. Vaezi MF, Richter JE, Stasney CR, et al. Treatment of chronic posterior laryngitis with esomeprazole. Laryngoscope 2006;116:254–60.
19. Spantideas N, Drosou E, Bougea A, et al. Proton pump inhibitors for the treatment of laryngopharyngeal reflux. A systematic review. J Voice 2019. [Epub ahead of print].
20. Boeckxstaens G, El-Serag HB, Smout AJ, et al. Symptomatic reflux disease: the present, the past and the future. Gut 2014;63:1185–93.
21. Kahrilas PJ, Hughes N, Howden CW. Response of unexplained chest pain to proton pump inhibitor treatment in patients with and without objective evidence of gastro-oesophageal reflux disease. Gut 2011;60:1473–8.
22. Vakil N, van Zanten SV, Kahrilas P, et al, Global Consensus Group. The Montreal definition and classification of gastroesophageal reflux disease: a global evidence-based consensus. Am J Gastroenterol 2006;101:1900–20.
23. Kahrilas PJ, Jonsson A, Denison H, et al. Regurgitation is less responsive to acid suppression than heartburn in patients with gastroesophageal reflux disease. Clin Gastroenterol Hepatol 2012;10:612–9.
24. Vela MF, Camacho-Lobato L, Srinivasan R, et al. Simultaneous intraesophageal impedance and pH measurement of acid and nonacid gastroesophageal reflux: effect of omeprazole. Gastroenterology 2001;120:1599–606.
25. Fass R, Naliboff B, Higa L, et al. Differential effect of long-term esophageal acid exposure on mechanosensitivity and chemosensitivity in humans. Gastroenterology 1998;115:1363–73.
26. Spechler SJ, Jain SK, Tendler DA, et al. Racial differences in the frequency of symptoms and complications of gastro-oesophageal reflux disease. Aliment Pharmacol Ther 2002;16:1795–800.
27. Spechler SJ. Surgery for gastroesophageal reflux disease: esophageal impedance to progress? Clin Gastroenterol Hepatol 2009;7:1264–5.
28. Aziz Q, Fass R, Gyawali CP, et al. Functional esophageal disorders. Gastroenterology 2016;150:1368–79.
29. Charbel S, Khandwala F, Vaezi MF. The role of esophageal pH monitoring in symptomatic patients on PPI therapy. Am J Gastroenterol 2005;100:283–9.
30. Bautista JM, Wong WM, Pulliam G, et al. The value of ambulatory 24 hr esophageal pH monitoring in clinical practice in patients who were referred with persistent gastroesophageal reflux disease (GERD)-related symptoms while on standard dose anti-reflux medications. Dig Dis Sci 2005;50:1909–15.
31. Sifrim D, Mittal R, Fass R, et al. Review article: acidity and volume of the refluxate in the genesis of gastro-oesophageal reflux disease symptoms. Aliment Pharmacol Ther 2007;25:1003–17.
32. Mittal RK, Liu J, Puckett JL, et al. Sensory and motor function of the esophagus: lessons from ultrasound imaging. Gastroenterology 2005;128:487–97.
33. Wiener GJ, Richter JE, Copper JB, et al. The symptom index: a clinically important parameter of ambulatory 24-hour esophageal pH monitoring. Am J Gastroenterol 1988;83:358–61.
34. Weusten BL, Roelofs JM, Akkermans LM, et al. The symptom-association probability: an improved method for symptom analysis of 24-hour esophageal pH data. Gastroenterology 1994;107:1741–5.

35. Cheng E, Souza RF, Spechler SJ. Eosinophilic esophagitis: interactions with gastroesophageal reflux disease. Gastroenterol Clin North Am 2014;43:243–56.
36. Odiase E, Schwartz A, Souza RF, et al. New eosinophilic esophagitis concepts call for change in proton pump inhibitor management before diagnostic endoscopy. Gastroenterology 2018;154:1217–21.
37. Spechler SJ, Souza RF, Rosenberg SJ, et al. Heartburn in patients with achalasia. Gut 1995;37:305–8.
38. Smart HL, Foster PN, Evans DF, et al. Twenty four hour oesophageal acidity in achalasia before and after pneumatic dilatation. Gut 1987;28:883–7.
39. Kessing BF, Bredenoord AJ, Smout AJPM. Erroneous diagnosis of gastroesophageal reflux disease in achalasia. Clin Gastroenterol Hepatol 2011;9:1020–4.
40. Chang P, Friedenberg F. Obesity and GERD. Gastroenterol Clin North Am 2014; 43:161–73.
41. Teragawa H, Oshita C, Ueda T. History of gastroesophageal reflux disease in patients with suspected coronary artery disease. Heart Vessels 2019. [Epub ahead of print].
42. Bösner S, Haasenritter J, Becker A, et al. Heartburn or angina? Differentiating gastrointestinal disease in primary care patients presenting with chest pain: a cross sectional diagnostic study. Int Arch Med 2009;2:40.
43. Schmulson MJ, Drossman DA. What is new in Rome IV. J Neurogastroenterol Motil 2017;23:151–63.
44. Kessing BF, Conchillo JM, Bredenoord AJ, et al. Review article: the clinical relevance of transient lower oesophageal sphincter relaxations in gastro-oesophageal reflux disease. Aliment Pharmacol Ther 2011;33:650–61.
45. Li S, Shi S, Chen F, et al. The effects of baclofen for the treatment of gastroesophageal reflux disease: a meta-analysis of randomized controlled trials. Gastroenterol Res Pract 2014;2014:307805.
46. Vakil NB, Huff FJ, Bian A, et al. Arbaclofen placarbil in GERD: a randomized, double-blind, placebo-controlled study. Am J Gastroenterol 2011;106:1427–38.
47. Boeckxstaens GE, Beaumont H, Hatlebakk JG, et al. A novel reflux inhibitor lesogaberan (AZD3355) as add-on treatment in patients with GORD with persistent reflux symptoms despite proton pump inhibitor therapy: a randomised placebo-controlled trial. Gut 2011;60:1182–8.
48. Leiman DA, Riff BP, Morgan S, et al. Alginate therapy is effective treatment for GERD symptoms: a systematic review and meta-analysis. Dis Esophagus 2017;30:1–9.
49. Manabe N, Haruma K, Ito M, et al. Efficacy of adding sodium alginate to omeprazole in patients with nonerosive reflux disease: a randomized clinical trial. Dis Esophagus 2012;25:373–80.
50. Wang Y, Pan T, Wang Q, et al. Additional bedtime H2-receptor antagonist for the control of nocturnal gastric acid breakthrough. Cochrane Database Syst Rev 2009;(4):CD004275.
51. Hunt RH, Scarpignato C. Potassium-competitive acid blockers (P-CABs): are they finally ready for prime time in acid-related disease? Clin Transl Gastroenterol 2015;6:e119.
52. Tanabe T, Hoshino S, Kawami N, et al. Efficacy of long-term maintenance therapy with 10-mg vonoprazan for proton pump inhibitor-resistant reflux esophagitis. Esophagus 2019. [Epub ahead of print].
53. Weijenborg PW, de Schepper HS, Smout AJ, et al. Effects of antidepressants in patients with functional esophageal disorders or gastroesophageal reflux disease: a systematic review. Clin Gastroenterol Hepatol 2015;13:251–9.

54. Drossman DA, Tack J, Ford AC, et al. Neuromodulators for functional gastrointestinal disorders (disorders of gut-brain interaction): a rome foundation working team report. Gastroenterology 2018;154:1140–71.
55. Viazis N, Keyoglou A, Kanellopoulos AK, et al. Selective serotonin reuptake inhibitors for the treatment of hypersensitive esophagus: a randomized, double-blind, placebo-controlled study. Am J Gastroenterol 2012;107:1662–7.
56. Riehl ME, Kinsinger S, Kahrilas PJ, et al. Role of a health psychologist in the management of functional esophageal complaints. Dis Esophagus 2015;28:428–36.
57. Richter JE, Kumar A, Lipka S, et al. Efficacy of laparoscopic nissen fundoplication vs transoral incisionless fundoplication or proton pump inhibitors in patients with gastroesophageal reflux disease: a systematic review and network meta-analysis. Gastroenterology 2018;154:1298–308.
58. Morgenthal CB, Lin E, Shane MD, et al. Who will fail laparoscopic Nissen fundoplication? Preoperative prediction of long-term outcomes. Surg Endosc 2007;21: 1978–84.
59. Maret-Ouda J, Wahlin K, El-Serag HB, et al. Association between laparoscopic antireflux surgery and recurrence of gastroesophageal reflux. JAMA 2017;318: 939–46.
60. Saino G, Bonavina L, Lipham JC, et al. Magnetic sphincter augmentation for gastroesophageal reflux at 5 years: final results of a pilot study show long-term acid reduction and symptom improvement. J Laparoendosc Adv Surg Tech A 2015;25:787–92.
61. Bell R, Lipham J, Louie B, et al. Laparoscopic magnetic sphincter augmentation versus double-dose proton pump inhibitors for management of moderate-to-severe regurgitation in GERD: a randomized controlled trial. Gastrointest Endosc 2019;89:14–22.
62. Viswanath Y, Maguire N, Obuobi RB, et al. Endoscopic day case antireflux radiofrequency (Stretta) therapy improves quality of life and reduce proton pump inhibitor (PPI) dependency in patients with gastro-oesophageal reflux disease: a prospective study from a UK tertiary centre. Frontline Gastroenterol 2019;10: 113–9.
63. Lipka S, Kumar A, Richter JE. No evidence for efficacy of radiofrequency ablation for treatment of gastroesophageal reflux disease: a systematic review and meta-analysis. Clin Gastroenterol Hepatol 2015;13:1058–67.
64. Hunter JG, Kahrilas PJ, Bell RC, et al. Efficacy of transoral fundoplication vs omeprazole for treatment of regurgitation in a randomized controlled trial. Gastroenterology 2015;148:324–33.
65. Trad KS, Barnes WE, Simoni G, et al. Transoral incisionless fundoplication effective in eliminating GERD symptoms in partial responders to proton pump inhibitor therapy at 6 months: the TEMPO randomized clinical trial. Surg Innov 2015;22: 26–40.
66. Gawron AJ, Pandolfino JE. Ambulatory reflux monitoring in GERD–which test should be performed and should therapy be stopped? Curr Gastroenterol Rep 2013;15:316.

# Esophageal Evaluation for Patients Undergoing Lung Transplant Evaluation

## What Should We Do for Evaluation and Management

Zubair Malik, MD[a],*, Kartik Shenoy, MD[b]

### KEYWORDS

- Lung transplant • Gastroesophageal reflux • Esophageal motility
- Bronchiolitis obliterans • Scleroderma

### KEY POINTS

- Lung transplantation is lifesaving, but long-term survival is relatively low mainly due to chronic rejection, with bronchiolitis obliterans syndrome being the primary type.
- Gastroesophageal reflux disease and aspiration have been shown to cause or worsen bronchiolitis obliterans syndrome.
- Esophageal manometry and multichannel intraluminal impedance pH testing can help identify patients with acidic, weakly acidic, and nonacidic reflux.
- Aggressive management of reflux and aspiration, particularly with antireflux surgery, can improve lung function and survival in lung transplant recipients.

## INTRODUCTION

Lung transplantation is a high-risk solid organ transplant offered to patients with end-stage lung disease from a variety of different causes, which has dramatically increased in number over the past 20 years with more than 4500 lung transplants done in 2016.[1] Because of improvements in surgical techniques, immunosuppression, management of infections and ischemia-reperfusion injuries, and lung preservation, 1-year survival exceeds 80%, but long-term survival is not as high, with 5-year survival greater than 50%, and this has not changed much over the past 10 years.[1,2] Although lung

[a] Gastroenterology Section, Department of Medicine, Lewis Katz School of Medicine, Temple University, 3401 North Broad Street, 8th Floor Parkinson Pavilion, Philadelphia, PA 19140, USA;
[b] Department of Thoracic Medicine and Surgery, Lewis Katz School of Medicine, Temple University, 3401 North Broad Street, 7th Floor Parkinson Pavilion, Philadelphia, PA 19140, USA
* Corresponding author.
E-mail address: zubair.malik@tuhs.temple.edu
Twitter: @ZubairMalik_MD (Z.M.)

Gastroenterol Clin N Am 49 (2020) 451–466
https://doi.org/10.1016/j.gtc.2020.04.004
0889-8553/20/© 2020 Elsevier Inc. All rights reserved.

transplant can be lifesaving, chronic lung allograft dysfunction (CLAD), which encompasses all forms of chronic rejection including obstructive and restrictive forms of rejection, remains the biggest limiting factor to long-term survival.[3]

Bronchiolitis obliterans (BO) was first reported in 1984 and is defined as progressive obliteration of small airways that results from lymphocytic infiltrate of the submucosa of the airways, which invades into the basement membrane setting off an inflammatory cascade that leads to inflammation and fibrosis.[4-8] BO is diagnosed histologically by lung biopsy but due to its patchy nature biopsies have a low yield for detecting BO.[1,5] Bronchiolitis obliterans syndrome (BOS) is the clinical correlate of BO and is defined as a persistent decrease in forced expiratory volume in 1 second (FEV$_1$) of 20% of the 2 best postoperative measurements in the absence of any other cause.[4-6] Because of the significance of BOS, an early BOS stage was added in which the FEV1 is reduced to 81% to 90% and/or there is a drop in midexpiratory flow rate (BOS 0-P). BO and BOS are the most common types of CLAD, which are seen in 50% of lung transplantations at 5 years, and of those with BOS, 5-year survival is only 30% to 40%.

Several risk factors have been associated with the development of BOS, including cytomegalovirus infection, antibodies to class I human leukocyte antigen (HLA), and HLA mismatches. Acute rejection, which is divided into acute cellular rejection and lymphocytic bronchiolitis, has also been shown to be a risk factor to developing BOS, and the frequency and severity of acute rejection episodes are strongly associated with the development of BOS.[9] Recently there have been an increasing number of publications suggesting GERD can lead to BO.

## GASTROESOPHAGEAL REFLUX DISEASE AND LUNG DISEASE

Gastroesophageal reflux disease (GERD) is a common problem, affecting up to 20% of the general population and has been on the increase.[10,11] GERD is defined as retrograde movement of gastric content through the esophagogastric junction and into the esophagus resulting in symptoms and/or esophageal mucosal damage.[10,12] Symptoms of GERD include heartburn, regurgitation, chest pain, acid brash, or globus.[10] Mucosal damage that can occur from GERD includes esophagitis, Barrett's esophagus, and esophageal adenocarcinoma.[10] A phenomenon known as silent GERD exists and is defined as erosive esophagitis in the absence of GERD symptoms, and some studies have reported the prevalence of this at up to 43% of individuals with GERD can have silent reflux.[13-16] Several factors are implicated in the presence and severity of GERD, including incompetence of the lower esophageal sphincter, abnormal peristalsis of the esophagus, the presence and size of hiatal hernia, mixed gastroesophageal reflux, and the thoracoabdominal pressure gradient (TAPG).[17]

Several studies have shown an association between GERD and many different pulmonary disorders such as pulmonary fibrosis, asthma, chronic cough, cystic fibrosis, emphysema, bronchitis, and obstructive sleep apnea.[18-23] In fact, one previous case control study compared patients with and without erosive esophagitis and showed higher prevalence of pulmonary diseases including chronic obstructive pulmonary disease (COPD), pulmonary fibrosis, bronchiectasis, pulmonary collapse, chronic bronchitis, and asthma, suggesting a causal relationship with GERD to pulmonary disorders.[24]

Patients with idiopathic pulmonary fibrosis (IPF) in particular have very high rates of GERD. IPF is a specific form of chronic, progressive fibrosing interstitial pneumonia of unknown cause with relatively high mortality compared with incidence with a mean survival of 3 to 5 years.[25,26] A current hypothesis suggests that chronic microaspiration of refluxed gastric contents leads to IPF. Several studies have been performed looking at the prevalence of GERD in patients with IPF. Raghu and colleagues[27] performed 24-hour pH testing on 65 patients with IPF and showed that 87% of their patients not on acid suppressive therapy had a positive pH study but even more interesting was that 63% of patients on standard proton pump inhibitor (PPI) therapy had positive pH testing. Further studies demonstrated that there is more reflux in IPF compared with COPD and higher numbers of total and proximal reflux when compared with other lung diseases as well as healthy controls.[28,29]

Furthermore, patients with severe lung disease who are approaching lung transplant candidacy have even higher rates of GERD. D'Ovidio and colleagues[30] examined the prevalence of GERD in patients with end-stage lung disease being evaluated for lung transplant and noted that 63% of their patients (49/78) had positive symptoms of GERD, whereas 38% of their patients were positive for reflux by ambulatory pH testing, and many of them who were positive by pH testing did not have symptoms. In another study by Sweet and colleagues[31] of 109 patients with end-stage lung disease, 68% of their 109 patients had reflux on esophageal pH monitoring, with 37% having proximal esophageal reflux. Importantly in this group, it was noted that symptoms of reflux were not predictive of the presence of reflux with a sensitivity of 67% and specificity of 26%.[31] These studies and more obviate GERD and reflux evaluations in patients with pulmonary disorders and in particular those with IPF or those undergoing lung transplantation evaluation.

## ESOPHAGEAL DYSMOTILITY AND LUNG DISEASE

Not only is there increased reflux in patients with lung disease, but there have also been studies showing there is increased esophageal dysmotility as well. Esophageal dysmotility can lead to poor bolus clearance from the esophagus with retention of volume as well as difficulty in clearing that which is refluxed.[32] Because of the prolonged time in the esophagus, the retained contents can lead to microaspiration as described earlier. Masuda and colleagues[33] demonstrated that 55% of their lung transplant patients had esophageal dysmotility in their pretransplant testing mainly with ineffective esophageal motility (IEM) and esophagogastric junction outflow obstruction (EGJOO) but also noting jackhammer esophagus, diffuse esophageal spasm, and achalasia. In another study by Basseri and colleagues[22] 77% of lung transplant candidates had esophageal dysmotility, with these patients also having lower resting mean basal lower esophageal sphincter (LES) and upper esophageal sphincter pressures and a more negative intrathoracic pressure compared with normals. Patients with IPF in this study showed more aperistaltic contractions, lower intrathoracic pressure, and higher frequency of aperistaltic contractions.[22] This study, along with several other studies, show that esophageal dysmotility is prevalent in patients with lung disease, and again evaluation is needed, particularly in those undergoing evaluation for lung transplant.

The TAPG measured on manometry also seems to play an important role in the development of reflux in patients with lung disease. The TAPG is defined as intraabdominal pressure minus the intrathoracic pressure during inspiration, and the adjusted TAPG is the TAPG minus the resting LES pressure. Masuda and colleagues[34] showed that 59% of lung transplant recipients who were tested pretransplant with an adjusted TAPG greater than 0 mm Hg had pathologic reflux, whereas only 31% of patients with a TAPG of less than or equal to zero had reflux.[34] They also demonstrated that TAPG is higher in restrictive lung disease compared with obstructive lung diseases and the adjusted TAPG correlated with GERD among all patients.

## ASPIRATION AND GASTROESOPHAGEAL REFLUX DISEASE IN LUNG TRANSPLANT

Several studies have looked at effects of aspiration of gastric contents and bile acids in lung transplant. Animal models in rats and swine have been evaluated, which have studied the effects of chronic aspiration on acute and chronic rejection. These studies showed an increase in acute rejection with monocyte infiltration, fibrosis, and lung destruction as well as chronic rejection, increased shedding of allograft alloantigens, and increased activity of the indirect alloimmune response, which may contribute to fibrosis, obliterative bronchiolitis, and infection.[35–37] They also showed that the lungs that were exposed to chronic aspiration were firm and shrunken and were not as easy to ventilate when compared with the lungs that were not exposed to chronic aspiration.[35] The development of acute rejection, as mentioned earlier, is an important risk factor for developing BOS.[9]

Human studies have also looked at this relationship, and there has been a strong suggestion that there are negative effects on lung transplants in those with reflux and aspiration. Bronchoalveolar lavage (BAL) can be used to obtain fluid from the lungs and specifically can assess for the presence of pepsin and bile acids, which are used as markers of reflux and aspiration. Pepsin is a proteolytic enzyme found in the stomach that is active at an acidic pH, whereas bile acids are responsible for the digestion of fat and fat-soluble vitamins. Pepsin and bile acids should not be found in the lungs unless there is aspiration of gastric content.

D'Ovidio and colleagues[38] look at BAL fluid (BALF) in 120 lung transplant patients and noted there was increased BALF bile acids in patients with BOS compared with those that did not have BOS, as well as noting higher concentrations of bile acids in those who had early BOS compared with those who had late BOS. They also noted BALF bile acids correlated with BALF interleukin 8 (IL-8) and alveolar neutrophilia, which led to their conclusion that aspiration is associated with the development of BOS and is possibly mediated by IL-8 and alveolar neutrophilia.[38] The same group showed a high correlation between proximal reflux on pH testing and bile acids as well as impaired lung allograft innate immunity manifest by reduced surfactant collectins and altered phospholipids.[39]

Not all studies have shown a correlation between acid exposure and the development of BOS. Blondeau and colleagues[40] looked at 45 post–lung transplant patients who were evaluated with 24-hour pH testing as well as BALF analysis. They showed 49% of their patients had GERD by pH testing, lower than other studies, with about half of those patients with nonacid reflux, and that pepsin was found in BALF of all of their patients, but only 50% of their patients had BALF with bile acids.[40] They showed no difference in the development of BOS in patients with positive 24-hour pH studies or by pepsin but did show that 70% of patients with bile acid on BALF had BOS, whereas only 30% of those without bile acid on BALF had BOS.[40] The same group did show in another study that the number of weakly acidic reflux episodes and the volume of nocturnal exposure on pH testing were higher in lung transplant recipients with bile acids on BALF.[41] King and colleagues[42] also looked at 24-hour pH testing in lung transplant recipients and showed that acid exposure did not correlate with the development of BOS, but increased nonacidic reflux episodes measured by impedance increased the risk of BOS, with a hazard ratio of 2.8 in those whose impedance measurements were greater than the normal range.

The type of lung transplantation done also affects the development of GERD. Fisichella and colleagues[43] showed that patients who had bilateral lung transplant or retransplant had higher amounts of distal and proximal reflux, but they were unclear of the cause for this difference. Therefore, the type of lung transplantation should be considered during the evaluation.

## TESTING IN LUNG TRANSPLANT EVALUATION AND LUNG TRANSPLANT RECIPIENTS

Because of the significance of esophageal motility disorders and high prevalence of reflux in patients with lung diseases, and the high rates of reflux in lung transplant recipients that have correlated with both acute and chronic rejection, the routine use of esophageal testing in these patients has been advocated (**Table 1**).

High-resolution esophageal manometry consists of placement of a catheter with many closely spaced pressure sensors via the nare into the stomach. The catheter transmits intraluminal pressure data that are then converted into dynamic esophageal pressure topography.[44] Currently this topography is analyzed by using the Chicago Classification version 3.0, which is a formalized analytical scheme of assessment of the manometry data that has been devised and revised by a working group of experts in the field.[44] Manometry catheters with impedance are also available that can assess bolus transit with each swallow. Esophageal manometry is important in the assessment of these patients as noted by an expert multidisciplinary statement provided by the American Gastroenterological Association (AGA) in 2015. Manometry is used to determine the proper positioning of the pH probe, to rule out achalasia masquerading as GERD before surgical intervention, and to detect impairment or absence of esophageal peristalsis, particularly in those with scleroderma.[17] As discussed earlier, the TAPG can be determined via manometry as well and plays a crucial role in reflux. Also, a previous study noted that hyperventilation does have effects on esophageal motility and can lead to spasm or other nonspecific disorders, and patients with end-stage lung disease often have high respiratory rates, which may lead to their esophageal dysmotility.[45]

| Table 1 | | |
| --- | --- | --- |
| **Esophageal testing with benefits and drawbacks of each** | | |
| **Test** | **Benefits** | **Drawbacks** |
| High-resolution esophageal manometry | Placement of pH probe | No specific info on reflux or aspiration |
| | r/o EGJOO or achalasia | Rapid respirations can falsely elevate IRP |
| | r/o Esophageal dysmotility | Patient discomfort |
| Wireless capsule pH testing | Determine acidic reflux | Cannot determine weakly acidic or nonacidic reflux |
| | Good patient tolerability | Cannot determine proximal reflux episodes or volume |
| | 48–96 h testing | |
| Multichannel intraluminal impedance pH | Determine acidic, nonacidic, and weakly acidic reflux | Worse patient tolerability |
| | Can determine proximal reflux and volume | 24 h testing |
| Upper GI series or barium esophagram | Can give a sense of dysmotility or reflux | Cannot specify amount of reflux or type of motility disorders |
| Gastric emptying study | Assesses gastric emptying | Cannot identify reflux or aspiration |

*Abbreviations:* GI, gastrointestinal; IRP, integrated relaxation pressure.

Many different patterns of esophageal motility and dysmotility are seen in patients who have lung disease and who have undergone a lung transplant. Normal manometry is the most common, although this was noted in less than half of the lung transplant evaluation patients, with the second most common finding being IEM (**Fig. 1**).[22,33] All other forms of dysmotility have been noted in the lung transplant patients, but EGJOO and achalasia when discovered need to need to have special attention paid to these diagnosis. EGJOO and achalasia both can lead to volume retention in the esophagus, which can lead to aspiration. In those with severe lung disease, often times during esophageal manometry, there is a high respiratory rate, which can lead to the

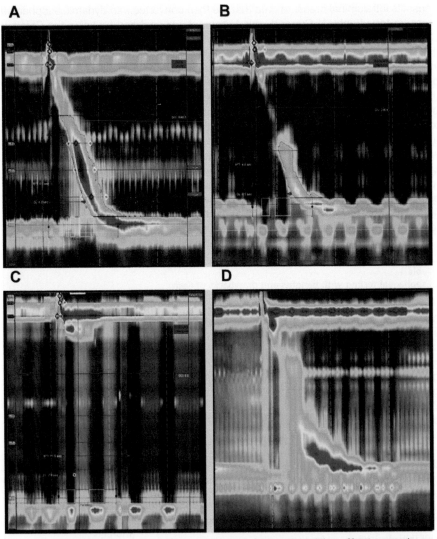

**Fig. 1.** Esophageal manometry patters. (*A*) Normal manometry. (*B*) Ineffective esophageal motility. (*C*) Absent peristalsis. (*D*) EGJ outflow obstruction but seen in rapid respirations with strong diaphragm component. (*Courtesy of* Temple University Hospital GI Motility Lab, Philadelphia, PA.)

diagnosis of EGJOO or achalasia, when there may be normal peristalsis instead of EGJOO or absent peristalsis instead of achalasia with a falsely elevated integrated relaxation pressure due to pressure from the diaphragm and rapid respirations (see **Fig. 1**). Individuals who read esophageal manometry need to pay attention to the respiratory rate for those with EGJOO or achalasia and consider further testing with barium esophagram, endoscopy, or possibly even a nuclear medicine esophageal transit scan, but this study is only available at limited centers. If true EGJOO or achalasia are diagnosed, early intervention is needed to try to prevent aspiration injury and BOS.

Ambulatory pH testing can be done by 2 methods. Wireless telemetry capsule–based pH testing is done by placing a wireless monitor 6 cm above the gastroesophageal junction, which can take readings for 48 to 96 hours.[46] This wireless capsule measures pH only, but does not measure intraluminal impedance; therefore it can only detect acidic reflux but will not detect weakly acidic or nonacidic reflux.[46] Although the wireless capsule does not measure impedance, it is more tolerable than catheter-based testing. On the other hand, transnasal catheter–based pH testing is a 24-hour test, which initially was done with pH monitoring only, but later multichannel intraluminal impedance pH (MII-pH) testing was developed allowing for measurement of both acidic as well as nonacidic reflux.[46] MII-pH allows for the measurement of movement of fluid, independent of pH, and can also assess the amount of proximal reflux.[46] Despite its lower tolerance, the increased information from the catheter-based testing is crucial in lung transplant patients. Lo and colleagues[47,48] showed that impedance testing was better at predicting early allograft injury post–lung transplant when compared with pH alone, and they concluded that impedance testing was being underutilized. Once again it is important for the physician who is interpreting the study to closely analyze the study and note true reflux on pH versus stasis, as this may be important in determining the care and treatment of these patients.

Although not routinely tested, gastric emptying studies to rule out gastroparesis may play a role in the evaluation of patients undergoing transplant. A recent study by Jehangir and colleagues[49] showed that in a group of patients with gastroparesis, those with GERD had more severe 4-hour gastric retention, decreased lower esophageal sphincter resting pressures, and more esophageal motility disorders. This study suggests that gastroparesis can worsen esophageal motility and GERD. Lung transplant itself has been associated with the development of gastroparesis as well, as Hooft and colleagues[50] showed that 5.8% of their transplant patients had delayed gastric emptying before transplant, but 53% of patient's posttransplant had delayed gastric emptying, with other reports of postoperative gastroparesis ranging from 23% to 91%. When combined, high rates of postoperative gastroparesis may contribute to esophageal dysmotility and reflux, which possibly could play a role in the development of lung transplant rejection.

Currently, there are no standard recommendations in patients with end-stage lung disease and lung transplant patients on who should be tested for GERD and when the optimal timing of the testing should be. Posner and colleagues[51] demonstrated that esophageal motility improves after transplant but GERD does not in a study of 76 patients who had esophageal manometry and MII-pH before and after lung transplant. They also showed that in those with GERD, there was less improvement in pulmonary function at 1 year.[51] Masuda and colleagues[33] also demonstrated that esophageal motility increased after lung transplant.[33] They also showed that pretransplant reflux was worse in restrictive lung diseases compared with obstructive lung diseases, and there was a high TAPG in patients with restrictive lung disease as well but also showed no difference in pretransplant versus posttransplant reflux. This study suggests that reflux is the key factor in lung injury, but the timing of reflux testing either pre- or posttransplant does not change these results. In regard to testing, the AGA panel of experts who met in 2015 to discuss GERD and the lung transplant patient made 2 recommendations based on evidence available to them at the time. (1) They recommended that all patients with IPF and scleroderma and end-stage lung disease, regardless of symptoms, be screened for GERD by manometry and pH monitoring and possibly a bronchoscopy with analysis of BALF for pepsin or bile acids. (2) Every patient early after lung transplant, regardless of symptoms, should be screened for GERD by esophageal manometry, pH monitoring, and possibly with bronchoscopy and BALF analysis for pepsin or bile acids. Other groups have suggested that all patients undergoing lung transplant evaluation should have routine esophageal manometry and impedance testing, with some groups including an upper gastrointestinal (GI) series or barium esophagram as well, to identify early patients with reflux and dysmotility and intervene on them earlier to try to prevent early allograft injury.[47,48,52] Other groups will do pretransplant testing but also advocate for repeat MII-pH testing in those who did not have preoperative GERD on MII-pH, as the evidence as discussed earlier discusses increased reflux and gastroparesis posttransplant.[52]

## TREATMENT

Standard medical treatment of GERD consists of PPI or histamine-2 blockers (H2B) (**Table 2**). Sometimes prokinetic medications are used to try to improve esophageal and gastric motility. Several studies have looked at the usefulness of antireflux medications and their effect on lung diseases as well as lung transplant outcomes.

Jo and colleagues,[53] using the Australia IPF registry, evaluated 587 patients with IPF and looked to see if the use of antacids, either PPI or H2Bs, or the diagnosis or

**Table 2**
**Treatment modalities for gastroesophageal reflux disease and aspiration in patients with end-stage lung disease and post–lung transplant**

| Treatment Modality | Benefits | Drawbacks |
|---|---|---|
| PPIs | Reduce acidic reflux<br>May reduce BOS | Does not reduce total reflux<br>May not reduce BOS |
| H2Bs | May improve symptoms | Does not reduce total reflux<br>Does not improve lung function or reduce BOS |
| Promotility agent (azithromycin) | Reduces BOS<br>Reduces reflux and aspiration | Unknown mechanism of action<br>Is an antibiotic<br><br>Limited studies |
| Other promotility agents | May improve gastric emptying, which may reduce reflux | Limited studies<br>May not improve symptoms of gastroparesis |
| Laprascopic antireflux surgery (LARS) | Decreased reflux and aspiration<br>Decreased acute and chronic rejection<br>Improved lung function<br><br>Improved mortality | Requires general anesthesia<br><br>Small rates of morbidity and mortality with the procedure<br>Ideal timing of procedure not know |

symptoms of GERD affected outcome. They showed no difference in disease progression or survival regardless of antacid treatment, diagnosis of GERD, or GERD symptoms. Although this did not show any benefit in all comers, MII-pH was not used, and the authors suggest that tailoring the treatment of GERD in IPF is still warranted, but may not be beneficial in all patients with IPF.[53] Other studies though, such as the one by Lee and colleagues,[54] demonstrated GERD medications led to longer survival times and lower radiologic fibrosis scores in patients with IPF.

Blondeau and colleagues[40] noted that the use of PPI was not related to BOS development, but a more recent retrospective analysis of 188 post–lung transplant patients by Lo and colleagues[55] showed that lower body mass index and use of PPI independently predicted against rejection and that persistent PPI use was more protective than intermittent PPI use or H2B use. PPIs have been shown to have antiinflammatory properties separate from their role in acid suppression, and this study suggests that there may be antiinflammatory properties of PPI that can help protect against lung transplant rejection.[55]

Tamhankar and colleagues[56] previously studied the effects of PPI on reflux. Although the use of PPI significantly decreased the number of acid reflux episodes, the number of total reflux episodes did not significantly differ, showing that PPIs reduce acid but not reflux episodes. Borges and colleagues[57] showed that patients with IPF with increased bolus exposure time on MII-pH had worse pulmonary outcomes over a 1-year period. These findings are important, particularly in the lung transplant patients, as many studies have shown that the total reflux, not the acidic reflux, can play a role in the development or worsening of BOS. Therefore, other methods are needed to decrease total reflux, not just acidic reflux.

Azithromycin, a macrolide antibiotic, has been shown to have promotility effects on both the esophagus and stomach.[58] Previous studies have shown a beneficial effect of azithromycin on BOS, showing reduced IL-8 and airway neutrophilia.[59] Mertens and colleagues[60] further investigated the effects of azithromycin on reflux and aspiration by looking at MII-pH and BALF. They showed that patients on azithromycin had significantly lower reflux episodes, less proximal reflux events, decreased bolus exposure, and reduced concentration of bile acids in BALF. The benefits of prokinetic agents may be due to the high prevalence of gastroparesis after lung transplant. Although data for other prokinetic agents are limited, a previous small limited study by Sodhi and colleagues[61] in combined heart and lung transplant patients stated that these patients with symptomatic gastroparesis did not respond well to prokinetic agents. Because of the limited studies, unknown mechanism of action, and antibiotic usage, routine azithromycin is currently not recommended for all lung transplant patients.

With the mixed data on improvement of BOS or other lung injury with medication management alone, more definitive therapy to reduce reflux was sought by using fundoplication. Patti and colleagues established that there is a correlation between MII-pH and laparoscopic antireflux surgery (LARS) and that LARS improved pulmonary symptoms. Linden and colleagues then showed that in patients with IPF awaiting lung transplantation, LARS was done safely without any perioperative complications and in those with IPF and LARS, oxygen requirements remained unchanged over a 15-month average follow-up, but in those with IPF without LARS there was a statistically significant deterioration in oxygen requirement.[62] Other studies have demonstrated improvement in $FEV_1$ and longer survival times after LARS in patients with IPF and end-stage lung disease.[54,63]

Several early studies done out of Duke University explored the safety and efficacy of LARS in the lung transplant population.[64,65] They showed that the surgery was safe without any mortality, there was improvement in lung function, and that 61% of patients with BOS at the time of fundoplication had improvement of their symptoms including 50% of them who no longer met criteria for BOS.[64,65] Since then many studies have reported on different outcomes with LARS in the lung transplant population. Fisichella and colleagues[66,67] reported in 2 different studies that with LARS there was decreased aspiration based on BALF evaluation and that the pulmonary leukocyte concentrations and proinflammatory mediators on BALF returned to normal after LARS. The group from Duke also reported from their early studies that early fundoplication, within 90 days of transplant, compared with late fundoplication done after 90 days, increased survival and decreased the incidence of BOS.[68]

With this in mind, further studies were undertaken to determine the safety, efficacy, and optimal timing of LARS. Several studies looked at the safety of fundoplication in transplant patients compared with nontransplant patients and showed longer length of stay and higher readmission rates but showed no difference in operative times or complications, respiratory complications, or mortality.[69,70] Lo and colleagues[71] evaluated patients who had pretransplant LARS, early posttransplant LARS (<6 months), and late posttransplant LARS and showed that both the pretransplant LARS and the early posttransplant LARS groups had similar outcomes, but the late post-LARS group had increased risk of early allograft injury. A more recent study looked at outcomes out to 5 years in early (<6 months after transplant) versus late (>6 months after transplant) LARS in lung transplant patients and showed no significant difference in actuarial survival rates at 1, 3, and 5 years (90%, 70%, 70% vs 91%, 66%, 66%) but did show decreased $FEV_1$ in the late LARS group at 3 and 5 years.[72]

The debate still remains as to the optimal timing of LARS in end-stage lung disease and in posttransplant patients, but with the abovementioned data it seems that LARS in either the pretransplant setting or early posttransplant setting provides the most benefit. Although studies have shown that pretransplant LARS has been safe, it is imperative to evaluate each patient on an individual basis with a multidisciplinary team approach, which involves the pulmonologists, transplant surgeons, thoracic surgeons, and gastroenterologist, to discuss the safety and tolerance of the procedure based on a patient's lung function and comorbidities. It is for these reasons that the AGA group recommended that if the presence of GERD and aspiration is established, LARS should be considered if the patient can tolerate an operation under general anesthesia and that if GERD is detected a fundoplication should be performed as soon as the diagnosis is established before the development of BOS.[17]

Treatment of underlying gastroparesis may be important as well. Management of gastroparesis is similar to gastroparesis patients without a transplant with the use of antiemetics, prokinetics, acid suppression, and dietary adjustments. Although in the past the use of botulinum toxin A injections into the pylorus was shown to improve gastric emptying, but had no benefit over placebo, Hooft and colleagues[50] demonstrated that intrapyloric botulinum toxin A injections improved gastric emptying to normal in 70% of patients, with the remaining patients having improvement, but not normalization, of their gastric emptying study.[73] Minimal data exist on pyloromyotomy with and without fundoplication, but no current recommendations can be made based on this. If gastroparesis is seen with reflux, aggressive management should be the approach to try and prevent long-term injury.

## SCLERODERMA AND LUNG TRANSPLANTATION

Special considerations need to be taken for patients with scleroderma, an autoimmune collagen vascular disease that causes fibrosis of the small arteries and can manifest with cutaneous and/or visceral involvement. Scleroderma can affect the lungs in multiple ways directly and indirectly by causing interstitial lung disease, pulmonary hypertension, airway disease, pleural involvement, as well as muscle weakness, infections, GERD, and aspiration, among other complications.[74] Scleroderma can also affect the GI tract, primarily the esophagus, and manifests as ineffective esophageal motility or absent contractility that can lead to GERD, esophagitis, Barrett's, and pulmonary symptoms such as cough and wheezing (see **Fig. 1**).[75]

Medical therapy is limited in scleroderma lung disease, and lung transplant is a definitive therapy for its treatment, but because of concerns of esophageal dysmotility and GERD and aspiration, lung transplant has been controversial in patients with scleroderma. Several studies have looked at survival in scleroderma patients when compared with IPF and have shown similar outcomes between the groups, which were also similar even in patients with severe esophageal dysmotility.[76–78] GERD and aspiration are not uncommon in this group, but some studies have shown that LARS, even with partial fundoplication, can lead to dysphagia; therefore, Roux-en-Y esophagojejunostomy has been suggested as an alternative to fundoplication in these patients.[79,80] A more recent study by Goldberg and colleagues[81] showed that in patients with scleroderma with both ineffective motility and absent peristalsis, LARS, mainly partial Toupet fundoplication, was successful with improvement in symptoms and with persistent dysphagia in only 11% of patients, all of which resolved with endoscopic dilation. More research is needed into the optimal antireflux procedure in patients with scleroderma and hypomotility, but LARS may still be an option in these patients. Current recommendations in scleroderma lung disease are that patients should be assessed individually and can be carefully selected to undergo lung transplant.

Sometimes absent peristalsis is detected in patients without scleroderma. In these patients, sometimes the esophageal findings are the earliest findings of scleroderma and further rheumatologic workup is needed to rule out scleroderma. Also, a phenomenon known as scleroderma sine scleroderma exists in which skin findings are limited or absent, but with internal organ involvement, which may include the esophagus.[82] In these patients, GERD and esophageal management should be similar to those with scleroderma.

## SUMMARY

Lung transplantation for end-stage lung disease is a lifesaving procedure, but long-term survival is still low, with BOS being the biggest complication that leads to mortality. Advances in esophageal and pulmonary testing have shown a correlation between GERD and aspiration and allograft rejection, both acute and chronic rejection, but the mechanism of this injury is not well understood. Esophageal testing with esophageal manometry and MII-pH testing has been shown to play a significant role in helping to assess these patients and direct care to improve long-term outcomes in both end-stage lung disease and lung transplantation. Data with PPIs and other medical management of reflux have been mixed, but data with LARS have had positive results. With these data in mind, it is important that patients undergoing lung transplant evaluation or at least those with IPF or scleroderma and all patients posttransplant be evaluated for reflux with esophageal testing and if positive undergo LARS as early as possible to prevent long-term complications.

## DISCLOSURE

The authors have nothing to disclose.

## REFERENCES

1. Chambers DC, Yusen RD, Cherikh WS, et al. The registry of the international society for heart and lung transplantation: Thirty-fourth adult lung and heart-lung transplantation report-2017; focus theme: Allograft ischemic time. J HeartLung Transplant 2017;36(10):1047–59. Accessed June 22, 2019.
2. Christie JD, Edwards LB, Kucheryavaya AY, et al. The registry of the international society for heart and lung transplantation: 29th adult lung and heart-lung transplant report-2012. J HeartLung Transplant 2012;31(10):1073–86. Accessed June 22, 2019.
3. Costa J, Benvenuto LJ, Sonett JR. Long-term outcomes and management of lung transplant recipients. Best Pract Res Clin Anaesthesiol 2017;31(2):285–97. Available at: https://www.sciencedirect.com/science/article/pii/S152168961730023X.
4. Estenne M, Maurer JR, Boehler A, et al. Bronchiolitis obliterans syndrome 2001: an update of the diagnostic criteria. J HeartLung Transplant 2002;21(3):297–310. Accessed June 23, 2019.
5. Meyer KC, Raghu G, Verleden GM, et al. An international ISHLT/ATS/ERS clinical practice guideline: diagnosis and management of bronchiolitis obliterans syndrome. Eur Respir J 2014;44(6):1479–503. Accessed June 23, 2019.
6. Verleden SE, Sacreas A, Vos R. Advances in understanding bronchiolitis obliterans after lung transplantation. Chest 2016;150(1):219–25. Available at: https://www.clinicalkey.es/playcontent/1-s2.0-S0012369216485648.
7. Yousem SA. Lymphocytic bronchitis/bronchiolitis in lung allograft recipients. Am J Surg Pathol 1993;17(5):491–6. Accessed June 23, 2019.
8. Yousem SA, Duncan SR, Griffith BP. Interstitial and airspace granulation tissue reactions in lung transplant recipients. Am J Surg Pathol 1992;16(9):877–84. Accessed June 23, 2019.
9. Girgis RE, Tu I, Berry GJ, et al. Risk factors for the development of obliterative bronchiolitis after lung transplantation. J HeartLung Transplant 1996;15(12):1200–8. Accessed June 24, 2019.
10. Savarino E, Bredenoord AJ, Fox M, et al. Expert consensus document: advances in the physiological assessment and diagnosis of GERD. Nat Rev Gastroenterol Hepatol 2017;14(11):665. Available at: https://www.ncbi.nlm.nih.gov/pubmed/28951582.
11. Dent J, El-Serag HB, Wallander M-, et al. Epidemiology of gastro-oesophageal reflux disease: a systematic review. Gut 2005 May;54(5):710–7. https://doi.org/10.1136/gut.2004.051821.
12. Vakil N, van Zanten SV, Kahrilas P, et al. [The montreal definition and classification of gastroesophageal reflux disease: A global, evidence-based consensus paper]. Z Gastroenterol 2007;45(11):1125–40. Accessed June 21, 2019.
13. Fass R, Dickman R. Clinical consequences of silent gastroesophageal reflux disease. Curr Gastroenterol Rep 2006;8(3):195–201. Accessed June 22, 2019.
14. Suyu H, Liu Y, Jianyu X, et al. Prevalence and predictors of silent gastroesophageal reflux disease in patients with hypertension. Gastroenterol Res Pract 2018;2018:7242917. Accessed June 22, 2019.
15. Lee D, Lee KJ, Kim KM, et al. Prevalence of asymptomatic erosive esophagitis and factors associated with symptom presentation of erosive esophagitis. Scand J Gastroenterol 2013;48(8):906–12. Accessed June 22, 2019.
16. Choi JY, Jung H, Song EM, et al. Determinants of symptoms in gastroesophageal reflux disease: Nonerosive reflux disease, symptomatic, and silent erosive reflux

disease. Eur J Gastroenterol Hepatol 2013;25(7):764–71. Accessed June 22, 2019.

17. Patti MG, Vela MF, Odell DD, et al. The intersection of GERD, aspiration, and lung transplantation. J Laparoendosc Adv Surg Tech 2016;26(7):51–505. Available at: https://www.liebertpub.com/doi/abs/10.1089/lap.2016.0170.

18. Tobin RW, Pope CE, Pellegrini CA, et al. Increased prevalence of gastroesophageal reflux in patients with idiopathic pulmonary fibrosis. Am J Respir Crit Care Med 1998;158(6):1804–8. Accessed June 23, 2019.

19. Harding SM, Richter JE. The role of gastroesophageal reflux in chronic cough and asthma. Chest 1997;111(5):1389–402. Accessed June 23, 2019.

20. Feigelson J, Girault F, Pecau Y. Gastro-oesophageal reflux and esophagitis in cystic fibrosis. Acta Paediatr Scand 1987;76(6):989–90. Accessed June 23, 2019.

21. Gaude GS. Pulmonary manifestations of gastroesophageal reflux disease. Ann Thorac Med 2009;4(3):115–23. Accessed Jun 23, 2019.

22. Basseri B, Conklin JL, Pimentel M, et al. Esophageal motor dysfunction and gastroesophageal reflux are prevalent in lung transplant candidates. Ann Thorac Surg 2010;90(5):1630–6. Accessed June 20, 2019.

23. Casanova C, Baudet JS, del Valle Velasco M, et al. Increased gastro-oesophageal reflux disease in patients with severe COPD. Eur Respir J 2004; 23(6):841–5. Accessed June 24, 2019.

24. el-Serag HB, Sonnenberg A. Comorbid occurrence of laryngeal or pulmonary disease with esophagitis in united states military veterans. Gastroenterology 1997;113(3):755–60. Accessed June 23, 2019.

25. Raghu G, Rochwerg B, Zhang Y, et al. An official ATS/ERS/JRS/ALAT clinical practice guideline: treatment of idiopathic pulmonary fibrosis. An update of the 2011 clinical practice guideline. Am J Respir Crit Care Med 2015;192(2):3. Accessed June 23, 2019.

26. Wang Z, Bonella F, Li W, et al. Gastroesophageal reflux disease in idiopathic pulmonary fibrosis: uncertainties and controversies. Respiration 2018;96(6):571–87. Available at: https://www.karger.com/Article/FullText/492336.

27. Raghu G, Freudenberger TD, Yang S, et al. High prevalence of abnormal acid gastro-oesophageal reflux in idiopathic pulmonary fibrosis. Eur Respir J 2006; 27(1):136–42. Accessed June 23, 2019.

28. Gavini S, Finn RT, Lo W-, et al. Idiopathic pulmonary fibrosis is associated with increased impedance measures of reflux compared to non-fibrotic disease among pre-lung transplant patients. Neurogastroenterol Motil 2015;27(9): 1326–32. Accessed June 23, 2019.

29. Savarino E, Carbone R, Marabotto E, et al. Gastro-oesophageal reflux and gastric aspiration in idiopathic pulmonary fibrosis patients. Eur Respir J 2013;42(5): 1322–31. Accessed June 23, 2019.

30. D'Ovidio F, Singer LG, Hadjiliadis D, et al. Prevalence of gastroesophageal reflux in end-stage lung disease candidates for lung transplant. Ann Thorac Surg 2005; 80(4):1254. Available at: http://ats.ctsnetjournals.org/cgi/content/abstract/80/4/1254. Accessed June 16, 2019.

31. Sweet MP, Herbella FAM, Leard L, et al. The prevalence of distal and proximal gastroesophageal reflux in patients awaiting lung transplantation. Ann Surg 2006;244(4):491–7. Accessed June 23, 2019.

32. Kahrilas PJ, Dodds WJ, Hogan WJ. Effect of peristaltic dysfunction on esophageal volume clearance. Gastroenterology 1988;94(1):73–80. Accessed June 24, 2019.

33. Masuda T, Mittal SK, Kovács B, et al. Foregut function before and after lung transplant. J Thorac Cardiovasc Surg 2019. https://doi.org/10.1016/j.jtcvs.2019.02.128. Available at: https://www.sciencedirect.com/science/article/pii/S0022522319307950.

34. Masuda T, Mittal SK, Kovacs B, et al. Thoracoabdominal pressure gradient and gastroesophageal reflux: insights from lung transplant candidates. Dis Esophagus 2018;31(10). https://doi.org/10.1093/dote/doy025. Accessed June 23, 2019.

35. Hartwig MG, Appel JZ, Li B, et al. Chronic aspiration of gastric fluid accelerates pulmonary allograft dysfunction in a rat model of lung transplantation. J Thorac Cardiovasc Surg 2006;131(1):209–17. Accessed June 24, 2019.

36. Li B, Hartwig MG, Appel JZ, et al. Chronic aspiration of gastric fluid induces the development of obliterative bronchiolitis in rat lung transplants. Am J Transplant 2008;8(8):1614–21. Accessed June 24, 2019.

37. Meltzer AJ, Weiss MJ, Veillette GR, et al. Repetitive gastric aspiration leads to augmented indirect allorecognition after lung transplantation in miniature swine. Transplantation 2008;86(12):1824–9. Accessed June 24, 2019.

38. D'Ovidio F, Mura M, Tsang M, et al. Bile acid aspiration and the development of bronchiolitis obliterans after lung transplantation. J Thorac Cardiovasc Surg 2005;129(5):1144–52. Accessed June 24, 2019.

39. D'Ovidio F, Mura M, Ridsdale R, et al. The effect of reflux and bile acid aspiration on the lung allograft and its surfactant and innate immunity molecules SP-A and SP-D. Am J Transplant 2006;6(8):1930–8. Accessed June 24, 2019.

40. Blondeau K, Mertens V, Vanaudenaerde BA, et al. Gastro-oesophageal reflux and gastric aspiration in lung transplant patients with or without chronic rejection. Eur Respir J 2008;31(4):707–13. Accessed June 24, 2019.

41. Blondeau K, Mertens V, Vanaudenaerde BA, et al. Nocturnal weakly acidic reflux promotes aspiration of bile acids in lung transplant recipients. J HeartLung Transplant 2009;28(2):141–8. Accessed June 25, 2019.

42. King BJ, Iyer H, Leidi AA, et al. Gastroesophageal reflux in bronchiolitis obliterans syndrome: A new perspective. J HeartLung Transplant 2009;28(9):870–5. Accessed June 25, 2019.

43. Fisichella PM, Davis CS, Shankaran V, et al. The prevalence and extent of gastroesophageal reflux disease correlates to the type of lung transplantation. Surg Laparosc Endosc Percutan Tech 2012;22(1):46–51. Accessed June 25, 2019.

44. Yadlapati R. High-resolution esophageal manometry: Interpretation in clinical practice. Curr Opin Gastroenterol 2017;33(4):301–9. Accessed June 25, 2019.

45. Cooke RA, Anggiansah A, Wang J, et al. Hyperventilation and esophageal dysmotility in patients with noncardiac chest pain. Am J Gastroenterol 1996;91(3):480–4. Accessed June 29, 2019.

46. Katz PO, Gerson LB, Vela MF. Guidelines for the diagnosis and management of gastroesophageal reflux disease. Am J Gastroenterol 2013;108(3):308. Available at: https://journals.lww.com/ajg/fulltext/2013/03000/Guidelines_for_the_Diagnosis_and_Management_of.6.aspx. Accessed June 25, 2019.

47. Lo W, Burakoff R, Goldberg HJ, et al. Pre-lung transplant measures of reflux on impedance are superior to pH testing alone in predicting early allograft injury. World J Gastroenterol 2015;21(30):9111–7. Available at: https://www.wjgnet.com/1007-9327/full/v21/i30/9111.htm. Accessed June 16, 2019.

48. Hathorn KE, Chan WW, Lo W. Role of gastroesophageal reflux disease in lung transplantation. World J Transplant 2017;7(2):103–16. Accessed Jun 22, 2019.

49. Jehangir A, Parkman HP. Reflux symptoms in gastroparesis: Correlation with gastroparesis symptoms, gastric emptying, and esophageal function testing. J Clin

Gastroenterol 2019. https://doi.org/10.1097/MCG.0000000000001190. Accessed June 25, 2019.

50. Hooft N, Smith M, Huang J, et al. Gastroparesis is common after lung transplantation and may be ameliorated by botulinum toxin-A injection of the pylorus. J HeartLung Transplant 2014;33(12):1314–6. Accessed June 25, 2019.
51. Posner S, Finn RT, Shimpi RA, et al. Esophageal contractility increases and gastroesophageal reflux does not worsen after lung transplantation. Dis Esophagus 2019. https://doi.org/10.1093/dote/doz039. Accessed June 20, 2019.
52. Castor JM, Wood RK, Muir AJ, et al. Gastroesophageal reflux and altered motility in lung transplant rejection. Neurogastroenterol Motil 2010;22(8):841–50. Accessed June 26, 2019.
53. Jo HE, Corte TJ, Glaspole I, et al. Gastroesophageal reflux and antacid therapy in IPF: Analysis from the australia IPF registry. BMC Pulm Med 2019;19(1):84. Accessed June 20, 2019.
54. Lee JS, Ryu JH, Elicker BM, et al. Gastroesophageal reflux therapy is associated with longer survival in patients with idiopathic pulmonary fibrosis. Am J Respir Crit Care Med 2011;184(12):1390–4. Accessed June 28, 2019.
55. Lo W, Goldberg HJ, Boukedes S, et al. Proton pump inhibitors independently protect against early allograft injury or chronic rejection after lung transplantation. Dig Dis Sci 2018;63(2):403–10. Accessed June 24, 2019.
56. Tamhankar AP, Peters JH, Portale G, et al. Omeprazole does not reduce gastroesophageal reflux: new insights using multichannel intraluminal impedance technology. J Gastrointest Surg 2004;8(7):898. Accessed June 25, 2019.
57. Borges LF, Jagadeesan V, Goldberg H, et al. Abnormal bolus reflux is associated with poor pulmonary outcome in patients with idiopathic pulmonary fibrosis. J Neurogastroenterol Motil 2018;24(3):395–402. Accessed June 27, 2019.
58. Peeters TL. Erythromycin and other macrolides as prokinetic agents. Gastroenterology 1993;105(6):1886–99. Accessed June 26, 2019.
59. Verleden GM, Vanaudenaerde BM, Dupont LJ, et al. Azithromycin reduces airway neutrophilia and interleukin-8 in patients with bronchiolitis obliterans syndrome. Am J Respir Crit Care Med 2006;174(5):566–70. Accessed June 26, 2019.
60. Mertens V, Blondeau K, Pauwels A, et al. Azithromycin reduces gastroesophageal reflux and aspiration in lung transplant recipients. Dig Dis Sci 2009;54(5):972–9. Accessed June 26, 2019.
61. Sodhi SS, Guo J, Maurer AH, et al. Gastroparesis after combined heart and lung transplantation. J Clin Gastroenterol 2002;34(1):34–9. Accessed June 27, 2019.
62. Linden PA, Gilbert RJ, Yeap BY, et al. Laparoscopic fundoplication in patients with end-stage lung disease awaiting transplantation. J Thorac Cardiovasc Surg 2006;131(2):438–46. Accessed June 27, 2019.
63. Hoppo T, Jarido V, Pennathur A, et al. Antireflux surgery preserves lung function in patients with gastroesophageal reflux disease and end-stage lung disease before and after lung transplantation. Arch Surg 2011;146(9):1041–7. Accessed June 28, 2019.
64. Lau CL, Palmer SM, Howell DN, et al. Laparoscopic antireflux surgery in the lung transplant population. Surg Endosc 2002;16(12):1674–8. Accessed June 28, 2019.
65. Davis RD, Lau CL, Eubanks S, et al. Improved lung allograft function after fundoplication in patients with gastroesophageal reflux disease undergoing lung transplantation. J Thorac Cardiovasc Surg 2003;125(3):533–42. Accessed June 28, 2019.
66. Fisichella PM, Davis CS, Lundberg PW, et al. The protective role of laparoscopic antireflux surgery against aspiration of pepsin after lung transplantation. Surgery 2011;150(4):598–606. Accessed June 28, 2019.

67. Fisichella PM, Davis CS, Lowery E, et al. Pulmonary immune changes early after laparoscopic antireflux surgery in lung transplant patients with gastroesophageal reflux disease. J Surg Res 2012;177(2):65. Accessed June 28, 2019.

68. Cantu E, Appel JZ, Hartwig MG, et al. J. Maxwell chamberlain memorial paper. early fundoplication prevents chronic allograft dysfunction in patients with gastroesophageal reflux disease. Ann Thorac Surg 2004;78(4):1151. Accessed June 28, 2019.

69. O'Halloran EK, Reynolds JD, Lau CL, et al. Laparoscopic nissen fundoplication for treating reflux in lung transplant recipients. J Gastrointest Surg 2004;8(1): 132–7. Accessed June 28, 2019.

70. Kilic A, Shah AS, Merlo CA, et al. Early outcomes of antireflux surgery for united states lung transplant recipients. Surg Endosc 2013;27(5):1754–60. Accessed June 28, 2019.

71. Lo W, Goldberg HJ, Wee J, et al. Both pre-transplant and early post-transplant antireflux surgery prevent development of early allograft injury after lung transplantation. J Gastrointest Surg 2016;20(1):118 [discussion: 118]. Accessed June 28, 2019.

72. Biswas Roy S, Elnahas S, Serrone R, et al. Early fundoplication is associated with slower decline in lung function after lung transplantation in patients with gastroesophageal reflux disease. J Thorac Cardiovasc Surg 2018;155(6):2771.e1. Available at: http://www.sciencedirect.com/science/article/pii/S002252231830357X. Accessed June 16, 2019.

73. Friedenberg FK, Palit A, Parkman HP, et al. Botulinum toxin A for the treatment of delayed gastric emptying. Am J Gastroenterol 2008;103(2):416–23. Accessed June 27, 2019.

74. Solomon JJ, Olson AL, Fischer A, et al. Scleroderma lung disease. Eur Respir Rev 2013;22(127):6–19. Accessed June 28, 2019.

75. Tang DM, Pathikonda M, Harrison M, et al. Symptoms and esophageal motility based on phenotypic findings of scleroderma. Dis Esophagus 2013;26(2): 197–203. Accessed June 28, 2019.

76. Crespo MM, Bermudez CA, Dew MA, et al. Lung transplant in patients with scleroderma compared with pulmonary fibrosis. short- and long-term outcomes. Ann Am Thorac Soc 2016;13(6):784–92. Accessed June 28, 2019.

77. Sottile PD, Iturbe D, Katsumoto TR, et al. Outcomes in systemic sclerosis-related lung disease after lung transplantation. Transplantation 2013;95(7):975–80. Accessed June 28, 2019.

78. Miele CH, Schwab K, Saggar R, et al. Lung transplant outcomes in systemic sclerosis with significant esophageal dysfunction.A comprehensive single-center experience. Ann Am Thorac Soc 2016;13(6):793–802. Accessed June 28, 2019.

79. Gasper WJ, Sweet MP, Golden JA, et al. Lung transplantation in patients with connective tissue disorders and esophageal dysmotility. Dis Esophagus 2008; 21(7):650–5. Accessed June 28, 2019.

80. Kent MS, Luketich JD, Irshad K, et al. Comparison of surgical approaches to recalcitrant gastroesophageal reflux disease in the patient with scleroderma. Ann Thorac Surg 2007;84(5):1716. Accessed June 28, 2019.

81. Goldberg MB, Abbas AE, Smith MS, et al. Minimally invasive fundoplication is safe and effective in patients with severe esophageal hypomotility. Innovations (Phila) 2016;11(6):396–9. Accessed June 28, 2019.

82. Kucharz EJ, Kopeć-Mędrek M. Systemic sclerosis sine scleroderma. Adv Clin Exp Med 2017;26(5):875–80. Accessed June 29, 2019.

# Tailoring Endoscopic and Surgical Treatments for Gastroesophageal Reflux Disease

Charles T. Bakhos, MD, MS[a,b],*, Abbas E. Abbas, MD, MS[a],
Roman V. Petrov, MD, PhD[a]

## KEYWORDS

- Transoral • Incisionless • Fundoplication • Reflux • Esophagus • Manometry
- Dysphagia

## KEY POINTS

- Gastroesophageal reflux disease (GERD) remains quite prevalent, and its complex pathophysiology involves an incompetent esophagogastric junction.
- Esophageal dysmotility is commonly present in GERD patients, potentially complicating the choice of surgical fundoplication (partial or complete).
- There is no strong evidence supporting tailoring of the surgical fundoplication according to the degree of esophageal dysmotility, except in cases of aperistalsis.
- Endoscopic antireflux procedures currently are available, but there is a lack of data on its merits in the specific setting of esophageal dysmotility.
- Fundoplication can be offered to a select group of patients with complete esophageal aperistalsis after thorough and comprehensive multidisciplinary assessment; alternatively, Roux-en-Y gastric bypass can be contemplated after a careful nutritional evaluation.

## INTRODUCTION

Gastroesophageal reflux disease (GERD) remains quite prevalent worldwide, with estimated incidence rates of 18% to 28% in North America, 9% to 26% in Europe, 12% in Australia, and 23% in South America.[1] Pharmacologic therapy with proton pump inhibitors (PPIs) is the mainstay management modality of this common disease and accounts for at least half of the overall treatment cost.[2] Medications, however, can lose efficacy over time and are associated with side effects, such as small intestinal

---

Funding: None.
[a] Department of Thoracic Medicine and Surgery, Temple University Hospital, Lewis Katz School of Medicine, 3401 North Broad Street, C501, 5th Floor, Parkinson Pavilion, Philadelphia, PA 19140, USA; [b] Department of Surgery, Einstein Medical Center, Klein 101, Philadelphia, PA 19141, USA
* Corresponding author.
*E-mail address:* Charles.bakhos@tuhs.temple.edu

Gastroenterol Clin N Am 49 (2020) 467–480
https://doi.org/10.1016/j.gtc.2020.04.005
gastro.theclinics.com

bacterial overgrowth and osteoporosis; more recently, concerns have been raised regarding increased risk of cardiac events, Alzheimer dementia, acute interstitial nephritis, and increased overall mortality.[3,4] Surgical fundoplication has an established role in the management of hiatal hernia and GERD, since the first full posterior fundoplication was described by Nissen and Rosetti[5] (**Fig. 1**A). Significant variations have been introduced since then, including the partial 270$\underline{o}$ fundoplication (Toupet) and the anterior 180$\underline{o}$ wrap (Dor) (**Fig. 1**B, C). The advent of minimally invasive laparoscopic and robotic approaches further popularized the surgical treatment option, especially in patients with severe or uncontrolled symptoms despite medications and those desiring to discontinue them because of side effects or other reasons. More recently, magnetic sphincteric augmentation (LINX® (Torax Medical Inc, Shoreview, MN)) demonstrated comparable short-term outcomes in the management of patients with GERD and hiatal hernias smaller than 2 cm.[6] Additionally, endoluminal approaches, such as transoral incisionless fundoplication (TIF), were developed as an even less invasive option for patients with GERD and moderate symptoms.[7] The choice of surgery depends on many factors, including patient symptoms, esophageal function, and comorbid conditions, such as the presence of hiatal herniation, gastroparesis, esophagitis, and esophageal dysmotility. Esophageal motility disorders can complicate the choice of fundoplication, from a fear of creating or worsening obstructive symptoms, such as dysphagia and regurgitation.

This report reviews the pathophysiology of GERD, with a particular focus on the impact of esophageal dysmotility. It also discusses the different surgical (extraluminal) and endoscopic (endoluminal) options for managing GERD in patients with baseline nonachalasia esophageal dysmotility disorders.

## PATHOPHYSIOLOGY OF GASTROESOPHAGEAL REFLUX DISEASE AND ESOPHAGEAL DYSMOTILITY

The pathophysiology of GERD is multifactorial and complex but mainly involves an incompetent esophagogastric junction (EGJ) as an antireflux barrier, in the form of transient lower esophageal sphincter (LES) relaxations and/or a hypotensive EGJ.[8] Additional conditions can contribute significantly to reflux development and/or further alteration of the antireflux barrier, such as the presence of hiatal hernia, xerostomia, and impaired saliva production, leading to reduction in the neutralization of the esophageal mucosa, delayed gastric emptying, and acid hypersecretion.[9] Esophageal

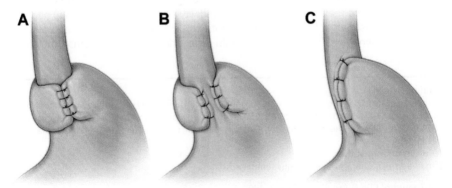

**Fig. 1.** (*A*) Nissen fundoplication (360° posterior). (*B*) Toupet fundoplication (270° posterior). (*C*) Dor fundoplication (180° anterior).

hypomotility in particular can lead to ineffective clearance of the refluxate and prolonged esophageal body acid exposure. For instance, Diener and colleagues[10] demonstrated more reflux episodes, longer acid exposure, and slower esophageal acid clearance in GERD patients with impaired esophageal motility compared with those with normal motility. The degree of esophageal mucosal injury seems to correlate with the progressive deterioration of esophageal motor function and impairment of acid clearance.[11] Whether esophageal dysmotility is a cause or consequence of reflux, however, is still debated, despite evidence that esophageal mucosal damage can lead to reduced esophageal compliance and an increased bolus progression resistance.[12,13]

For decades, conventional manometry was the mainstay diagnostic modality of esophageal motor function, with most reports using an average distal peristaltic amplitude of 30 mm Hg to define ineffective swallows. The recent advent of high-resolution manometry (HRM) allowed a more sophisticated analysis of this function and a better understanding of the morphology and vigor of the EGJ, which comprises both the LES and crural diaphragm.[14-16] Specifically, HRM characterizes esophageal peristalsis by the distal contractile integral (DCI), which measures the vigor of smooth muscle contraction taking into consideration the length, duration, and amplitude of contraction. For comparison purposes, a DCI threshold of 450 mm Hg/cm/s correlates with the average distal peristaltic amplitude of 30 mm Hg on conventional manometry.[17] Additionally, it is important the distinguish the different manometric parameters used to define hypomotility and appreciate the variation in the literature on esophageal dysmotility, GERD, and fundoplication. Not until recently were the 3 main patterns of abnormal esophageal motor function recognized in GERD.[9] The most frequent abnormal pattern is a weak or absent second segment, which manifests either as fragmented peristalsis (>5-cm break with DCI >450 mm Hg/cm/s in ≥50% of sequences) or as ineffective esophageal motility (IEM), where the DCI is less than 450 mm Hg/cm/s in greater than or equal to 50% of sequences. The most severe abnormality is absent contractility (often described as scleroderma-like esophagus), characterized by a DCI less than 100 mm Hg/cm/s in all sequences (**Fig. 2**). This pattern was found in 3.2% of 1081 patients who underwent HRM prior to antireflux surgery.[18]

### Esophageal Dysmotility in Systemic Sclerosis

Systemic sclerosis is a rare heterogeneous disease characterized by vasculopathy, excess deposition of collagen, and fibrosis with multiorgan involvement. The gastrointestinal tract, in particular the esophagus, is affected in up to 80% of patients.[19] From a manometry standpoint, scleroderma esophagus is characterized by a combination of absent esophageal body contractility and a hypotensive EGJ, both of which are found in more than 50% to 60% of patients with the systemic disease.[20] Scleroderma also is associated with gastric dysmotility and impaired saliva production, which can further compromise bolus transit and reflux clearance. Clinically, up to 80% of patients develop heartburn and dysphagia within 2 years of their diagnosis.[21] Erosive esophagitis and peptic strictures (up to 30%) often can develop in this context, further contributing to dysphagia symptoms.[19,21] Sclerodema often can affect the lungs too, in the forms of interstitial lung disease and pulmonary arterial hypertension: up to 90% of patients exhibit evidence of interstitial changes on high-resolution computed tomography scan, and between 40% to 75% of patients have pulmonary function test abnormalities.[22] The presence of concomitant pulmonary and esophageal involvement makes this patient population particularly challenging to manage, as discussed later, with reflux and aspiration from esophageal dysmotility further

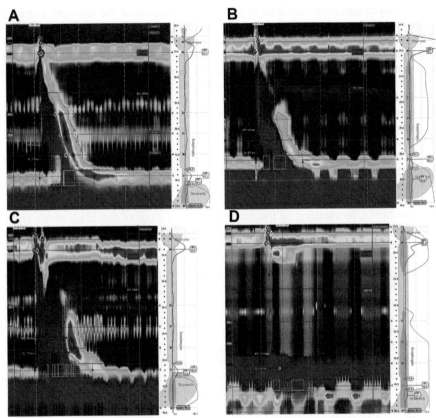

**Fig. 2.** HRM. (*A*) Normal esophageal motility. (*B*) IEM. (*C*) Fragmented peristalsis. (*D*) Failed peristalsis. BTT, bolus transit time; DL, distal latency; PIP, Pressure inversion point, SC, secondary contraction; UES, upper esophageal sphincter.

worsening the lung function and potentially jeopardizing the outcomes of lung transplantation when that is indicated.

## EFFECTS OF SURGICAL FUNDOPLICATION ON ESOPHAGEAL MOTILITY AND MANOMETRY PARAMETERS

As discussed previously, the pathophysiology of GERD mainly involves inappropriate and unprovoked transient LES relaxations. Surgical fundoplication with or without hiatal hernia repair is believed to change the mechanical properties and action of the EGJ that result in incomplete abolition of the high-pressure zone during LES relaxation and reduced triggering of transient sphincter relaxations.[23,24] Although the impact on esophageal motility is quite variable throughout the literature, most reports demonstrate an increase of the lower sphincter pressure after fundoplication, both in the clinical and experimental settings.[25,26] For instance, Stein and colleagues[27] showed normalization of the LES pressure, increased contraction amplitude, and reduced prevalence of low-amplitude contractions in 40 patients who underwent stationary manometry before and at a median of 30 months after Nissen fundoplication. Herbella and colleagues[28] evaluated 71 patients who underwent partial and total fundoplications; on postoperative manometry, the investigators found an increase in LES pressure and distal amplitude after both techniques but a higher rate of normalized peristalsis was seen among Nissen patients (86%).

In a randomized controlled trial of 200 patients who underwent either Nissen or Toupet fundoplication, repeat manometry at 4 months showed no significant difference in esophageal motor function in 85% of patients. The only noticeable finding was an increase in the LES resting pressures postoperatively, and that was more significant in the Nissen group compared with the Toupet group.[29] Another prospective non-randomized crossover study examined 60 patients who underwent a Nissen fundoplication (n = 20, normal peristalsis), Toupet fundoplication (n = 20, impaired motility) or continued medical therapy with PPI (n = 20).[30] On manometry evaluation after 6 months, a significant improvement of LES competence was seen in both surgical groups, but LES relaxation was complete after Toupet and incomplete after Nissen. On scintigraphic esophageal emptying for solid meals, there was no improvement after medical therapy but a significant improvement after Toupet and a significant deterioration after Nissen. Furthermore, there was a strong correlation between scintigraphic and manometric evaluation of peristalsis both preoperatively and postoperatively. On the other hand, a Swedish randomized study of 18 patients who underwent a 180° posterior fundoplication and 15 patients who underwent a Nissen did not report any significant change in esophageal motor function on repeat manometry after 3 years; although a significant increase in peristaltic amplitude in the middle and distal thirds of the esophagus was recorded compared with the preoperative findings, there was no corresponding effect on propagation speed and duration of contraction.[31]

Although all these studies are based on conventional manometry, Rerych and colleagues[32] recently reported on 25 patients with GERD who underwent HRM before and 3 to 5 months after laparoscopic Nissen fundoplication. The investigators found a significant increase in the mean and minimal basal EGJ pressure in the postoperative patients. Moreover, DCI was significantly higher postoperatively and, based on the DCI threshold of 450 mm Hg/s/cm, a trend from IEM to effective esophageal motility also was observed ($P = .07$).

## SURGICAL FUNDOPLICATION IN PATIENTS WITH INEFFECTIVE ESOPHAGEAL MOTILITY

Before reviewing the literature on fundoplication in the setting of esophageal dysmotility, it is important to re-emphasize the variability in manometric definition of esophageal hypomotility disorders and the nuances between conventional manometry and HRM. Despite well-known definitions of Nissen and Toupet fundoplications, there also are technical and operator-dependent variabilities in the degree of circumferential wrapping, with some reports describing 180o or 240o posterior fundoplication for instance. Other technical factors that may influence the postoperative neo-EGJ tightness, and outcomes include the length of the wrap (1.5–3 cm), tension of the fundoplication, and concomitant repair of giant hiatal hernias and/or large hiatus. Besides these technical factors, it is important to remember that dysphagia symptoms can be related to baseline peptic stricture or severe esophagitis and not just esophageal dysmotility. For instance, preoperative dysphagia has been shown to be a better predictor of postoperative dysphagia than conventional manometry parameters in a series of 156 laparoscopic Nissen fundoplication by Herron and colleagues.[33] Another series of 401 laparoscopic Toupet fundoplications found no association between preoperative LES pressure, distal esophageal pressure, or hypomotility on conventional manometry and postoperative dysphagia.[34] On the other hand, Blom and colleagues[35] found that patients with a normal preoperative LES (pressure >6 mm Hg; length >2 cm; and abdominal length >1 cm) had an almost 6-fold increase in the risk of developing post-Nissen dysphagia. Other early data using conventional manometry found that a distal esophageal contraction amplitude of 25 mm Hg in at least 70% of the swallows was sufficient to overcome the newly created fundoplication and lower the risk of postoperative dysphagia.[36] This led to the tailoring approach in GERD treatment, following the logic that esophageal contraction should overcome the outflow resistance imposed by the fundoplication.

For instance, Patti and colleagues[37] reported their tailored fundoplication experience in 240 patients with symptomatic GERD: 141 patients with esophageal hypomotility underwent a partial fundoplication, and 94 patients with normal motility underwent a laparoscopic Nissen fundoplication The incidence of postoperative symptomatic GERD was higher in the partial fundoplication group (19% vs 4%), whereas the incidence of postoperative dysphagia was similar between them at mean follow-up of 67 months. Novitsky and colleagues[38] demonstrated the safety of laparoscopic Nissen fundoplication in a multicenter review of 48 patients with GERD and esophageal dysmotility; the latter was defined by a contraction amplitude less than 30 mm Hg and/or greater than 70% nonperistaltic esophageal body contractions. Only 2 patients (4.2%) experienced persistent dysphagia, including 1 with severe preoperative dysphagia; only 1 patient required a reoperative fundoplication.[38] These results were comparable to those in another series by Tsereteli and coworkers, who found that the patients who experienced dysphagia post-Nissen were the same who had preoperative dysphagia, whether they were in the IEM group (n = 21) or normal motility group (n = 63).[39]

Two randomized trials also were conducted to investigate the need for tailoring fundoplication. Booth and colleagues[40] stratified 127 patients with established GERD into effective motility (n = 75) and IEM (n = 52) groups, based on preoperative conventional manometry. Dysphagia of any degree was more prevalent at 1 year in the Nissen group (n = 64) compared with the Toupet group (n = 63) (27% vs 9%, respectively; P = 0.018), but there were no differences in postoperative symptoms between the effective and IEM groups. Postoperative manometry was performed at 6 months in 75 of the 127 patients and showed no clear pattern of transition from normal preoperative motility to IEM or the other way around.[40] Strate and colleagues[41] also randomized 200 patients in a similar fashion and reported a higher incidence of dysphagia in the total group of Nissen patients than in the total group of Toupet patients, but there was no difference between the effective and IEM groups; furthermore, satisfaction with surgery was comparable between the latter 2 groups (83% vs 87%, respectively).

These studies suggest that tailoring antireflux surgery according to esophageal motility is not justified, because motility disorders do not seem to correlate with postoperative dysphagia. Furthermore, conventional manometry parameters do not reliably predict postfundoplication outcomes. Recent studies investigated whether HRM would guide the type of fundoplication and/or be a better predictor of postsurgical outcomes. Marjoux and colleagues[42] reported on 20 patients who underwent HRM before and after a laparoscopic Nissen fundoplication. Prolonged dysphagia was predicted only by postoperative elevated integrated relaxation pressure, probably reflecting a tighter wrap, and not by any preoperative metric.[42] A more recent study by Siegal and colleagues[43] included 94 patients who underwent HRM before a laparoscopic Nissen fundoplication. Among patients who did not have preoperative dysphagia, no HRM metric was associated with developing the symptom postoperatively. Among those with dysphagia prior to surgery, higher DCI, contraction front velocity, percent peristalsis, distal latency, and distal esophageal contraction amplitude were associated with resolution of dysphagia. Patients who had their dysphagia resolve were much more likely to have a DCI greater than or equal to 1000 mm Hg/s/cm. The investigators used statistical bootstrapping to power the study, and none of the patients had postoperative repeat HRM. More importantly, they did not include patients with baseline hypomotility in their study. Nevertheless, the findings imply that a stronger esophagus is better able to clear a bolus past the new fundoplication. This concept was investigated by Ayazi and colleagues,[44] who analyzed the esophageal outflow resistance imposed by a Nissen fundoplication. Esophageal manometry was performed in 53 healthy subjects and in 37 patients with symptomatic GERD but normal baseline esophageal motility, before/after Nissen fundoplication. The esophageal outflow resistance, reflected by the intrabolus pressure, was measured 5 cm above the LES. The investigators reported an increase in mean intrabolus pressure from 3.6 mm Hg to 12.0 mm Hg after Nissen and, as long the postoperative measurement was less than the 95% percentile value of 20 mm Hg, patients remained dysphagia-free.

While awaiting further studies to confirm these findings, preoperative manometry parameters cannot be reliably used to guide the type of fundoplication or predict the postoperative outcomes. This probably reflects the complexity of esophageal perception and symptom generation that potentially may involve factors other than circular muscle contraction.[45,46] This said, it may be prudent to offer a partial fundoplication to patients with impaired esophageal motility, especially that 2 recent meta-analyses showed comparable acid reflux control between laparoscopic Toupet and Nissen fundoplications.[47,48] On the other hand, magnetic sphincteric augmentation remains contraindicated in patients with GERD and known esophageal dysmotility (ie, manometry showing effective swallows <70%–80% and/or distal esophageal amplitude of <35 mm Hg).[6]

## SURGICAL FUNDOPLICATION IN PATIENTS WITH ESOPHAGEAL APERISTALSIS

Scleroderma patients with esophageal involvement were offered a variety of antireflux surgeries in the past, including combination of Collis gastroplasty with Nissen as well as an approach through the left chest with a Belsey Mark IV fundoplication. For instance, an early review by Mansour and Malone[49] reported encouraging results in terms of reflux control, but all patients demonstrated recurrence of esophagitis on endoscopic studies at mean follow-up of 7.4 years. Similarly, Orringer and co-workers[50,51] reported their experience with Collis-Belsey fundoplication in scleroderma patients and noted late recurrence of reflux symptoms in 41% of these patients over 42 months; the investigators then favored a Collis-Nissen repair, which demonstrated a 25% recurrence at 22 months postoperatively. In a different study, a Hill repair was performed on 29 patients with symptomatic GERD, 73% of which had preoperative non–stricture-related dysphagia. The investigators reported resolution of the dysphagia after surgery, despite persistence of the esophageal dysmotility on radionuclide esophageal transit studies that were performed on 20 of 29 patients postoperatively.[52]

The question of whether any fundoplication is safe in patients with complete esophageal peristalsis remains controversial, however, with many investigators considering it a contraindication, from the fear of creating pseudoachalasia.[53] In practice, however, these patients have few viable options, especially in the setting of severe scleroderma with concomitant esophageal and pulmonary involvement and the potential for lung transplantation. In that regard, Goldberg and colleagues[54] published their experience on 34 patients with GERD and esophageal hypomotility on HRM, 10 of which had systemic scleroderma (13 patients had scleroderma-like esophagus and 21 had ineffective peristalsis). Minimally invasive fundoplications included Toupet (n=30), Dor (n=2) and Nissen (n=2). Acid suppression was stopped in 24% (n = 8) of patients and continued at the same or reduced dose in 59% (n = 20). Only 1 patient required surgical revision at 4 months postoperatively, whereas persistent dysphagia was noted in 4 patients (11.7%) and was treated successfully with endoscopic dilation in all of them; 1 patient required pyloric botulinum toxin injection.[54] The authors did not systematically repeat esophageal motility evaluation or pH monitoring postoperatively and relied primarily on patient symptom queries. The authors are reviewing, however, more extensive experience in patients with reflux disease in the setting of esophageal dysmotility and scleroderma, especially those with interstitial lung disease awaiting or after lung transplantation. In general, the authors selectively offer a partial posterior fundoplication (180°–270°) to patients with esophageal aperistalsis, as long as they exhibit uncontrolled acid exposure on objective measurement and more prominent reflux symptoms than dysphagia.

The rest of the literature shows acceptable outcomes of fundoplication in the setting of esophageal aperistalsis, although overall it is limited and often patients are mixed along those with any degree of esophageal dysmotility. For instance, Watson and colleagues[55] reported on 26 patients with an aperistaltic esophagus who underwent a laparoscopic fundoplication (4 Nissen and 22 Dor). Using a standardized symptom assessment questionnaire, they noted control of reflux symptoms in 79% of patients at 5 years to 12 years, with no increase in overall dysphagia after surgery. Only 2 patients underwent reoperative surgery.[55] A recent series by Armijo and colleagues[56] reported 51 patients (9 with esophageal body amotility and 42 with severe hypomotility) who underwent a Toupet fundoplication with a hiatal hernia repair (31 patients had hiatal hernia >5 cm). At mean follow-up of 25 months (1–7 years), the investigators showed significant improvements of heartburn, regurgitation, and use of PPI and a lower rate of dysphagia postoperatively (26.7% vs 58.8% preoperatively, respectively), despite persistence of dysmotility on upper gastrointestinal studies.[56]

### Surgical Alternatives for Patients with Scleroderma Esophagus

Roux-en-Y gastric bypass (RYGBP) has been proposed as a viable surgical alternative for GERD patients with severe esophageal dysmotility or aperistalsis. RYGBP is known to reduce reflux in the morbidly obese population through different mechanisms: reduction of the excess weight loss, exclusion of the acid-producing mucosa of the fundus, and prevention of biliary reflux into the pouch and the esophagus as a result of the Roux limb.[57]

Yan and colleagues[58] recently reported a series of 14 patients with systemic sclerosis (scleroderma) and GERD who underwent 7 RYGBPs and 7 fundoplications (2 Nissen, 4 Toupet, and 1 Dor). All the RYGBP patients had symptom resolution or improvement, whereas only 3 patients reported partial improvement in the fundoplication group. Kent and colleagues[59] also examined their experience in scleroderma patients, with long-term follow-up available for 7 of 8 patients who underwent RYGBP and 7 of 10 patients who underwent fundoplication. Despite the small number of patients, the investigators reported a statistically lower incidence of postoperative dysphagia in the RYGBP group, who otherwise had more favorable scores on the GERD health-related quality-of-life (HRQL) questionnaire (mean of 4 vs 15.6 in the fundoplication group).

An important issue that has to be discussed in this setting, however, is the nutritional impact and weight loss associated with RYGBP in patients with significant upper gastrointestinal symptoms and generally limited baseline oral intake. Many of the patients discussed previously had a concurrent feeding tube placed at the time of surgery, and the Roux limb was made relatively short (<100 cm) to limit the malabsorption. Furthermore, patients with scleroderma also can feature small intestinal dysmotility and the possibility of bacterial overgrowth should also be considered before RYGBP.[19]

For complete thoroughness, other surgical options also have been reported in the literature. Biliary/duodenal diversion was described for complex/scleroderma esophagitis but is associated with high morbidity.[60,61] Esophagectomy with either gastric or colonic interposition also has been reported with variable success but is associated with significant morbidity and even mortality.[58,59,62]

## ENDOSCOPIC MANAGEMENT OF GASTROESOPHAGEAL REFLUX DISEASE

In discussing the contemporary surgical management of GERD, the role of endoscopic procedures designed to endoluminally reinforce the LES must be mentioned.

Currently, there are 2 basic approaches to endoscopic antireflux procedures: endoscopic fundoplication with full-thickness fastening of the fundus to the distal esophagus and endoscopic radiofrequency ablation (RFA) to induce nerve ablation and thickening of the LES. Other techniques previously attempted but no longer available included submucosal injection of biopolymer or polytetrafluoroethylene and mucosal plication.

The more widely used endoscopic plication device is the EsophyX (EndoGastric Solutions, Redmond, Washington). It utilizes a pin and suction technique to create a 270o anterior wrap using 3 to 5 polypropylene fasteners. Contraindications for this procedure include a hiatal hernia larger than 3 cm, prior fundoplication, and severe esophagitis.[63] A recent meta-analysis with pooled data from 18 prospective studies, including 5 randomized controlled trials, demonstrated a decrease in the total number of reflux episodes and, unlike with surgical fundoplication, the patients did not report gas-bloat symptoms. There was no significant difference, however, in the esophageal acid exposure time and, on follow-up, most patients had resumed PPIs. Additionally, the overall complication rate was 2.4%, some of which were severe, including perforation and bleeding.[64] In a study by Ebright and colleagues,[7] TIF was performed on 21 patients with esophageal dysmotility, including 20 patients with nonspecific disorders and 1 with scleroderma. They found that when compared with those with normal motility, patients with esophageal dysmotility had a difference neither in overall symptomatic improvement in GERD-HRQL scores nor in overall satisfaction. They concluded that TIF may be a viable antireflux option for patients with impaired motility, similar to a partial fundoplication.[7]

The Stretta device (Mederi Therapeutics, Norwalk, Connecticut) applies RFA to the LES using a balloon catheter assembly. The system applies RFA through 4 needle tips, which project perpendicularly from the balloon to administer a series of lesions from above to just below the squamocolumnar junction. This somehow decreases the compliance of the LES, likely by a combination of nerve ablation, fibrosis, and increase in wall thickness. The system has been approved by the Food and Drug Administration since 2001 and has been evaluated by several long-term studies. One clinical trial with 10-year follow-up reported normalization of GERD-HRQL scores in 72% of 217 patients, 41% cessation of PPIs, and 85% complete resolution of Barrett esophagus (28 of 33 patients).[65]

Besides these endoluminal procedures, endoscopic technology potentially can be used to tailor the fundoplication. One such device is the endoluminal functional lumen imaging probe (EndoFLIP; Crospon, Carlsbad, California), which can provide real-time information about the physical characteristics of the EGJ. The device is composed of a balloon with sensors, which can detect the real-time cross-sectional diameter, cross-sectional area, and distensibility index (DI). Studies have shown that patients who have DI less than 0.5 $mm^2$/mm Hg after the fundoplication have significant dysphagia, often requiring revision of the wrap.[66] This may be a helpful adjunct to use in the setting of esophageal dysmotility. For instance, in a study by Kim and colleagues,[67] the Endo-FLIP was used in 40 patients during laparoscopic hiatal hernia repair to tailor the size of the crural closure and tightness of the fundoplication. After fundoplication, the average minimal diameter decreased to 5.97 mm ± 0.6 mm, from 8.92 mm ± 1.93 mm, and DI decreased to 1.26 $mm^2$/mm Hg ± 0.38 $mm^2$/mm Hg, from 2.88 $mm^2$/mm Hg ± 1.55 $mm^2$/mm Hg ($P$<.0001). After 1 month, none of the patients had reflux or significant dysphagia.[67]

## SUMMARY

Esophageal dysmotility is quite common in the setting of GERD, covering a wide spectrum of ineffective motility, fragmented peristalsis, and complete absence of contractility. Essentially, most of the literature demonstrates the safety of fundoplication in cases of moderate hypomotility and that[1] surgical outcomes cannot be reliably predicted by preoperative manometry parameters[2]; more emphasis should be placed on baseline symptoms. Both Toupet and Nissen fundoplications seem to achieve comparable reflux control without significant worsening of the obstructive symptoms. Fundoplication in the setting of complete esophageal peristalsis remains controversial, although a tailored partial wrap can be selectively offered to patients after a multidisciplinary assessment and thorough counseling. RYGBP also can be considered cautiously in cases of scleroderma-like esophagus as an alternative to fundoplication, taking into account nutritional status. More data are needed on the merits of endoscopic approaches to GERD in the setting of esophageal dysmotility, either as a partial endoluminal fundoplication or as an intraprocedural functional measurement that can better guide the type of wrap.

## ACKNOWLEDGMENTS

Herit Vachhani, MD (gastroenterology fellow, Temple University Hospital).

## DISCLOSURE

None of the authors have any disclosures.

## REFERENCES

1. El-Serag HB, Sweet S, Winchester CC, et al. Update on the epidemiology of gastroesophageal reflux disease: a systematic review. Gut 2014;63:871–80.
2. Shaheen NJ, Hansen RA, Morgan DR, et al. The burden of gastrointestinal and liver diseases, 2006. Am J Gastroenterol 2006;101:2128–38.
3. Schnoll-Sussman F, Katz PO. Clinical implications of emerging data on the safety of proton pump inhibitors. Curr Treat Options Gastroenterol 2017;15(1):1–9.
4. Xie Y, Bowe B, Yan Y, et al. Estimates of all cause mortality and cause specific mortality associated with proton pump inhibitors among US veterans: cohort study. BMJ 2019;365:l1580.
5. Nissen R, Rossetti M. Modern operations for hiatal hernia and reflux esophagitis: gastropexy and fundoplication. Archivio Chir Torace 1959;13:375–87.

6. Skubleny D, Switzer NJ, Dang J, et al. LINX® magnetic esophageal sphincter augmentation versus Nissen fundoplication for gastroesophageal reflux disease: a systematic review and meta-analysis. Surg Endosc 2017;31(8):3078–84.
7. Ebright MI, Sridhar P, Litle VR, et al. Endoscopic fundoplication: effectiveness for controlling symptoms of gastroesophageal reflux disease. Innovations (Phila) 2017;12(3):180–5.
8. Dodds WJ, Dent J, Hogan WJ, et al. Mechanisms of gastroesophageal reflux in patients with reflux esophagitis. N Engl J Med 1982;307:1547–52.
9. Gyawali CP, Roman S, Bredenoord AJ, et al, International GERD Consensus Working Group. Classification of esophageal motor findings in gastro-esophageal reflux disease: conclusions from an international consensus group. Neurogastroenterol Motil 2017;29(12).
10. Diener U, Patti MG, Molena D, et al. Esophageal dysmotility and gastroesophageal reflux disease. J Gastrointest Surg 2001;5(3):260–5.
11. Meneghetti AT, Tedesco P, Damani T, et al. Esophageal mucosal damage may promote dysmotility and worsen esophageal acid exposure. J Gastrointest Surg 2005;9(9):1313–7.
12. Bremner RM, DeMeester TR, Crookes PF, et al. The effect of symptoms and nonspecific motility abnormalities on outcomes of surgical therapy for gas- troe-sophageal reflux disease. J Thorac Cardiovasc Surg 1994;107:1244–9.
13. Jiang LQ, Ye BX, Wang MF, et al. Acid exposure in patients with gastroesophageal reflux disease is associated with esophageal dysmotility. J Dig Dis 2019; 20(2):73–7.
14. Pandolfino JE, Kim H, Ghosh SK, et al. High-resolution manometry of the EGJ: an analysis of crural diaphragm function in GERD. Am J Gastroenterol 2007;102: 1056–63.
15. Kahrilas PJ, Bredenoord AJ, Fox M, et al, International High Resolution Manom-etry Working Group. The Chicago Classification of esophageal motility disorders, v3.0. Neurogastroenterol Motil 2015;27(2):160–74.
16. Gyawali CP, Kahrilas PJ, Savarino E, et al. Modern diagnosis of GERD: the Lyon Consensus. Gut 2018;67(7):1351–62.
17. Xiao Y, Kahrilas PJ, Kwasny MJ, et al. High-resolution manometry correlates of ineffective esophageal motility. Am J Gastroenterol 2012;107(11):1647–54.
18. Chan WW, Haroian LR, Gyawali CP. Value of preoperative esophageal function studies before laparoscopic antireflux surgery. Surg Endosc 2011;25:2943–9.
19. Denaxas K, Ladas SD, Karamanolis GP. Evaluation and management of esophageal manifestations in systemic sclerosis. Ann Gastroenterol 2018;31(2):165–70.
20. Roman S, Hot A, Fabien N, et al, Reseau Sclerodermie des Hospices Civils de Lyon. Esophageal dysmotility associated with systemic sclerosis: a high-resolution manometry study. Dis Esophagus 2011;24:299–304.
21. Abu-Shakra M, Guillemin F, Lee P. Gastrointestinal manifestations of systemic sclerosis. Semin Arthritis Rheum 1994;24:29.
22. Schoenfeld SR, Castelino FV. Interstitial lung disease in scleroderma. Rheum Dis Clin North Am 2015;41(2):237–48.
23. Ireland AC, Holloway RH, Toouli J, et al. Mechanisms underlying the antireflux ac-tion of fundoplication. Gut 1993;34:303–8.
24. Lundell L, Abrahamsson H, Ruth M, et al. Lower esophageal sphincter character-istics and esophageal acid exposure following partial or 360 degrees fundoplica-tion: results of a prospective, randomized, clinical study. World J Surg 1991;15: 115–20.

25. Bell RCW, Hanna P, Powers B, et al. Clinical and manometric results of laparoscopic partial (Toupet) and complete (Rosetti-Nissen) fundoplication. Surg Endosc 1996;10:724–8.

26. Freys SM, Fuchs KH, Heimbucher J, et al. Tailored augmentation of the lower esophageal sphincter in experimental antireflux operations. Surg Endosc 1997; 11:1183–8.

27. Stein HJ, Bremner RM, Jamieson J, et al. Effect of Nissen fundoplication on esophageal motor function. Arch Surg 1992;127:788–91.

28. Herbella FA, Tedesco P, Nipomnick I, et al. Effect of partial and total laparoscopic fundoplication on esophageal body motility. Surg Endosc 2007;21(2):285–8.

29. Fibbe C, Layer P, Keller J, et al. Esophageal motility in reflux disease before and after fundoplication: a prospective, randomized, clinical, and manometric study. Gastroenterology 2001;121:5–14.

30. Wykypiel H, Hugl B, Gadenstaetter M, et al. Laparoscopic partial posterior (Toupet) fundoplication improves esophageal bolus propagation on scintigraphy. Surg Endosc 2008;22:1845–51.

31. Rydberg L, Ruth M, Lundell L. Does oesophageal motor function improve with time after successful antireflux surgery? Results of a prospective, randomised clinical study. Gut 1997;41:82–6.

32. Rerych K, Kurek J, Klimacka-Nawrot E, et al. High-resolution manometry in patients with gastroesophageal reflux disease before and after fundoplication. J Neurogastroenterol Motil 2017;23(1):55–63.

33. Herron DM, Swanstrom LL, Ramzi N, et al. Factors predictive of dysphagia after laparoscopic Nissen fundoplication. Surg Endosc 1999;13(12):1180–3.

34. Cole SJ, van den Bogaerde JB, van der Walt H. Preoperative esophageal manometry does not predict postoperative dysphagia following anti-reflux surgery. Dis Esophagus 2005;18:51–6.

35. Blom D, Peters JH, DeMeester TR, et al. Physiologic mechanism and preoperative prediction of new-onset dysphagia after laparoscopic Nissen fundoplication. J Gastrointest Surg 2002;6(1):22–7 [discussion: 27–8].

36. Kahrilas PJ, Dodds WJ, Hogan WJ. Effect of peristaltic dysfunction on esophageal volume clearance. Gastroenterology 1988;94:73–80.

37. Patti MG, Robinson T, Galvani C, et al. Total fundoplication is superior to partial fundoplication even when esophageal peristalsis is weak. J Am Coll Surg 2004; 198:863–9 [discussion: 869–70].

38. Novitsky YW, Wong J, Kercher KW, et al. Severely disordered esophageal peristalsis is not a contraindication to laparoscopic Nissen fundoplication. Surg Endosc 2007;21(6):950–4.

39. Tsereteli Z, Sporn E, Astudillo JA, et al. Laparoscopic Nissen fundoplication is a good option in patients with abnormal esophagealmotility. Surg Endosc 2009; 23(10):2292–5.

40. Booth MI, Stratford J, Jones L, et al. Randomized clinical trial of laparoscopic total (Nissen) versus posterior partial (Toupet) fundoplication for gastro-oesophageal reflux disease based on preoperative oesophageal manometry. Br J Surg 2008;95(1):57–63.

41. Strate U, Emmermann A, Fibbe C, et al. Laparoscopic fundoplication: Nissen versus Toupet two-year outcome of a prospective random- ized study of 200 patients regarding preoperative esophageal motil- ity. Surg Endosc 2008;22:21–30.

42. Marjoux S, Roman S, Juget-Pietu F, et al. Impaired post- operative EGJ relaxation as a determinant of post laparoscopic fundoplication dysphagia: a study with

high-resolution manometry before and after surgery. Surg Endosc 2012;26: 3642–9.

43. Siegal SR, Dunst CM, Robinson B, et al. Preoperative high-resolution manometry criteria are associated with dysphagia after Nissen fundoplication. World J Surg 2019;43(4):1062–7.

44. Ayazi S, DeMeester SR, Hagen JA, et al. Clinical significance of esophageal outflow resistance imposed by a Nissen fundoplication. J Am Coll Surg 2019; 229(2):210–6.

45. Xiao Y, Kahrilas PJ, Nicodème F, et al. Lack of correlation between HRM metrics and symptoms during the manometric protocol. Am J Gastroenterol 2014;109(4): 521–6.

46. Kapadia S, Osler T, Lee A, et al. The role of preoperative high resolution manometry in predicting dysphagia after laparoscopic Nissen fundoplication. Surg Endosc 2018;32(5):2365–72.

47. Tian ZC, Wang B, Shan CX, et al. A meta-analysis of randomized controlled trials to compare long-term outcomes of Nissen and Toupet fundoplication for gastroesophageal reflux disease. PLoS One 2015;10:e0127627.

48. Du X, Hu Z, Yan C, et al. A meta-analysis of long follow- up outcomes of laparoscopic Nissen (total) versus Toupet (270 degrees) fundoplication for gastroesophageal reflux disease based on randomized controlled trials in adults. BMC Gastroenterol 2016;16:88.

49. Mansour K, Malone C. Surgery for scleroderma of the esophagus: a 12-year experience. Ann Thorac Surg 1988;46:513–4.

50. Orringer MB, Dabich L, Zarafonetis CJD, et al. Gastroesophageal reflux in esophageal scleroderma: diagnosis and implications. Ann Thorac Surg 1976;22(2): 120–30.

51. Orringer MB, Orringer JS, Dabich L, et al. Combined Collis gastroplasty-fundoplication operations for scleroderma reflux esophagitis. Surgery 1981; 90(4):624–30.

52. Russell CO, Pope CE, Gannan RM, et al. Does surgery correct esophageal motor dysfunction in gastro- esophageal reflux. Ann Surg 1981;194:290–6.

53. Yadlapati R, Hungness ES, Pandolfino JE. Complications of antireflux surgery. Am J Gastroenterol 2018;113(8):1137–47.

54. Goldberg MB, Abbas AE, Smith MS, et al. Minimally invasive fundoplication is safe and effective in patients with severe esophageal hypomotility. Innovations (Phila) 2016;11(6):396–9.

55. Watson DI, Jamieson GG, Bessell JR, et al. Laparoscopic fundoplication in patients with an aperistaltic esophagus and gastroesophagealreflux. Dis Esophagus 2006;19(2):94–8.

56. Armijo PR, Hennings D, Leon M1, et al. Surgical management of gastroesophageal reflux disease in patients with severe esophageal dysmotility. J Gastrointest Surg 2019;23(1):36–42.

57. Madalosso CA, Gurski S, Callegari-Jacques RR, et al. The impact of gastric bypass on gastroesophageal reflux disease in patients with morbid obesity. Ann Surg 2010;251:244–8.

58. Yan J, Strong AT, Sharma G, et al. Surgical management of gastroesophageal reflux disease in patients with systemic sclerosis. Surg Endosc 2018;32(9): 3855–60.

59. Kent MS, Luketich JD, Irshad K, et al. Comparison of surgical approaches to recalcitrant gastroesophageal reflux disease in the patient with scleroderma. Ann Thorac Surg 2007;84(5):1710–5 [discussion 1715–6].

60. Peix J, Maroun J, Tekinel O, et al. Treatment of sclerodermic esophagitis: value of duodenal diversion. Ann Chir 1993;47(4):302–6.
61. Fekete F, Kabbej M, Sauvenet A. Total duodenal diversion in the treatment of complex peptic esophagitis. Chirurgie 1996;121:326.
62. Orringer M, Orringer J. Esophagectomy: definitive treatment for esophageal neuromotor dysfunction. Ann Thorac Surg 1982;34:237–48.
63. Mayor MA, Fernando HC. Endoluminal approaches to gastroesophageal reflux disease. Thorac Surg Clin 2018;28(4):527–32.
64. Huang X, Chen S, Zhao H, et al. Efficacy of transoral incisionless fundoplication (TIF) for the treatment of GERD: a systematic review with meta-analysis. Surg Endosc 2017;31(3):1032–44.
65. Fass R, Cahn F, Scotti DJ, et al. Systematic review and meta-analysis of controlled and prospective cohort efficacy studies of endoscopic radiofrequency for treatment of gastroesophageal reflux disease. Surg Endosc 2017;31(12):4865–82.
66. Ilczyszyn A, Botha AJ. Feasibility of esophagogastric junction distensibility measurement during Nissen fundoplication. Dis Esophagus 2014;27:637–44.
67. Kim MP, Meisenbach LM, Chan EY. Tailored fundoplication with endoluminal functional lumen imaging probe allows for successful minimally invasive hiatal hernia repair. Surg Laparosc Endosc Percutan Tech 2018;28:178–82.

# Endoscopic and Surgical Treatments for Achalasia
## Who to Treat and How?

Romulo A. Fajardo, MD[a], Roman V. Petrov, MD[b],*,
Charles T. Bakhos, MD[b], Abbas E. Abbas, MD[b]

## KEYWORDS

- Achalasia • Gastroesophageal junction • Cardiomyotomy • Heller myotomy
- Peroral endoscopic myotomy

## KEY POINTS

- Achalasia is a progressive neurodegenerative disorder characterized by failure of relaxation of the LES and altered motility of the esophagus.
- Traditional surgical approach to relieve the obstruction at the LES includes cardiomyotomy, which is highly effective. Fundoplication is added to decrease the risk of postoperative reflux.
- Peroral endoscopic myotomy (POEM) is a new endoscopic procedure that allows division of the LES via transoral route.
- POEM has several advantages including less invasiveness, cosmesis, and tailored approach to the length on the myotomy. However, it is associated with increased rate of postprocedural reflux.
- Various endoscopic interventions are used to manage post-POEM reflux. New POEM plus fundoplication (POEM + F) technique was recently introduced into clinical practice to specifically address this problem.

## INTRODUCTION

Achalasia is a neurodegenerative disorder characterized by progressive loss of normal function of the esophageal smooth muscle. Loss of ganglion cells of the myenteric plexus of the esophagus causes uncoordinated esophageal motility resulting in the failure of lower esophageal sphincter (LES) relaxation, accompanied by various alteration of normal peristalsis of the smooth muscle of the esophagus (**Fig. 1**). The cause of primary achalasia remains unknown. Secondary causes include infections,

[a] Department of General Surgery, Temple University Hospital, 3401 North Broad Street, C-401, Philadelphia, PA 19140, USA; [b] Department of Thoracic Medicine and Surgery, Lewis Katz School of Medicine at Temple University, 3401 North Broad Street, C-501, Philadelphia, PA 19140, USA
* Corresponding author.
*E-mail address:* Roman.Petrov@tuhs.temple.edu

Gastroenterol Clin N Am 49 (2020) 481–498
https://doi.org/10.1016/j.gtc.2020.05.003

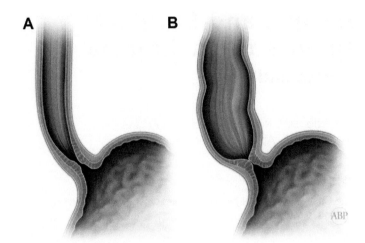

**Fig. 1.** Gastroesophageal junction. (*A*) Normal anatomy. (*B*) Achalasia. Failure of LES relaxation leads to an obstructive physiology, resulting in proximal esophageal dilation and tortuosity.

autoimmune disorders and malignancy. Clinical manifestations of achalasia include dysphagia to solids and liquids, regurgitation and substernal chest pain, leading in extreme cases to weight loss and malnutrition. Reflux is not characteristic for achalasia because of obstruction of the gastroesophageal junction by a hypertonic LES; however, stasis and fermentation of the retained food and secretions lead to frequent heartburn in these patients. Although restoration of normal esophageal function is impossible at present, over the last century a variety of treatments were introduced into clinical practice for the management of this chronic disease, aiming at palliation of symptoms by obliterating the LES and relieving the obstruction. This article discusses the endoscopic and surgical treatments of achalasia.

## HISTORY OF SURGICAL THERAPY FOR ACHALASIA

A landmark publication on the topic occurred in 1914 when German physician Ernst Heller (1877–1964) published the first report on esophagocardiomyotomy as a way of relieving dysphagia in case of achalasia.[1] Initially confronted with disbelief that an extramucosal myotomy could correct impaired esophageal function, the operation proved to be incredibly effective in alleviating symptoms and complications of achalasia. The procedure, which took place on April 14, 1913, was an extramucosal esophagomyotomy on a 49-year-old man with a 30-year history of dysphagia. In Heller's original report, he quoted a then-recent publication by Heyrovsky[2] describing success with side-to-side esophagogastrostomy, bypassing the spastic LES.

During the conduct of the procedure, Heller abandoned his initial plan of performing a side-to-side anastomosis by Heyrovsky and instead performed the transabdominal double vertical extramucosal esophagomyotomy. The procedure was a huge success with an immediate and durable resolution of the dysphagia. The patient resumed full oral intake the next day after the surgery, maintaining good health and nutrition at 8 years follow-up.[3] According to Heller, Gottstein first expressed the concept of extramucosal myotomy in 1901, theorizing that a procedure similar to a pyloromyotomy could be performed at the gastric cardia. However, despite this early theoretic speculation, an esophagomyotomy was not performed in practice until Heller.[3,4] Despite a variety of other contemporary procedures for achalasia, extramucosal cardiomyotomy has rapidly gained wide acceptance, becoming a standard of care, whereas other operations of esophagogastrostomy fell out of favor mainly because of side effects from regurgitation of gastric contents and subsequent severe esophagitis.[5–9]

For decades since this initial description, surgical therapy has remained the gold standard of achalasia treatment because medical therapy failed to provide substantial and sustainable relief. Currently, medical therapy is reserved for poor surgical candidates unable to tolerate invasive procedures. Medications include nitrates, calcium channel blockers and other agents, such as sildenafil, atropine, terbutaline, and theophylline. The premise of medical therapy is to relax the smooth muscle of the LES to reduce LES pressure and dysphagia, although clinical applications have been limited secondary to systemic side effects.

For these reasons endoscopic and surgical therapy for achalasia prevails and the role of pharmacologic treatment of esophageal achalasia is limited particularly to early stage disease, high surgical risk elderly patients, or for the temporary bridging of symptoms in patients waiting for definitive therapy. This is especially evident now with the recent development of new minimally invasive surgical and endoscopic interventions for the management of achalasia.[10–12]

## SURGICAL THERAPY FOR ACHALASIA

After Heller's initial description, open extramucosal esophagomyotomy for many years had remained the principal therapy for achalasia. Although the procedure enjoyed overall excellent results with few complications, a traditional open approach via either a thoracotomy or a laparotomy required a prolonged hospital stay, delayed recovery, and elevated levels of surgical pain.[13]

With the advent of minimally invasive technology in 1980s to 1990s, the laparoscopic approach was rapidly adopted in foregut surgery. Just a few years after initial introduction of laparoscopic cholecystectomy, in 1991 a group led by Cuschieri reported on the first experience of laparoscopic cardiomyotomy in a single patient with manometrically confirmed achalasia. The patient enjoyed complete relief of dysphagia postoperatively with minimal postoperative discomfort and required only 3 days of hospital stay, a significant advantage over the traditional open approach.[14] This procedure was introduced in the United States by Pellegrini and colleagues.[13] In 1992 authors published their results of a minimally invasive esophagomyotomy. They approached the gastroesophageal junction through the left chest rather than through a transabdominal approach. The authors operated on 17 patients with radiographically confirmed achalasia with success of the thoracoscopic approach in 15 patients. In two patients, a second laparoscopic procedure was required likely because of the incomplete myotomy secondary to limited extension onto the gastric cardia via the chest. Authors believed that the thoracoscopic approach had an advantage of less disruption of the elements of the antireflux mechanism reducing the incidence of postoperative gastroesophageal reflux, obviating an antireflux procedure. Authors postulated that the laparoscopic Heller myotomy should be reserved only for patients with previously failed thoracoscopic myotomy or "hostile" chest with previous surgical intervention.[13] However, in a follow-up publication on the topic reporting on their 8-year experience, the group demonstrated a 60% incidence of gastroesophageal reflux after the thoracoscopic procedure as opposed to 17% after laparoscopic myotomy with fundoplication. Clearly, with the experience, the authors switched their preference as only 35 patients had thoracoscopy and most patients (133 of 168) underwent laparoscopic cardiomyotomy with the fundoplication.[15] They cited three main advantages of the laparoscopic approach with the fundoplication-more effective relief of dysphagia, shorter hospital stay and significantly decreased postoperative reflux, declaring it the primary treatment modality for esophageal achalasia.[15]

Relieving obstruction in patients with achalasia via anatomic disruption of the LES with cardiomyotomy leads to substantial gastroesophageal reflux (**Fig. 2**). With increasing volume of Heller myotomies being performed laparoscopically, a great deal of controversy was raised regarding the role of an antireflux procedure after a cardiomyotomy for control of reflux. In a meta-analysis of 21 studies on laparoscopic Heller myotomy with and without antireflux procedure from 1991 to 2001, Lyass and colleagues[16] did not observe any difference in pathologic acid exposure between these two patient groups making no recommendation regarding the role of antireflux in this patient population. However, a prospective double-blind trial randomizing 43 patients with achalasia by Richards and colleagues[17] demonstrated a substantial decrease in pathologic reflux in combined procedure with Heller myotomy and Dor fundoplication (**Fig. 3**A) versus Heller myotomy alone. Six months postoperatively, 24-hour pH demonstrated a decrease in reflux from 47.6% (10 of 21 patients) after Heller myotomy alone to 9.1% (2 of 22 patients) with the combined approach, laying the ground for standardization of adding fundoplication to cardiomyotomy.[17]

In a follow-up publication to address the shortcoming of limited time observation, authors analyzed the long-term (mean, 11.8 years) results on the same patient cohort.[18] In the analysis, 27 of the original 41 patients (66%) were studied on the patient-reported measures of dysphagia and gastroesophageal reflux using the Dysphagia Score and the Gastroesophageal Reflux Disease-Health-Related Quality of Life (GERD-HRQL) questionnaires. The authors demonstrated that Dysphagia Scores and GERD-HRQL scores were slightly worse but not statistically significant for the Heller myotomy alone group versus combined procedure of the myotomy with fundoplication. With this long-term follow-up, most patients post-treatment still required dietary modifications and antireflux medications and about 40% of participants required additional endoscopic interventions for dysphagia. One patient in each group required redo Heller myotomy ultimately followed by esophagectomy. Authors concluded that long-term patient-reported outcomes between the two interventions were comparable.[18] It is likely that due to limited number of patients, this study was underpowered and failed to demonstrate the difference between these groups.

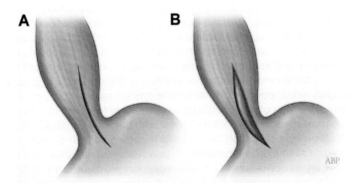

**Fig. 2.** Heller cardiomyotomy. (*A*) placement of the incision across the LES. (*B*) Completed myotomy with disruption of the lower esophageal sphincter.

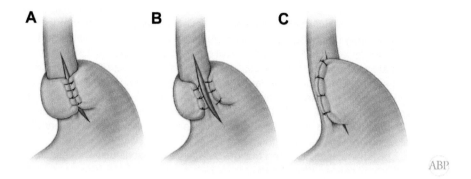

**Fig. 3.** Types of fundoplication. (*A*) Nissen fundoplication. (*B*) Toupet fundoplication. (*C*) Dor fundoplication.

Despite convincing evidence of benefits of the fundoplication drawn from Richards and colleagues[17] trial, increasing controversy persisted as to the preferred type of fundoplication after cardiomyotomy. In a review of more than 5000 patients from 75 papers, the mean incidence of symptomatic reflux was demonstrated at 8.6%.[19] The most commonly performed antireflux procedures were the anterior 180-degree Dor fundoplication and the 360-degree Nissen fundoplication (**Fig. 3**A, C). However, the concern surrounding the Nissen procedure was the risk of obstructive physiology with a complete circumferential wrap in the aperistaltic esophagus.[20]

This concern was proven true in a prospective randomized trial, comparing long-term outcomes of Dor versus floppy-Nissen fundoplication after laparoscopic Heller myotomy for achalasia. After excluding nine patients in the initial cohort of 153 patients, 144 patients were randomized to one of the two treatment groups. With a mean follow-up of 125 months, there were no differences in clinical (5.6% vs 0%) or instrumental (2.8% vs 0%) rates of gastroesophageal reflux. However, patients undergoing Nissen fundoplication had significantly higher rates of dysphagia (2.8% vs 15%). Authors supported the use of the Dor fundoplication as the preferred method of reflux control in patients with achalasia after Heller myotomy.[20]

With these data suggesting better functional outcomes with a partial wrap for reflux control, further discussion centered on the use of a posterior (Toupet) versus an anterior (Dor) fundoplication (**Fig. 3**B, C). The potential disadvantage of a posterior approach is the angulation of the gastroesophageal junction, hypothetically creating an impediment to the bolus passage and extensive retroesophageal dissection, potentially leading to induction of reflux.[21] However, evidence from GERD literature suggested an advantage of posterior partial fundoplication for reflux control. In a randomized controlled trial comparing the anterior and posterior laparoscopic partial fundoplications in 95 patients with GERD, reflux control was better after the posterior fundoplication. In this group of patients during the first postoperative year acid exposure was significantly lower in the Toupet group in comparison with the Dor group.[22]

Several subsequent studies comparing the efficacy of an anterior versus posterior partial fundoplication after a cardiomyotomy has produced conflicting results, essentially leaving the choice of fundoplication to the individual surgeon's preferences.[21,23] In the first randomized trial comparing Dor with Toupet fundoplication after laparoscopic Heller myotomy, 60 patients were assigned to one of these two approaches. Postoperatively, reflux was assessed with 24-hour pH monitoring at 6 and 12 months.

Abnormal acid reflux was reported in 41.7% of the Dor group versus 21.1% of the Toupet group; however, the differences were not statistically significant.[23] In another trial, 42 patients with newly diagnosed achalasia were randomized to undergo either a Toupet or a Dor fundoplication following a classical open or laparoscopic cardiomyotomy. Results were assessed during the first postoperative year with Eckardt scores, EORTC QLQ-OES18 scores, HRQL questionnaires, barium esophagram, and ambulatory 24-hour pH monitoring. The analysis showed dramatic improvement of Eckardt scores with both procedures, but the EORTC QLQ-OES18 scores and esophageal emptying were significantly better in the Toupet group, yet no differences were observed in HRQL evaluations or 24-hour pH monitoring.[21]

In another prospective randomized trial of 73 patients with achalasia with either Dor or Toupet fundoplication after laparoscopic Heller myotomy, postoperative high-resolution manometry at 6 and 24 months showed similar lower esophageal pressure patterns with both procedures. Abnormal acid exposure was significantly lower in Dor (6.9%) as opposed to Toupet patients (34%) at 6 months, but equivalent at 12 or 24 months. Nevertheless, there was no difference in postoperative symptom scores at 1, 6, or 24 months. Authors again left the choice of the procedure to the surgeon's preferences, concluding the choice of fundoplication does not affect the long-term outcome.[24] A retrospective study of 97 patients comparing long-term rates of dysphagia, reflux symptoms, and patient satisfaction between the anterior and posterior approach also showed effective resolution of the dysphagia with both procedures (89% Toupet vs 93% Dor) but substantially higher reflux rates with anterior fundoplication (11% after Toupet vs 35% after Dor fundoplication; $P<.05$), although overall patient satisfaction was 88% in both groups.[25]

Robotic surgery was a logical evolution of minimally invasive surgery with computer-enhanced technology (**Fig. 4**). Improved binocular visualization, tremor filtration, instrument articulation, and other embedded safety features potentially conved an outcome benefit. Several studies reported on the outcomes of a robotic versus a laparoscopic Heller myotomy. A retrospective multicenter trial involving 121 patients demonstrated similar operative outcomes and operative times between the two approaches. There was, however, decreased incidence of intraoperative esophageal mucosal perforations with the use of the surgical robot (0% vs 16%). Both patient groups did well with 92% versus 90% relief of their dysphagia at 18- and 22-month follow-up.[26] Similarly, in another study of 61 patients, a lower rate of esophageal perforations and a better quality of life based on the Short Form-36 Health Status Questionnaire and disease-specific GERD activity index (GRACI) were demonstrated in the robotic group.[27] A meta-analysis published in 2010 concluded that the risk of perforation is lower in robotic myotomy.[28] Although results are overall positive in these studies in favor of a robotic approach, most authors compared robotic outcomes with earlier laparoscopic procedures and a learning curve may have been attributable for the difference.

## ENDOSCOPIC THERAPY FOR ACHALASIA

The results of pharmacologic treatments for achalasia including botulinum toxin injection have been unsupported and are only recommended to patients unfit for interventions under general anesthesia.[11,12] The first randomized control study, comparing laparoscopic cardiomyotomy and fundoplication with botulinum toxin injections in patients with esophageal achalasia demonstrated that although at 6 months the results in the two groups were comparable, at 12 months, symptom recurrence in the Botox group was 40% versus 13% in the

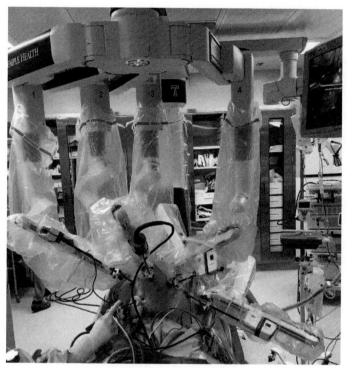

**Fig. 4.** DaVinci Xi robot docket for Heller myotomy procedure.

surgical group.[29] Authors concluded that laparoscopic myotomy is safe, offering better and longer lasting symptomatic control over serial botulinum toxin injections, reserving the latter to patients unfit for surgery or as a bridge to surgical management.

Endoscopic pneumatic dilation until recently was considered the most effective nonsurgical treatment of achalasia (**Fig. 5**).[30] Pneumatic dilators are preferred over rigid dilators because they not only stretch but also produce disruption of the LES muscle fibers. Varying rates of success are reported in the literature. Postdilation symptom-free rates range from 40% to 78% at 5 years to 12% to 58% at 15 years.[31] Even some authors have reported success rates at 5 years to be up to 97% and 93% at 10 years with repeat on-demand dilatations, although it is generally accepted that sustainable long-term results cannot be expected from this therapy.[30] Predictors of treatment failure include patients younger than 40 years, presence of pulmonary symptoms and failure to respond to the initial dilation treatment. Complications from esophageal dilation include esophageal perforation, intramural hematoma, and gastroesophageal reflux. In a meta-analysis of 1065 patients treated by experienced physicians, esophageal perforations occurred in 1.6% of patients. Up to 40% of patients developed active and even ulcerated esophagitis after serial dilations, likely because of uncontrolled reflux, although only 4% were symptomatic. Endoscopic pneumatic dilation currently is considered the most effective therapy among nonoperative treatment choices, but is associated with a high risk of complications and should be considered in select patients who refuse surgery or are poor operative candidates.[30]

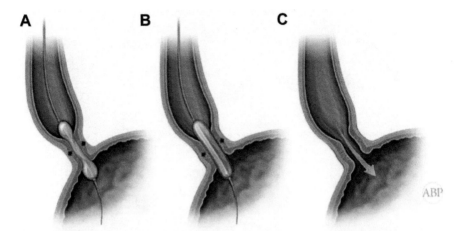

**Fig. 5.** Pneumatic dilation of the gastroesophageal junction. (*A*) Placement of the balloon across the gastroesophageal junction. (*B*) Inflation of the balloon, leading to the disruption of the fibers of the LES. (*C*) Relieved obstruction of the LES.

## PERORAL ENDOSCOPIC MYOTOMY

As a new development in the therapy for achalasia, in 2008 Inoue and colleagues[32] introduced a concept of natural orifice transluminal endoscopic surgery for the treatment of achalasia, called peroral endoscopic myotomy (POEM). In 2010, the authors published their first series of POEM for the treatment of achalasia.[33] All cases of achalasia were considered for POEM including tortuous dilated sigmoid esophagus, which is considered a relative contraindication to surgical myotomy. POEM could also be performed in patients that have failed previous therapies, such as botulinum toxin injection, pneumatic dilation, or Heller myotomy.

The standard POEM procedure consists of four sequential steps: (1) mucosal incision, (2) submucosal tunneling, (3) myotomy itself and (4) closure of the mucosotomy defect (**Fig. 6**). A 2-cm mucosal incision is made after creating a submucosal cushion

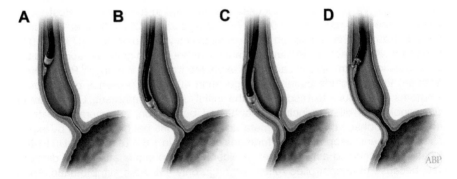

**Fig. 6.** POEM procedure. (*A*) Mucosotomy and initial submucosal entry. (*B*) Dissection of the submucosal tunnel. (*C*) Division of the esophageal muscle (myotomy). (*D*) Closure of the mucosotomy. (*From* Petrov RV, Fajardo RA, Bakhos CT, Abbas AE. Peroral endoscopic myotomy: techniques and outcomes. Shanghai Chest 2020.)

with saline and blue dye mixture, providing entrance to the submucosal space. Subsequently, the submucosal dissection, which extends 3 cm distal to the gastroesophageal junction, creates the submucosal tunnel. Once the tunnel has been completed, the myotomy is performed, starting 3 to 5 cm distally to the site of mucosotomy. The length of the myotomy may be adjusted depending on the achalasia subtype. Next, after a careful inspection of the mucosa for any inadvertent mucosal injuries, closure of the mucosotomy is performed with either endoscopic hemostatic clips or endoscopic suturing (ie, Overstitch, Apollo Endosurgery, Austin, TX).[34]

From a procedural perspective, POEM offers a significant advantage by adapting the extent and location of the myotomy according to patients' specific characteristics and the type of the achalasia.[34] The impact of the differential length of the myotomy in different types of achalasia was studied by Kane and colleagues.[35] The group reported using high-resolution esophageal manometry in 40 POEM cases to define myotomy length. The authors found significantly improved postoperative Eckardt scores in the group with tailored (longer) myotomy length in patients with subtype III achalasia.[35]

The POEM procedure has enjoyed rapid and wide adoption worldwide becoming the primary and preferred treatment of achalasia with thousands of procedures performed since its initial description. Data from largely single-center studies and small case series suggest that POEM is a safe alternative to Heller myotomy. POEM was popularized in the United States by Swanstrom and colleagues[36] who published the first report in 2012 with results of this technique in 18 patients with esophageal achalasia. At a mean follow-up of 11 months, all patients had excellent outcomes, with a median Eckardt score of 0 (range, 0–3). Endoscopy-proven esophagitis was observed in 28% of patients, whereas pH monitoring demonstrated pathologic reflux in 46%. In an international multicenter study involving 70 patients at 12 months, 82% were in remission with esophagitis shown in 42% of patients after POEM.[37] In an analysis of 94 patients after POEM at a mean follow-up of 11 months, excellent results were observed in 94.5% with postoperative pH monitoring displaying pathologic reflux in 53.4% of patients.[38] Analysis of outcomes of 80 patients with achalasia at a mean follow-up of 29 months revealed a success rate of 77.5% with esophagitis present in 37.5% of patients.[39] Authors reported on the outcomes of personal series of POEM procedures. Out of 80 cases of submucosal endoscopy there were 37 patients undergoing POEM procedure - 22 (59%) patients with type I or II, 10 (27%) with type III achalasia and 5 (14%) with jackhammer esophagus. Three (8%) patients had end stage achalasia with sigmoid esophagus. Two (5%) patients had prior surgical myotomy and all had at least one previous endoscopic intervention. Length of the myotomy was defined by the manometry findings. Average length for type I or II achalasia was $8\pm2$ cm and for type III achalasia average length of the myotomy was $21\pm2$ cm. For Nutcracker esophagus myotomy was performed up to the LES with preservation of the sphincter. Average length of the myotomy was $18\pm2$ cm. Technical success rate was 100% and clinical success, defined as Eckardt score <2, was 97%. Postoperatively 11 (30%) patients are taking PPIs for GERD.[40]

Despite its wide success, the safety of the POEM procedure is still debated. This question was addressed in a large retrospective multicenter review of adverse events from 12 centers, including almost 2000 patients. The study demonstrated low overall prevalence of any adverse events, such as inadvertent mucosotomy, esophageal leak, complications related to insufflation, submucosal hematoma, and cardiopulmonary complications at 7.5% (156 events in 137 patients). Most of the adverse events were mild in 6.4% cases with only 0.5% being severe. The most common adverse event in this study was an inadvertent mucosotomy, which occurred in 51 (2.8%) patients.

Sigmoid-type esophagus, triangular tip knife, an inexperienced operator (<20 cases performed), and nonspray coagulation were significant predictors of adverse event occurrences.[34] It is also noteworthy to mention that the wide range of reported complication rates with POEM (0%–72%) is mainly attributable to the lack of consensus on terminology in the literature. For instance, whereas some authors report asymptomatic gas-related events, such as subcutaneous emphysema, pneumoperitoneum, pneumothorax, or pneumomediastinum as an incidental finding, others give them a grading of a full adverse event.[34,40,41]

Since its inception, the POEM procedure has frequently been compared with other well-established modalities for the treatment of achalasia. In a randomized controlled trial of 133 patient with achalasia treatment success was observed in 92% of patients after POEM procedure versus 54% after pneumatic dilation. Two serious adverse events, including one perforation, occurred after pneumatic dilation, whereas none occurred in the POEM group.[42] In another retrospective study, comparing outcomes of 71 patients with newly diagnosed achalasia undergoing POEM or pneumatic dilation, POEM demonstrated a durable effect, whereas the effect of pneumatic dilation progressively decreased starting at 6 months.[43] Although the difference was demonstrated in all three subtypes of achalasia, statistical significance was only reached in type III achalasia.

## GASTROESOPHAGEAL REFLUX AFTER PERORAL ENDOSCOPIC MYOTOMY

Postoperative gastroesophageal reflux remains a concern after any type of myotomy for achalasia because of mechanical disruption of the LES. Since the basis of the POEM procedure is identical to the Heller myotomy in mechanical disruption of the LES, post-POEM gastroesophageal reflux has been naturally reported. In a retrospective case-control study of 282 patients that aimed to identify the prevalence of reflux after POEM, clinical success was demonstrated at 94%. At a median follow-up of 12 months, an abnormal DeMeester score was reported in 58%, with reflux esophagitis present in 23% on upper endoscopy. Despite that, reflux was symptomatic only in 40% of patients.[44]

The comparative incidence of postoperative gastroesophageal reflux among laparoscopic or robotic Heller myotomy and POEM was assessed in a systematic review and meta-analysis including almost 8000 patients from 74 published reports. Primary outcomes were the improvement of dysphagia and the rate of postoperative gastroesophageal reflux. Analysis demonstrated symptomatic improvement in dysphagia in 93.5% for POEM and 91% for laparoscopic Heller myotomy at 12 months and 92.7% versus 90.0% at 24 months, respectively. However, POEM patients were more likely to develop gastroesophageal reflux (odds ratio, 1.69), erosive esophagitis (odds ratio, 9.31), and abnormal pH monitoring values (odds ratio, 4.30).[45]

Although POEM is associated with increased rates of reflux and acid exposure it is successfully managed with long-term proton pump inhibitor (PPI) use in most cases. However, given the known association between long-standing GERD, Barrett esophagus, and esophageal adenocarcinoma and the increasing adverse effects of long-term PPI use, high incidences of post-procedural esophageal acid exposure is a significant concern.[46–49] In previously published randomized control trials, transoral incisionless fundoplication has shown superiority over high-dose medical therapy in relieving GERD symptoms with efficacy rates comparable with surgical Nissen fundoplication.[50–52] Recently a case series of transoral incisionless fundoplication for management of post-POEM GERD was presented, a logical adjunct to the POEM procedure, allowing to keep patients in the realm of endoscopic therapy, while definitively addressing the reflux. Authors demonstrated a 100% success rate with discontinuation of PPI therapy in all five presented patients and resolution of all cases of esophagitis with mean follow-up time of 27 months.[53] Recently Gutierrez and colleagues[54] reported on the TIF procedure performed simultaneously with POEM to address post POEM reflux problem.

Although surgical Heller myotomy achieves high success and low complication rates, in cases of procedure failure, performing a redo Heller myotomy is a tedious and complex procedure.[55] POEM has been reported as a successful rescue endoscopic therapy for patients who have had failed previous Heller operation. In a case series of eight patients with recurrent dysphagia after failed Heller myotomy, three patients underwent redo laparoscopic Heller myotomy with fundoplication and five patients underwent redo myotomy with POEM. All patients achieved significant improvement in symptoms and Eckardt scores at an average follow-up of 5 months.[56] In a retrospective cohort study of 180 patients with achalasia who underwent POEM at 13 tertiary care centers worldwide, technical success rates were demonstrated at 98% in prior Heller myotomy group and 100% in non-Heller myotomy group. However, a significantly lower proportion of patients in the Heller myotomy group achieved clinical success (81%) than in the non-Heller myotomy group (94%), suggesting other etiologies for failure. There were no significant differences in rates of adverse events and symptomatic reflux between the two groups.[41] In another publication, POEM after failed Heller was performed in 46 patients with 100% technical success rate and 85% clinical success rate; eight (17%) patients developed adverse events, all managed endoscopically without surgical conversion.[57] In a systematic review of 289 patients requiring repeat intervention after previous Heller myotomy, 36 patients were treated with POEM. Analysis demonstrated a technical success rate in excess of 98% with a 39% rate of insignificant adverse events.[58] An important feature of the POEM procedure is an ability to localize the myotomy in any aspect of the esophageal wall, frequently away from the previous plane of dissection-an advantage unavailable in the redo laparoscopic approach.

## CHRONIC AND END-STAGE ACHALASIA

Persistent obstruction of the gastroesophageal junction with chronic retention of food bolus leads to progressive dilation and elongation of the esophagus resulting in a sigmoid appearance in end-stage achalasia (**Fig. 7**A–D). Even with modern therapy, esophageal function deteriorates over time in 10% to 15% of individuals with achalasia, and up to 5% develop end-stage achalasia with sigmoidal features.[59] Some authors have recommended a surgical myotomy for the primary treatment of sigmoid esophagus, reserving esophagectomy for patients with failure of surgical myotomy. Others prefer primary esophagectomy. The appropriate surgical intervention for sigmoidal esophagus in the setting of chronic achalasia remains controversial.[60] In a retrospective analysis of minimally invasive myotomy (MIM) and minimally invasive esophagectomy (MIE) in the treatment of 30 patients with sigmoidal esophagus, 24 (80%) patients had undergone MIM and only 6 (20%) patients proceeded straight to MIE. There was no mortality with a median hospital stay of 2 days for MIM and 7 days for MIE. At a mean follow-up of 30 months, nine patients (37.5%) had failed MIM and required either redo myotomy in one case (11%) or an esophagectomy in the rest of eight patients (89%). Previous myotomy, younger age (mean, 53 years vs 66 years in MIM success), and duration of symptoms (mean, 25 years) were significant predictors of failure of MIM.[61] Currently, there are no randomized data available to

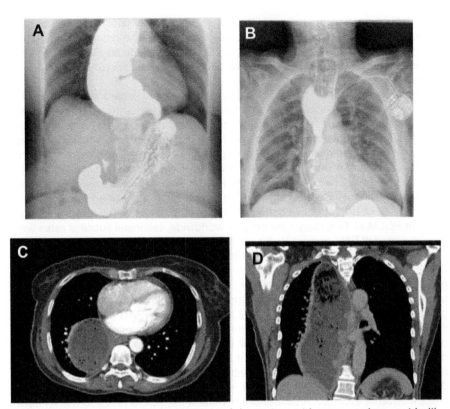

**Fig. 7.** End-stage achalasia. (A) Esophagram of the patient with megaesophagus with dilation and tortuosity of the entire organ. (B) Esophagram of the patient with proximal megaesophagus and distal corkscrew appearance of the type III achalasia. (C) Axial computed tomography image of the patient with megaesophagus. (D) Coronal reconstruction image of the patient with megaesophagus.

definitively establish indications for primary MIM or MIE in the setting of advanced achalasia with sigmoid esophagus.[59]

Esophagogastrostomy is an alternative to myotomy procedure, establishing an anastomosis in end-stage achalasia between the dilated esophagus and the stomach to relieve the obstruction. The first description of the technique of an esophagogastrostomy in the care of end-stage achalasia was published more than a century ago.[2,6] It all but disappeared from the clinical practice because of unacceptably high rate of reflux complications. Laparoscopic-stapled cardioplasty, a modern adaptation of this open technique, in a case series of seven patients with persistent achalasia was recently published. All but one patient had successful resolution of symptoms, with four patients developing post-procedure reflux, which was controlled with chronic PPI use.[62] A similar procedure was reported in another series of three individuals with end-stage type IV achalasia. All patients had significant improvement in their symptoms and two required chronic PPI therapy for reflux postoperatively.[59]

POEM has also effectively been applied for the treatment of end-stage achalasia. All major series reporting on the POEM procedure include a subset of patients with end-stage achalasia that were successfully treated.[34,40] In the report of 32 consecutive patients with sigmoid-type achalasia, technical success was achieved in all patients with a treatment success rate of 96.8% at a 30-month average follow-up with a significant decrease in LES pressure and Eckardt scores. Authors noted that morphologic changes of the esophagus made endoscopic tunneling more challenging and time-consuming but did not prevent successful POEM. Clinical reflux was observed in 25.8% of these patients post-procedure.[63]

## ACHALASIA: A RISK FACTOR FOR CARCINOMA

Currently, there are no generally accepted recommendations on follow-up for patients with achalasia. The real burden of achalasia at the malignancy genesis is still a controversial issue.[64] There have been several factors leading to an increased risk of esophageal carcinoma in patients with achalasia. Continuous chemical irritation caused by saliva and food decomposition in the esophagus could induce chronic hyperplastic esophagitis, dysplasia, and eventually carcinoma. In a systematic review and meta-analysis of 11,978 patients with achalasia from 40 selected studies, the absolute risk increase was 308 cases for squamous cell carcinoma and 18 cases for adenocarcinoma per 100,000 patients per year. These data potentially make an even stronger argument for performing a fundoplication after myotomy, to avoid reflux and Barrett esophagus- a known risk factor for carcinogenesis.[64]

## FUTURE DIRECTION

With POEM becoming the minimally invasive endoscopic treatment of choice for achalasia, the problem of gastroesophageal reflux post-POEM has been heightened.[44,64] In 2019, Inoue and colleagues[64] reported their first experience of combined endoscopic fundoplication added to the standard POEM procedure (POEM + F). The post-POEM fundoplication stage consisted of three steps: (1) entry into the peritoneal cavity, (2) distal and proximal anchoring of the endoloop with clips, and (3) closure of the endoloop. The fundoplication was technically feasible in all 21 cases. No immediate or delayed complications occurred. The partial rotation and traction of the anterior gastric wall toward the gastroesophageal junction created a visually identifiable wrap that mimicked a surgical partial fundoplication (**Fig. 8**). Acknowledging limited experience, authors believe that POEM + F may help mitigate the post-POEM incidence of gastroesophageal reflux and serve as a minimally invasive endoscopic alternative to the surgical Heller-Dor procedure.[65]

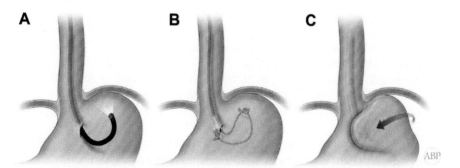

**Fig. 8.** Endoscopic fundoplication step of the POEM + F procedure by Inoue and colleagues. (*A*) Peritoneal cavity entry. (*B*) Anchoring of the endoloop with endoclips. (*C*) Closure of the endoloop with creation of the fundoplication. (*From* Petrov RV, Fajardo RA, Bakhos CT, Abbas AE. Peroral endoscopic myotomy: techniques and outcomes. Shanghai Chest 2020.)

LES electrical stimulation has been described to improve GERD symptoms and reduce esophageal acid exposure while enhancing the LES tone without impairing relaxation.[66,67] In 2015, Rodriguez and colleagues[66] reported the first clinical use of electrical LES stimulation in the care of post-POEM GERD not responsive to PPI use. In this case report, patients had a significant reduction of GERD-HRQL reflux (26 vs 7), regurgitation scores (24 vs 3), and a reduced total number of reflux episodes (82 vs 14) 3 months after implantation of the device.[66]

Another possible alternative therapeutic approach is the transplantation of neural progenitor cells. Researchers have demonstrated that stem cells with neurogenic potentiation can successfully survive, migrate, and differentiate into neurons and glia within the aganglionic organ. There has been preliminary evidence indicating that transplanted cell-based therapies can lead to a functional recovery of aganglionic disease, such as esophageal achalasia, although no strong evidence has been reported.[68]

## SUMMARY

Achalasia has featured a century-long history of ever evolving surgical therapy, with myotomy remaining the mainstay management modality. Heller myotomy, currently performed laparoscopically or robotically, offers successful relief of the obstruction in patients with achalasia. Fundoplication is currently routinely added to surgical myotomy to decrease incidence of postoperative reflux. POEM is a new endoscopic technique and is being rapidly adopted into clinical practice. High rates of post-POEM reflux are addressed with either medical therapy or other endoscopic procedures. Recently introduced POEM + F procedure holds promise as a potentially future procedure of choice. Despite the long history of such a challenging problem as achalasia, recent developments in minimally invasive techniques offer new hope for patients with better outcomes, faster recovery, and most importantly improved long-term functional results.

## ACKNOWLEDGEMENTS

This research was funded in part through the NIH/NCI Cancer Center Support Grant P30 CA006927.

## REFERENCES

1. Heller E. Extramukose Kardioplastik beimchronischen Kardiospasmus mit Dilatation des Oesophagus. Mitteilungen aus den Grenzgebieten der Medizin und Chirurgie 1914;27:141.
2. Heyrovsky H. Casuistik und Therapie der idiopathischen Dilatation der Speiserohre: Oesophagogastroanastomose. Arch Klin Chir 1913;100:703–15.
3. Payne WS. Heller's contribution to the surgical treatment of achalasia of the esophagus. 1914. Ann Thorac Surg 1989;48(6):876–81.
4. Steichen FM, Ravitch MM. Ernst Heller, M.D., 1877-1964. N Y State J Med 1965; 65(19):2500–2.
5. Wendel W. Zur Chirurgie des Oesophagus. Arch Klin Chir 1910;93:311–29.
6. Grondahl N. Cardiaplastik ved cardiospasmus. Nord Kirurgisk Forenings 1916; 11:236–40.
7. Barrett NR, Franklin RH. Concerning the unfavourable late results of certain operations performed in the treatment of cardiospasm. Br J Surg 1949;37(146): 194–202, illust.

8. Ripley HR, Olsen AM, Kirklin JW. Esophagitis after esophagogastric anastomosis. Surgery 1952;32(1):1–9.
9. Fisichella PM, Patti MG. A one hundred year journey: the history of surgery for esophageal achalasia. In: Fisichella PM, Herbella FAM, Patti MG, editors. Achalasia: diagnosis and treatment. Switzerland: Springer International Publishing; 2016. p. 3–9.
10. Bassotti G, Annese V. Review article: pharmacological options in achalasia. Aliment Pharmacol Ther 1999;13(11):1391–6.
11. Traube M, Dubovik S, Lange RC, et al. The role of nifedipine therapy in achalasia: results of a randomized, double-blind, placebo-controlled study. Am J Gastroenterol 1989;84(10):1259–62.
12. Vaezi MF, Richter JE, Wilcox CM, et al. Botulinum toxin versus pneumatic dilatation in the treatment of achalasia: a randomised trial. Gut 1999;44(2):231–9.
13. Pellegrini C, Wetter LA, Patti M, et al. Thoracoscopic esophagomyotomy. Initial experience with a new approach for the treatment of achalasia. Ann Surg 1992;216(3):291–6 [discussion: 296–9].
14. Shimi S, Nathanson LK, Cuschieri A. Laparoscopic cardiomyotomy for achalasia. J R Coll Surg Edinb 1991;36(3):152–4.
15. Patti MG, Pellegrini CA, Horgan S, et al. Minimally invasive surgery for achalasia: an 8-year experience with 168 patients. Ann Surg 1999;230(4):587–93 [discussion: 593–4].
16. Lyass S, Thoman D, Steiner JP, et al. Current status of an antireflux procedure in laparoscopic Heller myotomy. Surg Endosc 2003;17(4):554–8.
17. Richards WO, Torquati A, Holzman MD, et al. Heller myotomy versus Heller myotomy with Dor fundoplication for achalasia: a prospective randomized double-blind clinical trial. Ann Surg 2004;240(3):405–12 [discussion: 412–5].
18. Kummerow Broman K, Phillips SE, Faqih A, et al. Heller myotomy versus Heller myotomy with Dor fundoplication for achalasia: long-term symptomatic follow-up of a prospective randomized controlled trial. Surg Endosc 2018;32(4): 1668–74.
19. Andreollo NA, Earlam RJ. Heller's myotomy for achalasia: is an added anti-reflux procedure necessary? Br J Surg 1987;74(9):765–9.
20. Rebecchi F, Giaccone C, Farinella E, et al. Randomized controlled trial of laparoscopic Heller myotomy plus Dor fundoplication versus Nissen fundoplication for achalasia: long-term results. Ann Surg 2008;248(6):1023–30.
21. Kumagai K, Kjellin A, Tsai JA, et al. Toupet versus Dor as a procedure to prevent reflux after cardiomyotomy for achalasia: results of a randomised clinical trial. Int J Surg 2014;12(7):673–80.
22. Hagedorn C, Jonson C, Lonroth H, et al. Efficacy of an anterior as compared with a posterior laparoscopic partial fundoplication: results of a randomized, controlled clinical trial. Ann Surg 2003;238(2):189–96.
23. Rawlings A, Soper NJ, Oelschlager B, et al. Laparoscopic Dor versus Toupet fundoplication following Heller myotomy for achalasia: results of a multicenter, prospective, randomized-controlled trial. Surg Endosc 2012;26(1):18–26.
24. Torres-Villalobos G, Coss-Adame E, Furuzawa-Carballeda J, et al. Dor vs toupet fundoplication after laparoscopic Heller myotomy: long-term randomized controlled trial evaluated by high-resolution manometry. J Gastrointest Surg 2018;22(1):13–22.
25. Kiudelis M, Kubiliute E, Sakalys E, et al. The choice of optimal antireflux procedure after laparoscopic cardiomyotomy: two decades of clinical experience in one center. Wideochir Inne Tech Maloinwazyjne 2017;12(3):238–44.

26. Horgan S, Galvani C, Gorodner MV, et al. Robotic-assisted Heller myotomy versus laparoscopic Heller myotomy for the treatment of esophageal achalasia: multicenter study. J Gastrointest Surg 2005;9(8):1020–9 [discussion: 1029–30].

27. Huffmanm LC, Pandalai PK, Boulton BJ, et al. Robotic Heller myotomy: a safe operation with higher postoperative quality-of-life indices. Surgery 2007;142(4): 613–8 [discussion: 618–20].

28. Maeso S, Reza M, Mayol JA, et al. Efficacy of the Da Vinci surgical system in abdominal surgery compared with that of laparoscopy: a systematic review and meta-analysis. Ann Surg 2010;252(2):254–62.

29. Zaninotto G, Annese V, Costantini M, et al. Randomized controlled trial of botulinum toxin versus laparoscopic Heller myotomy for esophageal achalasia. Ann Surg 2004;239(3):364–70.

30. Stefanidis D, Richardson W, Farrell TM, et al. SAGES guidelines for the surgical treatment of esophageal achalasia. Surg Endosc 2012;26(2):296–311.

31. Katsinelos P, Kountouras J, Paroutoglou G, et al. Long-term results of pneumatic dilation for achalasia: a 15 years' experience. World J Gastroenterol 2005;11(36): 5701–5.

32. Inoue H, Minami H, Satodate H, et al. First clinical experience of submucosal endoscopic myotomy for esophageal achalasia with no skin incision. Gastrointest Endosc 2009;69:AB122.

33. Inoue H, Minami H, Kobayashi Y, et al. Peroral endoscopic myotomy (POEM) for esophageal achalasia. Endoscopy 2010;42(4):265–71.

34. Haito-Chavez Y, Inoue H, Beard KW, et al. Comprehensive analysis of adverse events associated with per oral endoscopic myotomy in 1826 patients: an international multicenter study. Am J Gastroenterol 2017;112(8):1267–76.

35. Kane ED, Budhraja V, Desilets DJ, et al. Myotomy length informed by high-resolution esophageal manometry (HREM) results in improved per-oral endoscopic myotomy (POEM) outcomes for type III achalasia. Surg Endosc 2019; 33(3):886–94.

36. Swanstrom LL, Kurian A, Dunst CM, et al. Long-term outcomes of an endoscopic myotomy for achalasia: the POEM procedure. Ann Surg 2012;256(4):659–67.

37. Von Renteln D, Fuchs KH, Fockens P, et al. Peroral endoscopic myotomy for the treatment of achalasia: an international prospective multicenter study. Gastroenterology 2013;145(2):309–11.e1-3.

38. Familiari P, Gigante G, Marchese M, et al. Peroral endoscopic myotomy for esophageal achalasia: outcomes of the first 100 patients with short-term follow-up. Ann Surg 2016;263(1):82–7.

39. Werner YB, Costamagna G, Swanstrom LL, et al. Clinical response to peroral endoscopic myotomy in patients with idiopathic achalasia at a minimum follow-up of 2 years. Gut 2016;65(6):899–906.

40. Petrov RV, Fajardo RA, Bakhos CT, et al. Peroral endoscopic myotomy: techniques and outcomes. Shanghai Chest 2020. https://doi.org/10.21037/shc. 2020.02.02.

41. Ngamruengphong S, Inoue H, Ujiki MB, et al. Efficacy and safety of peroral endoscopic myotomy for treatment of achalasia after failed Heller myotomy. Clin Gastroenterol Hepatol 2017;15(10):1531–7.e3.

42. Ponds FA, Fockens P, Lei A, et al. Effect of peroral endoscopic myotomy vs pneumatic dilation on symptom severity and treatment outcomes among treatment-naive patients with achalasia: a randomized clinical trial. JAMA 2019;322(2): 134–44.

43. Meng F, Li P, Wang Y, et al. Peroral endoscopic myotomy compared with pneumatic dilation for newly diagnosed achalasia. Surg Endosc 2017;31(11):4665–72.
44. Kumbhari V, Familiari P, Bjerregaard NC, et al. Gastroesophageal reflux after peroral endoscopic myotomy: a multicenter case-control study. Endoscopy 2017;49(7):634–42.
45. Schlottmann F, Luckett DJ, Fine J, et al. Laparoscopic Heller myotomy versus peroral endoscopic myotomy (POEM) for achalasia: a systematic review and meta-analysis. Ann Surg 2018;267(3):451–60.
46. Johansson J, Hakansson HO, Mellblom L, et al. Prevalence of precancerous and other metaplasia in the distal oesophagus and gastro-oesophageal junction. Scand J Gastroenterol 2005;40(8):893–902.
47. Hvid-Jensen F, Pedersen L, Drewes AM, et al. Incidence of adenocarcinoma among patients with Barrett's esophagus. N Engl J Med 2011;365(15):1375–83.
48. Freedberg DE, Kim LS, Yang YX. The risks and benefits of long-term use of proton pump inhibitors: expert review and best practice advice from the American Gastroenterological Association. Gastroenterology 2017;152(4):706–15.
49. Zoll B, Jehangir A, Malik Z, et al. Gastric electric stimulation for refractory gastroparesis. J Clin Outcomes Manag 2019;26(1):27–38.
50. Richter JE, Kumar A, Lipka S, et al. Efficacy of laparoscopic Nissen fundoplication vs transoral incisionless fundoplication or proton pump inhibitors in patients with gastroesophageal reflux disease: a systematic review and network meta-analysis. Gastroenterology 2018;154(5):1298–308.e7.
51. Hunter JG, Kahrilas PJ, Bell RC, et al. Efficacy of transoral fundoplication vs omeprazole for treatment of regurgitation in a randomized controlled trial. Gastroenterology 2015;148(2):324–33.e5.
52. Trad KS, Fox MA, Simoni G, et al. Transoral fundoplication offers durable symptom control for chronic GERD: 3-year report from the TEMPO randomized trial with a crossover arm. Surg Endosc 2017;31(6):2498–508.
53. Tyberg A, Choi A, Gaidhane M, et al. Transoral incisional fundoplication for reflux after peroral endoscopic myotomy: a crucial addition to our arsenal. Endosc Int Open 2018;6(5):E549–52.
54. Brewer Gutierrez OI, Benias PC, Khashab MA. Same- Session Per-Oral Endoscopic Myotomy Followed by Transoral Incisionless Fundoplication in Achalasia: Are We There Yet? Am J Gastroenterol 2020;115:162.
55. Mandovra P, Kalikar V, Patel A, et al. Redo laparoscopic Heller's cardiomyotomy for recurrent achalasia: is laparoscopic surgery feasible? J Laparoendosc Adv Surg Tech A 2018;28(3):298–301.
56. Vigneswaran Y, Yetasook AK, Zhao JC, et al. Peroral endoscopic myotomy (POEM): feasible as reoperation following Heller myotomy. J Gastrointest Surg 2014;18(6):1071–6.
57. Tyberg A, Seewald S, Sharaiha RZ, et al. A multicenter international registry of redo per-oral endoscopic myotomy (POEM) after failed POEM. Gastrointest Endosc 2017;85(6):1208–11.
58. Fernandez-Ananin S, Fernandez AF, Balague C, et al. What to do when Heller's myotomy fails? Pneumatic dilatation, laparoscopic remyotomy or peroral endoscopic myotomy: a systematic review. J Minim Access Surg 2018;14(3):177–84.
59. Griffiths EA, Devitt PG, Jamieson GG, et al. Laparoscopic stapled cardioplasty for end-stage achalasia. J Gastrointest Surg 2013;17(5):997–1001.
60. Orringer MB, Orringer JS. Esophagectomy: definitive treatment for esophageal neuromotor dysfunction. Ann Thorac Surg 1982;34(3):237–48.

61. Schuchert MJ, Luketich JD, Landreneau RJ, et al. Minimally invasive surgical treatment of sigmoidal esophagus in achalasia. J Gastrointest Surg 2009;13(6): 1029–35 ]discussion: 1035–6].

62. Dehn TC, Slater M, Trudgill NJ, et al. Laparoscopic stapled cardioplasty for failed treatment of achalasia. Br J Surg 2012;99(9):1242–5.

63. Hu JW, Li QL, Zhou PH, et al. Peroral endoscopic myotomy for advanced achalasia with sigmoid-shaped esophagus: long-term outcomes from a prospective, single-center study. Surg Endosc 2015;29(9):2841–50.

64. Tustumi F, Bernardo WM, da Rocha JRM, et al. Esophageal achalasia: a risk factor for carcinoma. A systematic review and meta-analysis. Dis Esophagus 2017; 30(10):1–8.

65. Inoue H, Ueno A, Shimamura Y, et al. Peroral endoscopic myotomy and fundoplication: a novel NOTES procedure. Endoscopy 2019;51(2):161–4.

66. Rodriguez L, Rodriguez P, Gomez B, et al. Two-year results of intermittent electrical stimulation of the lower esophageal sphincter treatment of gastroesophageal reflux disease. Surgery 2015;157(3):556–67.

67. Rieder E, Paireder M, Kristo I, et al. Electrical stimulation of the lower esophageal sphincter to treat gastroesophageal reflux after POEM. Surg Innov 2018;25(4): 346–9.

68. Furuzawa-Carballeda J, Torres-Landa S, Valdovinos MA, et al. New insights into the pathophysiology of achalasia and implications for future treatment. World J Gastroenterol 2016;22(35):7892–907.

# GASTRIC

# Enhancing Scintigraphy for Evaluation of Gastric, Small Bowel, and Colonic Motility

Alan H. Maurer, MD[a,b],*

## KEYWORDS

- Solid meal gastric emptying • Liquid meal gastric emptying
- Gastric accommodation • Antro-pyloro motility • Small bowel transit • Colon transit

## KEY POINTS

- Gastric emptying scintigraphy now has standards for not only solid but also liquid meal emptying. Advanced gastric regional analysis methods now permit more complete assessments of fundic accommodation and antropyloroduodenal motility.
- Whole-gut scintigraphy studies also now are standardized and available to measure small bowel and colon transit after oral administration of a single mixed solid-liquid gastric emptying meal.
- New American Medical Association Current Procedural Terminology codes and commercially developed software now make these new scintigraphic gastrointestinal motility studies more routinely available.

## INTRODUCTION

The advantages of scintigraphy for studying gastrointestinal (GI) motility have remained the same since the first application of a radiolabeled meal to measure gastric emptying (GE) more than 55 years ago.[1] Scintigraphy is noninvasive, does not affect normal physiology, and provides accurate quantification of the bulk transit of an orally administered radiolabeled solid or liquid meal. Compared with radiographic methods, scintigraphy involves low radiation exposure, is quantifiable, and uses common foods rather than barium or nonphysiologic radiopaque markers or wireless capsules.

GE involves coordination of different regions of the stomach. Initial proximal fundic relaxation (accommodation) is followed by tonic fundic contractions. Next, antral

a Department of Radiology, Nuclear Medicine Section, Lewis Katz School of Medicine, Temple University Hospital, 3401 North Broad Street, Philadelphia, PA 19140, USA; b Department of Medicine, Gastroenterology Section, Lewis Katz School of Medicine, Temple University Hospital, 3401 North Broad Street, Philadelphia, PA 19140, USA
* Department of Radiology, Nuclear Medicine Section, Lewis Katz School of Medicine, Temple University Hospital, 3401 North Broad Street, Philadelphia, PA 19140.
E-mail address: amaurer@temple.edu

Gastroenterol Clin N Am 49 (2020) 499–517
https://doi.org/10.1016/j.gtc.2020.04.006

**gastro.theclinics.com**

contractions triturate solids to 1 mm to 2 mm so that antral contractions, coordinated with pyloric relaxation, permit emptying of the solid particulates. GE scintigraphy (GES), which utilizes a radiolabeled solid and/or liquid meal, has remained the gold standard for measuring GE because the retained meal radioactive counts are directly proportional to the amount of the meal remaining without geometric assumptions on gastric shape needed by other imaging modalities. Previously, GES lacked standardization, but professional society guidelines now provide performance standards.[2,3]

Patients with functional dyspepsia (FD) often do not have well-defined GI symptoms and present with symptoms that include any pain or discomfort thought to originate in the upper GI tract. The goal of diagnosing delayed GE typically has been to identify patients who will benefit from a prokinetic drug or other treatment to alleviate symptoms. Any functional GE study for patients with suspected gastroparesis or FD is indicated only after an anatomic cause for symptoms has been excluded. The pathophysiology in FD is multifactorial and appears to include delayed GE, impaired fundal accommodation, and/or visceral hypersensitivity.[4–6] Analysis of proximal stomach (fundal) emptying as part of standard GES as well as dynamic antral scintigraphy to assess antral contractions may unmask a subset of patients with normal GE but impaired fundal accommodation or antral motility.[7]

GES also may be indicated in the absence of FD symptoms for patients with gastroesophageal reflux disease (GERD) not responding to acid suppressants (to see whether delayed GE contributes to reflux); those suspected of having a diffuse GI motility disorder; and diabetics with poor glycemic control. GES also can be used to assess patients for dumping syndrome, where GE is rapid. Classically, this occurs after surgery but also is described in patients with cyclic vomiting syndrome and FD.[8]

Because the correlation between severity of FD and delayed GE has been weak, with only approximately 40% of patients with a working diagnosis of FD showing delayed GE,[9] GES has been expanded beyond the simple measurement of total GE to provide details on fundic and antral motility. This review focuses on the advances made over the past 5 years to 10 years to improve the conventional GES test, which measured only total GE as well as the enhancements to expand the capabilities of GI scintigraphy for evaluation of not only the stomach but also the small bowel and colon.

## STANDARDIZATION AND ALTERNATIVE MEAL ENHANCEMENTS

For many years, lack of standardization on how to perform a GES study led to difficulty in comparing GE results from site to site. In the current guidelines endorsed by the American Neurogastroenterology and Motility Society (ANMS) and the Society of Nuclear Medicine and Molecular Imaging (SNMMI),[2,3] a low-fat egg white meal (Egg Beaters [ConAgra Foods; Downers, Illinois]) or equivalent generic egg white meal is described. This currently is the recommended solid meal GE test based on a prior multicenter study.[10] Advantages of this test include ease of preparation, good tolerability by a majority of patients, and validated multicenter normal values for men and women. For many years, most imaging centers measured GE only out to 90 minutes or 120 minutes. The importance of imaging GE for up to 4 hours to maximize the detection of gastroparesis now has been recognized as a requirement in the current guidelines.[11]

Although the reporting values for delayed GE of the current standardized test meal have been established as a part of a large multicenter study (>60% retained at 2 hours and >10% retained at 4 hours),[10] the values for rapid GE have not been studied as rigorously. The current ANMS and SNMMI guidelines suggest rapid solid meal GE is present if gastric retention is less than 70% at 0.5 hour or less than 30% at 1 hour.[2,3]

As a note of caution to referring physicians, however, despite these published standards, many nuclear medicine/radiology departments are not following established procedure guidelines, which may invalidate study results. Recently the Intersocietal Accreditation Commission looked at compliance with the SNMMI guidelines 8 years after publication. They found 69.3% (127 laboratories studied) were not compliant with the standards for the meal and only 3.1% were compliant with all 14 variables studied.[12]

### Solid Meal Enhancements

The currently recommended GES solid test meal, discussed previously, has a low fat content and thus produces different results than higher-fat or caloric meals that have been tested.[13] Some have suggested that the currently recommended 2-egg sandwich meal is not of a sufficient caloric or solid consistency to adequately stress the stomach. This may account for the finding of a normal GES study in patients where there is high clinical suspicion of a GE abnormality. Parker and colleagues[14] have published normal values for use of a larger (400-mL) mixed liquid-solid meal. This, however, has not yet been more widely tested and validated.

Patients who cannot tolerate the current egg-based solid meal can be tested with the nutritional supplement Ensure Plus (Abbott;Chicago, Illinois).[15,16] The advantages of this substitute meal are that it uses the same imaging protocol as and that it has normal GE values similar to those of the solid egg-based meal. A rice-based solid meal substitute that is gluten-free and vegan has documented normal values but may not be widely available.[17]

### Liquid Meal Enhancements

Measurement of GE rates of a non-nutrient, water meal is not well established; however, there is some evidence that a subset of patients with gastroparesis can have normal solid GE but abnormal GE of water. A water-only GE test was compared with the standard solid meal and showed a delay in water GE in 32% of patients with normal solid GE.[18,19] The potential advantages of a water-only meal are meal tolerability, shorter acquisition time, and increased sensitivity. Currently, however, there are only single-center data to support the use of a non-nutrient, water meal. Its use has not been validated in multicenter studies.

Because water has no caloric value, it likely is clinically more relevant to utilize a nutrient liquid meal for patients referred for GES who cannot tolerate the standard solid meal. The GE characteristics of Ensure Plus are similar to those of the standard solid meal but with a slightly faster emptying rate.[15,20] A recent study of 21 normal subjects with Ensure Plus confirmed that it can serve as an acceptable alternative meal. The mean (95% upper reference limit) percentages for gastric retention were 69.9% (87.1%) at 1 hour, 35.1% (64.3%) at 2 hours, 13.5% (23.2%) at 3%, and 8.9% (13.5%) at 4 hours.[16]

### COMBINED SOLID WITH LIQUID MEAL ENHANCEMENTS

GES of solids typically is used only to evaluate for FD and suspected gastroparesis. Although it has been stated that GE of liquid meals would be less sensitive for diagnosing delayed GE,[21] as discussed previously, recent reports show liquid GE can be abnormal with solid GE being normal.

Another recent consensus guideline that incorporates GE with small bowel transit (SBT) and colon transit (CT) now includes standards for measuring GE of liquid (water) in the presence of the solid radiolabeled egg white sandwich meal.[22] In a large study, which analyzed 449 patients who underwent GES with assessment of both solid and liquids in the presence of solids, liquid GE was significantly correlated to solid GE: 30 minutes (r = 0.652; P<.001), 60 minutes (r = 0.624; P<.001), and 120 minutes (r = 0.766; P<.001). Sixty patients (57 nondiabetic) had normal solid GE but delayed liquid emptying, which was 26% of the 228 patients with normal solid GE.[21] Thus, while GE of liquids correlates well with GE of solids it can also help to identify patients with delay GE missed by a solid meal only GE test. The National Institutes of Health Gastroparesis Consortium has published preliminary results using GE of liquids in the presence of solids in 136 patients. More than 40% of gastroparetic patients with delayed solid emptying were shown to have delayed liquid GE.[23]

## ENHANCEMENTS IN GLUCOSE CONTROL DURING GASTRIC EMPTYING STUDIES

Most nuclear medicine departments fast patients overnight before a GES study but do not check a prestudy blood glucose level (BGL). BGL typically is tightly controlled in normal subjects. Typically, after a meal, blood glucose rises and then returns to pre-meal levels as postprandial glucoregulatory mechanisms occur. The GI tract and GE play an important role in regulating BGL.

Prior studies have shown that the relationship of GE and BGL is complex and can differ in normal controls compared with patients with diabetes. There is a well-recognized relationship between the BGL and its effect on the rate of GE and vice versa, such that the rate of GE also acts to control BGLs. If GE is too fast and post-prandial BGL increases, there is a slowing of GE.[24] Hypoglycemia accelerates GE to increase BGLs.[25]

A recent systematic review has concluded that evidence supports that acute, severe hyperglycemia marked hyperglycemia with BGL 16–20 mmol/L [288–360 mg/dL] delays GE relative to euglycemia in patients with type 1 diabetes mellitus.[26] Modest hyperglycemia (BGL 8 mmol/L [145 mg/dL]) also delays GE; however, the effect is small and not greater than day-to-day variation in GE in patients with type 1 diabetes mellitus.[27] The effects of differing levels of hyperglycemia in normal subjects are not well documented. Insulin-induced hypoglycemia has been shown to accelerate the GE of both solids and liquids in long-standing type 1 diabetes mellitus.[28]

Although it is recognized that the relationship of BGL and GE is complicated, it has been an accepted concept that BGL, especially in diabetic patients, should be checked and controlled during measurement of GE. This recently has been questioned in an editorial showing how varying methods can effect study results.[29] This editorial was in response to a recent study showing that higher fasting BGLs were associated with faster, not slower, gastric emptying.[30] One major variable to consider in conflicting reports is that at least 2 studies suggest that it is liquid and not solid emptying that is primarily affected by BGL.[31,32]

The SNMMI guideline recommends that the prestudy fasting BGL should be less than or equal to 200 mg/dL.[3] A recent American Gastroenterological Association (AGA) practice guideline states, "markedly uncontrolled (>200 mg/dL) glucose levels may delay GE and aggravate symptoms of gastroparesis (strong recommendation, high level of evidence)" and recommends deferring GE testing until relative euglycemia is achieved. This guideline states, "Patients with diabetes should have blood glucose measured before starting the GE test, and hyperglycemia treated with test started after blood glucose is <275 mg/dL (Strong recommendation, moderate-high level of evidence)."[33]

A review with suggestions on how to best achieve euglycemic status for patients on diabetic medications undergoing GES is now available.[34] Some of these recommendations are summarized.

### General Prestudy Recommendations

A. All patients are instructed to be fasted (nothing by mouth) after midnight the night prior to the study. Patients can take any nondiabetic, oral medications with water at home prior to coming for their GE study.
B. All patients should have a BGL test done prior to beginning the study.

### Nondiabetic and Type 2 Diabetes Mellitus Patients

A. If fasting BGL is less than 200 mg/dL, study proceeds. If it is greater than 200 mg/dL and the patient cannot return when controlled to less than 200 mg/dL, there is an option to give a small dose of rapid-acting insulin to bring BGL under control.
B. If fasting BGL is less than 275 mg/dL by AGA guideline or close to 200 mg/dL by SNMMI guideline, the site can make a determination to have the GE study proceed. No monitoring is needed during the study. Patients on oral diabetic drugs, which are antihyperglycemic and not hypoglycemic (sulfonylureas, glinides or meglitinides, and DPP-4), typically need not discontinue medication (discussed later).
C. If fasting BGL is significantly greater than 200 mg/dL by SNMMI or greater than 275 mg/dL per AGA, the following options can be considered:
   a. The study may be canceled and the patient rescheduled to return on another date with better control.
   b. An option is to continue despite poor control if the patient's BGL is chronically poorly controlled, because it might be useful to assess the patient at usual baseline and then compare it with another when the BGL is better controlled.
   c. Rapid-acting insulins may be used for acute control, because they peak at 1 hour to 1.5 hours. Wait to begin study and check a BGL at 0.5 hour to 1.0 hour and, if controlled, proceed with GE study.
D. If a diabetic patient is on sulfonylurea or meglitinide medication, it should be held for the morning of the GE test. If the pretest BGL is less than 200 mg/dL to 275 mg/dL, the patients should take the medication with the GE test meal and proceed. If greater than 200 mg/dL to 275 mg/dL, the patient should take medication and be given supplemental short-acting insulin to achieve control.
E. If a diabetic patient is on GLP-1 receptor analogs, these need to be discontinued because they slow GE. Some of these are taken once weekly, others once or twice daily. The GE study should be timed for at least 5 days to 7 days after last medication dose if weekly and 24 hours after last dose if daily or twice daily. Note that these patients may experience acute hyperglycemia off the agent and need insulin to control BGL using insulin.

### Type 1 Diabetes Mellitus Patients

A. Using single basal insulin dose: if a patient is on a correct basal insulin dosage, there is no peak to the insulin effect and the dose needs no dose adjustment. If a patient is on glargine, detemir, or degludec, it could be considered that the GE test meal has less caloric content than the patient's typical breakfast and the prior night or morning dose could be reduced by 20% to 40% prior to the GE test.
B. Using basal and short-acting insulin: because the caloric content of the test meal may be less than the patient's typical breakfast, it is suggested patient takes half the usual short-acting insulin with the GE test meal. The dose reduction can be made by comparing the calories of the patient's typical breakfast to the standard egg white, 2 pieces of white toast, and jam meal, which contains approximately 220 calories and 45 g carbohydrate.
C. Using NPH or premix insulins: use of these agents is decreasing but some diabetes patients may be on NPH or premix insulins. Patients are recommended to take half

their long-acting insulin dose before coming for the study. The patient then checks the BGL before the study and study proceeds if BGL is less than 200 mg/dL to 275 mg/dL. If BGL is greater than 200 mg/dLto 275 mg/dL, short-acting insulin for acute control could be considered. The patient then should check the BGL at end of the 4-hour study and take approximately half more of the long-acting insulin based on post-test BGL.

D. Insulin pump therapy: as discussed previously, depending on a patient's normal breakfast caloric content versus GE meal, reducing the basal insulin dose by 20% to 40% starting the morning of the test by putting in a temporarily basal infusion rate to start at the time of ingestion of the GE test meal can be suggested.

## ENHANCEMENTS IN SOLID MEAL INTRAGASTRIC MEAL DISTRIBUTION AND FUNDIC ACCOMMODATION

Gastric accommodation (GA), as first described by Cannon and Lieb in 1911,[35] is a postprandial reflex resulting in reduced proximal gastric tone that occurs with eating a meal. With GA, the fundus acts as a reservoir for ingested foods without significantly increasing intragastric pressure.

In addition to alterations in GE, impaired GA (IGA) and hypersensitivity to gastric distention have been shown to be associated with symptoms in idiopathic gastroparesis[36] and diabetic gastroparesis.[37] IGA has been reported in 40% of patients with FD.[38] Studies have shown an association between symptoms of nausea, early satiety, abnormal distention, and GERD with proximal gastric retention, whereas vomiting may be associated more with distal gastric retention.[39] A recent article by Chedid and colleagues[40] showed that unexplained upper GI symptoms may be explained in diabetics not only by delayed GE but also by rapid GE as well as IGA. IGA was found in 39% of patients. There is increasing recognition of the importance of assessing patients for IGA and of having a clinically available test to measure GA as new therapeutic approaches to treat IGA are being developed.[41]

The gastric balloon barostat has been considered the gold standard for assessing IGA. It is, however, invasive, uncomfortable for patients, and not widely available. In addition, the presence of the balloon is nonphysiologic and can exaggerate antral contractions[42] and alter GA.[43] These limitations of the gastric barostat have led to development of other modalities to assess GA.[44] Advanced 3-dimensional ultrasound has been compared with gastric barostat and correlates with symptoms of FD[45] and reflux esophagitis.[46] Ultrasound, although readily available, is very dependent on user experience and image quality. Magnetic resonance imaging (MRI) has been used to measure the GA response.[47–50] MRI potentially is capable of measuring accurate volumes and currently is under active investigation. Its high cost and lack of availability potentially limit its routine clinical use.

Two scintigraphic methods for measurement of GA have been reported. One uses conventional planar (2-dimensional) GES and examines intragastric solid meal distribution (IMD) immediately after meal ingestion. The second uses a 3-dimensional single-photon emission computed tomography (SPECT) acquisition and estimates gastric volume by imaging the gastric mucosa. The SPECT method, therefore, is not influenced by GE, is independent of intragastric content, and can assess both fasting and postprandial gastric volume during the first 10 minutes after meal ingestion. Measurements of gastric volume by SPECT differ significantly from the estimates of GA based on IMD measured immediately after food ingestion by the 2-dimensional method.

SPECT imaging of GA as proposed by Chedid[51] and studied by others[52–58] is probably the best validated method for measuring GA. SPECT GA imaging requires an intravenous injection of technetium Tc 99m pertechnetate to radiolabel the gastric mucosa and must be done as a separate study from a GES study. The SPECT method correlates well to the intragastric barostat balloon[59] and has excellent performance characteristics.[56] In another study by Chedid,[55] SPECT was performed in 214 patients with diverse symptoms with and without abnormal GE. GA was impaired in 43% of all patients, 47% of patients with FD, 44% of patients with postfundoplication syndromes, and 33% of diabetics with dyspepsia.[55] SPECT imaging also has been shown capable of measuring changes in gastric volume with pharmacologic interventions.[60] In addition, improvement in FD symptoms with low-dose antidepressants recently has been demonstrated with increased SPECT-measured GA.[61] SPECT GA imaging, however, currently is not approved for routine clinical use and is available only at a limited academic centers.

The use of standard GES and simple planar imaging is an attempt to make GA measurements more readily available than SPECT. Early studies using GES showed that rapid transit of a solid meal into the distal stomach, without normal GA, could be used as an index of IGA.[62,63] This assessed IMD as a part of a routine solid meal GES study. IMD has been defined as a measure of how much food is in the proximal portion of the stomach, compared with the food in the whole stomach. To utilize IMD as a measure of GA, the IMD immediately post–meal ingestion (t = 0 minutes), or $IMD^0$, has been calculated by simple anatomic division of the stomach in halves or thirds.[63,64]

The current evidence to support measurement of IGA based on 2-dimensional scintigraphy is more limited than for SPECT.[51,65] A recent study from the National Institutes of Health Gastroparesis Consortium, however, demonstrated that both a simple visual and quantitative assessment of $IMD^0$ as a measure of GA can be obtained from conventional GES.[66] This study showed that symptoms of early satiety correlated with IGA as assessed with quantitative measurement of $IMD^0$ from GES. It supports this simple measurement can serve as an index of the GA response. Another recent publication has shown that a solid meal GES test is capable of measuring in 1 test GE, GA, and antral motility.[67] This is discussed later.

A combined SPECT and conventional GES study can be performed using a dual-isotope method with technetium Tc 99m pertechnetate to radiolabel the gastric mucosa and indium indium 111 oxine to label the egg meal. Such combined studies have shown that the GA response lasts for up to 3 hours despite emptying of the majority of the meal (>80%).[68]

Ultimately, the ability to diagnose that dyspeptic symptoms are associated with IGA will have value if there is effective treatment of the IGA. Studies have been performed with sumatriptan, serotonin type 4 receptor agonists (tegaserod and cisapride), neurokinin-1 receptor antagonists (aprepitant), and serotonin type 1A agonists (buspirone). Recent data from Tack and colleagues[69] suggest that treatment with buspirone can improve symptoms of early satiety, postprandial fullness, early satiation, and upper abdominal bloating, which correlated with improved GA compared with placebo.[70]

## ENHANCED ASSESSMENT OF DYNAMIC ANTRAL AND ANTROPYLORODUODENAL MOTILITY
### Role in Gastric Motility

Conventional GES uses static images. Dynamic antral contraction scintigraphy (DACS) utilizes rapid image acquisitions, typically at 1 image per 3 seconds, to measure antral contractions. Early studies showed that by placing an antral region of interest (ROI) and utilizing Fourier analysis, the frequency of antral contractions and the strength of antral contractions using an antral ejection fraction can be measured.[71] Recent software updates to DACS show it also can be used to automate localization of the physiologic contracting antrum from the fundus and to measure the speed of antral contractions.[67] In 21 normal subjects, $IMD^0$ was calculated by segmenting the proximal stomach from the antrum using DACS. Using antral contractions (AC), defined $IMD^0$-AC was 0.85 ± 0.14, which was greater than the mean value for $IMD^0$ based on gastric division in halves ($IMD^0 = 0.75 \pm 0.15$ [$P = .004$]). Using DACS, sustained and periodic antral contractions started at a mean of 11.24 minutes ± 12.98 minutes after meal ingestion. Antral contraction frequency peaked 30 minutes after meal ingestion at 3.30 ± 0.71 contractions per minute, which also was the time when distal antral filling was greatest (36.65 ± 13.49%, based on proximal vs distal stomach division in halves, and 25.98 ± 15.10%, based on Fourier separation). The antral ejection fraction also peaked 30 minutes after meal ingestion (30.31 ± 13.69%). The average speed of contractions from 0 to 80 minutes after meal ingestion was 3.16 mm/s.

Imaging advances continue to be made in the acquisition and software for DACS, which promote a better understanding of the complexity of antral contractility. When the antral analysis ROI is placed in the prepyloric region, the cyclic variation of the radiolabeled food can document both antegrade and retrograde movements during the trituration process. With this type of regional analysis, midantrum contractions have been observed to increase in amplitude aborally, reaching a maximum just proximal to the prepyloric region.[72,73]

The clinical role for DACS ultimately will be determined by how it effects patient management. In patients with long-standing diabetes, GES with DACS has been able to demonstrate a prolonged lag phase with retention of food in the proximal stomach as well as a decrease in the amplitude of the antral contractions in diabetics.[71] This study also demonstrated that GES with DACS can characterize abnormalities of food distribution in the stomach and provides information on contractile function similar to that obtained from manometry. Another study utilizing DACS evaluated IMD and antral motor activity in patients with FD. Diminished residence of food in the proximal stomach and increased antral contractility were shown to play a role in dyspeptic symptoms.[7]

### Role in Antropyloroduodenal Motility

Small intestinal dysmotility also may contribute to delayed GE and symptoms of gastroparesis. A lack of antropyloroduodenal coordination (APDC) as well as small intestinal dysmotility may be important pathophysiology contributing to patient symptoms.[74,75] Expanding GES to include analysis of APDC may increase the diagnostic value of GES.

Using scintigraphy to assess duodenal contractility is particularly challenging because after trituration, solid particles of only 1 mm to 2 mm size are permitted to pass through the pylorus into the duodenum. With standard GES, the limited amount of radiopharmaceutical (technetium Tc 99m sulfur colloid) on these small particles reduces the signal available to the nuclear medicine camera from the small particles passing into the duodenum compared with the higher signal available from larger intragastric particles.

Utilizing a slightly higher dose of technetium Tc 99m sulfur colloid in the radiolabeled meal (185 MBq vs 37–74 MBq), a recent study has shown that duodenal bolus propagations (DBPs) of the food particles transiting through the pylorus into the duodenum can be measured in normal subjects.[76] Measuring DBP was accomplished by placing an ROI perpendicular to the duodenal sweep and imaging with DACS in an right anterior oblique projection.[76] At 60 minutes, antrum activity averaged 2.91 peaks/minute $\pm$ 0.66 peaks/minute and duodenum averaged 0.36 peaks/minute $\pm$ 0.18 peaks/minute. The ratios of duodenal peaks detected to antral peaks were 0.34/2.78 = 0.12 at 30 minutes, 0.36/2.91 = 0.12 at 60 minutes, and 0.19/2.82 = 0.07 at 120 minutes, showing that only a maximum 12% of antral contractions are followed by DBPs. Studies have suggested that cisapride is more effective in accelerating gastroduodenal emptying than metoclopramide or domperidone because it stimulates the largest number of gastropyloroduodenal contractions that enhance GE.[77] The investigators of this new APDC scintigraphy have suggested that this new method offers promise to assess APDC in patients with unexplained upper GI symptoms and will have value for measuring the response to therapies to improve APDC.

## ENHANCED WHOLE-GUT TRANSIT SCINTIGRAPHY

It often is difficult to determine whether a patient's symptoms originate in the upper or lower GI tract. GI transit scintigraphy is a unique, noninvasive, quantitative, and physiologic method of determining whether there is a motility disorder affecting the stomach, small bowel, or colon. SBT and CT studies can be performed alone or together with GES after the oral administration of a mixed solid-liquid radiolabeled meal. When combined in 1 study, this often is referred to as whole-gut transit scintigraphy (WGTS). A clinical guideline that includes all the technical standards for performing and interpreting WGTS has been approved by the SNMMI and the European Association of Nuclear Medicine.[22]

### Small Bowel Transit Scintigraphy

Measurement of SBT is complex because entry of a meal into the small intestine depends on GE and because small intestinal chyme spreads over a large distance as it progresses toward the colon. There is no simple small bowel peristaltic pattern. Antegrade and retrograde movements occur in the jejunum and ileum, with some areas progressing rapidly and others slowly. Jejunal peristaltic activity typically is more rapid, with slowing of peristalsis seen in the ileum.[78] The simplest approach to scintigraphic measurement of SBT is to measure orocecal transit time by imaging the leading edge of radiotracer transit through the bowel. Accurately defining the leading edge (the first visualized arrival of activity in the cecum), however, requires frequent (every 10–15 minutes) and prolonged imaging because of the stasis in the terminal ileum.

Because symptoms of small bowel dysmotility are similar to those of gastroparesis, SBT testing should be considered for those patients with persistent symptoms despite normal GE.[79] Although combining liquid (water) and solids to following the liquid transit through the small bowel previously was confined to the research setting, it recently has become clinically validated to assess SBT.[80,81] The current scintigraphic method for measuring SBT does not attempt to characterize complex peristaltic patterns or leading-edge transit but simply measures the overall bulk movement of an orally administered radiolabeled liquid meal as it progresses distally into the terminal ileum. Typically, the radiolabeled meal collects in a terminal ileal reservoir, also referred to as the ileocolonic junction. SBT is delayed if diffuse activity persists in multiple loops of small bowel at 6 hours and/or if little activity (<40%) has transited into the terminal ileum reservoir and/or cecum and colon. The wireless motility capsule has been shown to correlate well with scintigraphy for measuring SBT.[82]

Alternate methods of SBT scintigraphy have been used to document responsiveness to treatment in patients with functional GI disorders.[80] Using the percentage of colonic filling at 6 hours (reflecting orocecal transit), SBT was accelerated by the serotonin type 4 receptor agonist prokinetic medication tegaserod in 24 patients with constipation-predominant irritable bowel syndrome.[83] The prokinetic drug cisapride normalized SBT delays in chronic intestinal pseudo-obstruction patients.[84] In another study of 14 patients who had undergone small intestinal manometry to confirm dysmotility, including documentation of neuropathic findings in 8 of them and myopathic patterns in 6, scintigraphic SBT was markedly prolonged compared with that in healthy controls (median 328 minutes vs 218 minutes; $P<.01$).[85]

### Whole-Gut Transit Scintigraphy

As discussed previously, WGTS refers to a combined study that includes measurement of GE, small bowel transit (SBT), and CT after administration of a dual-isotope, solid-liquid meal.[81,86,87] The wireless motility capsule has been shown to correlate well with scintigraphy for measuring whole-gut transit.[82] WGTS studies are helpful for evaluating patients whose symptoms cannot be classified as either upper or lower GI in origin or where a functional and not an organic cause is suspected.[88] In a study of 108 patients with functional GI symptoms, 3 of 4 patients with dyspepsia and delayed SBT also exhibited delayed GES.[86] All 5 patients with constipation and delayed SBT also showed GE delays. In another investigation of 212 constipated patients, 9 individuals with slow-transit constipation and delayed SBT also had slow GE, confirming a generalized GI dysmotility.[89] Findings of these scintigraphy studies parallel investigations that use the wireless motility capsule, which also is able to measure whole-gut transit in a single diagnostic test. SBT delays were observed in 16% of 209 patients with suspected gastroparesis.[90]

In a scintigraphic study of patients referred for upper GI symptoms, constipation, or diarrhea, 40% were found to have an organic cause of symptoms, but 60% were diagnosed as functional.[87] The clinical utility of WGTS has been demonstrated. In 1 study, organic disease was found in many patients with an initial suspected functional disorder; the initial diagnosis was changed in 45% of patients and patient management was changed in 67% of patients.[86] Patients with diarrhea-predominant IBS have faster SBT and rapid colonic filling, whereas constipated patients have slower SBT and delayed colonic filling.[81,86,87,91] GI symptoms in patients with untreated celiac disease is associated with a wide range of WGTS dysmotility involving esophageal transit, GE, gallbladder emptying, SBT, and CT.[92]

WGTS is most helpful for evaluating patients with constipation. CT is slowed more commonly in patients with organic disease and is normal in patients with functional constipation. It is important to exclude significant upper GI dysmotility in such patients before surgery because subtotal colectomy may not correct their symptoms.[93] In a study of patients with severe idiopathic constipation with upper GI symptoms, 3 of 4 with upper GI symptoms had abnormal GE and SBT in addition to delayed CT.[94] Another study of patients with chronic diverse GI symptoms over a 5-year period who were referred for WGTS documented delayed CT in 63% of patients with constipation compared with only 29% with dyspepsia.[95]

## APPROPRIATE USE CRITERIA AND CURRENT PROCEDURAL TERMINOLOGY CODING ENHANCEMENTS FOR GASTROINTESTINAL SCINTIGRAPHY

Although the scintigraphic methods for measuring SBT and CT have been available for more than 20 years, they have not gained widespread clinical use. This, in part, was because there were no clinical guidelines on how they should be utilized. The Centers for Medicare & Medicaid Services (CMS) has just instituted its appropriate use criteria program to help enable physicians to order the most appropriate tests that utilize advanced diagnostic imaging. This includes GI scintigraphy.[96] In response to CMS requirements, professional societies, such as the Society of Nuclear Medicine (SNMMI) working with the AGA, the American College of Physicians, and the American College of Nuclear Medicine, have developed an appropriate use criteria guidance document

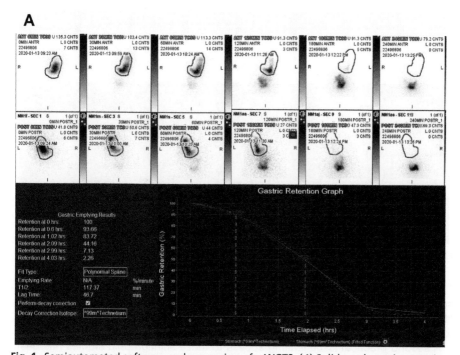

**Fig. 1.** Semiautomated software and processing of a WGTS. (*A*) Solid meal gastric emptying analysis. An automated software package opens the paired anterior and posterior solid (technetium Tc 99 m) images for all imaging times (0 hour, 0.5 hours, 1.0 hour, 2.0 hours, 3.0 hours, and 4 hours). A single ROI initially is placed manually over the total stomach at t = 0 minutes and then positioned automatically by the software over all other co-registered images to obtain the geometric mean of total gastric counts. The percentage of gastric retention at each timepoint are included in the results table as well as a graphic plot of the raw data. Computer-generated polynomial curve fitting functions then are applied to the emptying curve to produce standard measures of lag phase, rate of emptying, and half emptying time. The operator can choose the optimum curve fitting function from a pulldown menu. This example shows a polynomial fit to the data. (*B*) Liquid meal gastric emptying analysis. Similar to processing shown (*A*) for the solid-phase analysis, the liquid gastric emptying images are shown with computer-semiautomated positioned ROIs on the stomach for all time points. The automated analysis is now shown with an exponential curve fit, which is more appropriate for liquid emptying. (*C*) SBT analysis. An ROI (*arrows*) for total small bowel counts in the terminal ileum is placed in both anterior (Left Image) and posterior (Right Image) to obtain the percentage of the radiolabeled liquid meal in the terminal ileum at 6 hours. In this case, 77% of administered activity is in the terminal ileum consistent with normal SBT. (*D*) CT analysis. The 6 ROIs required to calculate the geometric mean of colon activity are shown. Once these are positioned at 24 hours, the computer groups the images and an automated final processing to calculate the geometric mean is performed for 24 hours, 48 hours, and 72 hours. (*Courtesy of* MIM Software Inc. Cleveland, OH.)

**B**

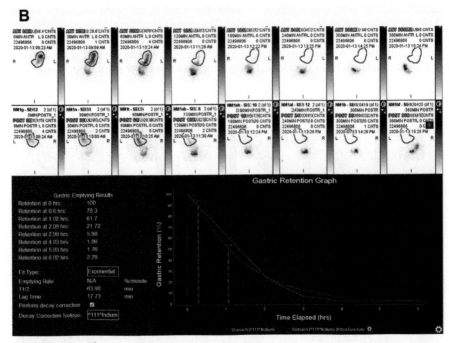

Fig. 1. (*continued*)

specifically on GI transit scintigraphy.[97] In this guidance an expert panel reviewed the literature and has established appropriateness ratings for a wide range of GI disorders to assist physicians on how best to utilize these studies.

A second practical issue limiting access to these scintigraphic studies has been the lack of Current Procedural Terminology (CPT) codes for reimbursement. Because they require significant time and complexity for their acquisition and processing without added reimbursement, this led many nuclear medicine imaging departments to not offer them. In 2016 the American Medical Association CPT codes were updated to include SBT and CT studies for reimbursement. The ability to now bill for these studies is anticipated to increase their availability in more imaging departments.

**C**

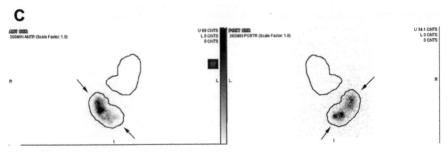

Fig. 1. (*continued*)

# D

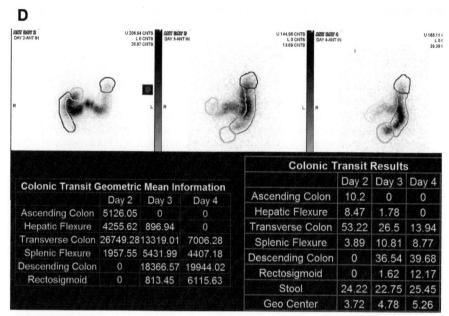

| Colonic Transit Geometric Mean Information | | | |
|---|---|---|---|
| | Day 2 | Day 3 | Day 4 |
| Ascending Colon | 5126.05 | 0 | 0 |
| Hepatic Flexure | 4255.62 | 896.94 | 0 |
| Transverse Colon | 26749.28 | 13319.01 | 7006.28 |
| Splenic Flexure | 1957.55 | 5431.99 | 4407.18 |
| Descending Colon | 0 | 18366.57 | 19944.02 |
| Rectosigmoid | 0 | 813.45 | 6115.63 |

| Colonic Transit Results | | | |
|---|---|---|---|
| | Day 2 | Day 3 | Day 4 |
| Ascending Colon | 10.2 | 0 | 0 |
| Hepatic Flexure | 8.47 | 1.78 | 0 |
| Transverse Colon | 53.22 | 26.5 | 13.94 |
| Splenic Flexure | 3.89 | 10.81 | 8.77 |
| Descending Colon | 0 | 36.54 | 39.68 |
| Rectosigmoid | 0 | 1.62 | 12.17 |
| Stool | 24.22 | 22.75 | 25.45 |
| Geo Center | 3.72 | 4.78 | 5.26 |

**Fig. 1.** (*continued*)

## ENHANCED SEMIAUTOMATED COMMERCIAL SOFTWARE FOR ANALYSIS

When joint society guidelines for GES were first established, one of the unresolved issues recognized was how to have industry develop software to support more universal access to processing of studies under the new standards.[2] The need for commercially available software is even more urgent as the software for enhanced measurements of fundic accommodation, DACS, DBT, SBT, and CT were developed typically only for local use at research centers. As new CPT codes and reimbursement have become available, more radiology/nuclear medicine equipment and software vendors have seen growing market demand for them to produce such software products. An example of commercially available, semiautomated software, which can provide enhanced computer-generated curve fitting and analysis of the data points of gastric retention over time, is shown in **Fig. 1**A, B. This can provide additional information on the half GE time, emptying rate, and the lag phase.[13] This same software package is able to generate the results of SBT and CT (**Fig. 1**C, D).

## SUMMARY

In conclusion, this review summarizes the exciting recent enhancements to GI transit scintigraphy at it continues to evolve on many technical and clinical levels. It permits assessments of global and regional (fundic and antral) gastric motility and in a single study (WGTS) provides measurements of not only solid and liquid gastric emptying but also SBT and CT. Improved quantification permits baseline assessments of motility and measures how patients may or may not respond to therapeutic interventions. With these enhancements, GI transit scintigraphy now provides for increased diagnostic information on physiologic solid and liquid test meal transit throughout the GI tract.

## DISCLOSURE

The author has nothing to disclose.

## REFERENCES

1. Griffith G, Owen G, Kirkman S, et al. Measurement of rate of gastric emptying using chromium-51. Lancet 1966;1(7449):1244–5.
2. Abell TL, Camilleri M, Donohoe K, et al. Consensus recommendations for gastric emptying scintigraphy: a joint report of the American Neurogastroenterology and Motility Society and the Society of Nuclear Medicine. Am J Gastroenterol 2008; 103(3):753–63.
3. Donohoe K, Maurer A, Ziessman H, et al. Procedure guideline for adult solid-meal gastric-emptying study 3.0. J Nucl Med Technol 2009;37(3):196–200.
4. Asano H, Tomita T, Nakamura K, et al. Prevalence of gastric motility disorders in patients with functional dyspepsia. J Neurogastroenterol Motil 2017;23(3):392–9.
5. Farre R, Vanheel H, Vanuytsel T, et al. In functional dyspepsia, hypersensitivity to postprandial distention correlates with meal-related symptom severity. Gastroenterology 2013;145(3):566–73.
6. Simren M, Tornblom H, Palsson OS, et al. Visceral hypersensitivity is associated with GI symptom severity in functional GI disorders: consistent findings from five different patient cohorts. Gut 2018;67(2):255–62.
7. Troncon LE, Herculano JR Jr, Savoldelli RD, et al. Relationships between intragastric food maldistribution, disturbances of antral contractility, and symptoms in functional dyspepsia. Dig Dis Sci 2006;51(3):517–26.
8. Hejazi RA, Lavenbarg TH, McCallum RW. Spectrum of gastric emptying patterns in adult patients with cyclic vomiting syndrome. Neurogastroenterol Motil 2010; 22(12):1298–302.e8.
9. Quartero AO, de Wit NJ, Lodder AC, et al. Disturbed solid-phase gastric emptying in functional dyspepsia: a meta-analysis. Dig Dis Sci 1998;43(9): 2028–33.
10. Tougas G, Eaker EY, Abell TL, et al. Assessment of gastric emptying using a low fat meal: establishment of international control values. Am J Gastroenterol 2000; 95(6):1456–62.
11. Guo J, Maurer A, Fisher R, et al. Extending gastric emptying scintigraphy from two to four hours detects more patients with gastroparesis. Dig Dis Sci 2001; 46:24–9.
12. Farrell M, Costello M, McKee J, et al. Compliance with gastric-emptying scintigraphy guidelines: an analysis of the intersocietal accreditation commission database. J Nucl Med Technol 2017;45(1):6–13.
13. Zinsmeister A, Bharucha A, Camilleri M. Comparison of calculations to estimate gastric emptying half-time of solids in humans. Neurogastroenterol Motil 2012; 24(12):1142–5.
14. Parker H, Tucker E, Hoad C, et al. Development and validation of a large, modular test meal with liquid and solid components for assessment of gastric motor and sensory function by non-invasive imaging. Neurogastroenterol Motil 2016;28: 554–68.
15. Sachdeva P, Kantor S, Knight LC, et al. Use of a high caloric liquid meal as an alternative to a solid meal for gastric emptying scintigraphy. Dig Dis Sci 2013; 58(7):2001–6.
16. Solnes LB, Sheikhbahaei S, Ziessman HA. EnsurePlus as an alternative to the standardized egg gastric-emptying meal. Clin Nucl Med 2019;44(6):459–61.

17. Somasundaram VH, Subramanyam P, Palaniswamy SS. A gluten-free vegan meal for gastric emptying scintigraphy: establishment of reference values and its utilization in the evaluation of diabetic gastroparesis. Clin Nucl Med 2014;39(11): 960–5.
18. Ziessman HA, Chander A, Clarke JO, et al. The added diagnostic value of liquid gastric emptying compared with solid emptying alone. J Nucl Med 2009;50(5): 726–31.
19. Ziessman HA, Okolo PI, Mullin GE, et al. Liquid gastric emptying is often abnormal when solid emptying is normal. J Clin Gastroenterol 2009;43(7):639–43.
20. Knight LC. Update on gastrointestinal radiopharmaceuticals and dosimetry estimates. Semin Nucl Med 2012;42(2):138–44.
21. Sachdeva P, Malhotra N, Pathikonda M, et al. Gastric emptying of solids and liquids for evaluation for gastroparesis. Dig Dis Sci 2011;56:1138–46.
22. Maurer A, Camilleri M, Donohoe K, et al. The SNMMI and EANM practice guideline for small-bowel and colon transit 1.0. J Nucl Med 2013;54:2004–13.
23. Pasricha P, Yates K, Clarke J, et al. Incidence and clinical significance of delayed gastric emptying for liquids in gastroparesis and chronic unexplained nausea and vomiting. Gastroenterology 2015;148. S-515.
24. Plummer M, Jones K, cousins C, et al. Hyperglycemia potentiates the slowing of gastric emptying iinduced by exopgenous GLP-1. Diabetes Care 2015;38(6): 1123–9.
25. Kar P, Jones K, Plummer M, et al. Antecedent hypoglycemia does not attenuate the acceleration of gastric emptying by hypoglycemia. J Clin Endocrinol Metab 2017;102:3953–60.
26. Halland M, Bharucha A. Perspectives in clinical gastroenterology and hepatology: Relationship between control of glycemia and gastric emptying disturbances in diabetes mellitus. Clin Gastroenterol Hepatol 2016;14:929–36.
27. Lartigue S, Bizais Y, desVarannes S, et al. Inter and intra subject variability of solid and liquid gastric emptying parameters: a scintigraphic study in healthy subjects and diabetic patients. Dig Dis Sci 1994;39:109–15.
28. Russo A, Stevens J, Chen R, et al. Insulin-induced hypolglycemia accelerates gastric emptying of solids and liquids in long-standing type 1 diabetes. J Clin Endocrinol Metab 2005;90(8):4489–95.
29. Pasricha P. Does the emptier have no clothes? Diabetes, gastric emptying, and the symdrome of gastroparesis. Clin Gastroenterol Hepatol 2015;13:477–9.
30. Bharucha A, Kudva Y, Basu A, et al. Relationship between glycemic control and gastric emptying in poorly controlled type 2 diabetes. Clin Gastroenterol Hepatol 2015;13:466–76.
31. Chang C, Kao C, Wang Y. Discrepant pattern of solid and liquid gsgtric emptying in Chinese patients with type II diabetes mellitus. Nucl Med Commun 1996; 17:60–5.
32. Horowitz M, Harding P, Maddox A, et al. Gastric and oesophageal emptying in patients with type 2(non-insulin-dependent) diabetes mellitus. Diabetologia 1989;32:151–9.
33. Camilleri M, Parkman H, Shafi M, et al. Clinical guideline: management of gastroparesis. Am J Gastroenterol 2013;108:18–37.
34. Sheik A, Anolik J, Maurer A. Update on serum glucose and metabolic management of clinical nuclear medicine studies: current status and proposed future directions. Semin Nucl Med 2019;49:411–21.
35. Cannon W, Lieb C. The receptive relaxation of the stomach. Am J Physiol 1911; 29:267–73.

36. Karamanolis G, Caenepeel P, Arts J, et al. Determinants of symptom pattern in idiopathic severely delayed gastric emptying: gastric emptying rate or proximal stomach dysfunction? Neurogastroenterol Motil 2007;56:29–36.

37. Kumar A, Attaluri A, Hashmi S, et al. Visceral hypersensitivity and impaired accommodation in refractory diabetic gastroparesis. Neurogastroenterol Motil 2008;20(6):635–42.

38. Kindt S, Tack J. Impaired gastric accomodation and its role in dyspepsia. Gut 2006;55:1685–91.

39. Gonlachanvit S, Maurer AH, Fisher RS, et al. Regional gastric emptying abnormalities in functional dyspepsia and gastro-oesophageal reflux disease. Neurogastroenterol Motil 2006;18(10):894–904.

40. Chedid V, Brandler J, Vijayvargiya P, et al. Characterization of upper gastrointestinal symptoms, gastric motor functions and associations in patients with diabetes at a referral center. Am J Gastroenterol 2019;114:143–54.

41. Bisschops B, Tack J. Dysaccommodation of the stomach: therapeutic nirvana? Neurogastroenterol Motil 2007;19:85–93.

42. Mundt M, Hausken T, Samsom M. Effect of intragastric barostat bag on proximal and distal gastric accommodation in response to liquid meal. Am J Physiol Gastrointest Liver Physiol 2002;282:G681–6.

43. deZwart I, deRoos A, Lamb H, et al. Gastric motility and emptying: evaluation of the barostat method with MRI. Gastroenterology 2003;124(Suppl.1):A673.

44. Ang D. Measurement of gastric accommodation: a reappraisal of conventional and emerging modalities. Neurogastroenterol Motil 2011;23:287–91.

45. Mundt M, Samsom M. Fundal dysaccommodation in functional dyspepsia: head-to-head comparison between the barostat and three-dimensional ultrasonographic technique. Gut 2006;55:1725–30.

46. Tefera S, Gilja O, Olafsdottir E, et al. Inragastric maldistribution of a liquid meal in patients with reflux oesophagitis assessed by three dimensional ultrasonography. Gut 2002;50:153–8.

47. Choi M, Kim B, Choo K, et al. Measurement of gastric accommodation and emptying of a solid meal by magnetic resonance imaging. Gastroenterology 2000;118:A388.

48. deZwart I, Mearadji B, Lamb H, et al. Gastric motility: comparison of assessment with real-time MR imaging or barostat measurement initial experience. Radiology 2002;224:592–7.

49. Faas H, Steingotter A, Feinle C, et al. Effects of meal consistency and ingested fluid volume on the intragastric distribution of a drug model—an MRI study. Gastroenterology 2001;120:A1491.

50. Mearadji B, Zwart Id. Assessment of gastric motility by combined real time MRI and barostat recording under fasting conditions. Gastroenterology 2001;120:A1485.

51. Chedid V, Halawi H, Brander J, et al. Gastric accommodation measurements by single photon emission computed tomography and two-dimensional scintigraphy in diabetic patients with upper gastrointestinal symptoms. Neurogastroenterol Motil 2019;31(6):e13581.

52. Kuiken SD, Samsom M, Camilleri M, et al. Development of a test to measure gastric accommodation in humans. Am J Physiol 1999;277:G1217–21.

53. Bouras E, Delgado-Aros S, Camilleri M, et al. Gastric accommodation measured noninvasively in post-fundoplication and nonulcer dyspepsia patients. Gut 2002;51:781–6.

54. Bouras E, Delgado-Aros S, Camilleri M, et al. SPECT imaging of the stomach: comparison with barostat, and effects of sex, age, body mass index, and fundoplication. Gut 2002;51:781–6.

55. Bredenoord A, Chial H, Camilleri M, et al. Gastric accommodation and emptying in evaluation of patients with upper gastrointestinal symptoms. Clin Gastroenterol Hepatol 2003;1:264–72.

56. Breen M, Camilleri M, Burton D, et al. Performance characteristics of the measurement of gastric volume using single photon emission computed tomography. Neurogastroenterol Motil 2011;23(4):308–15.

57. Burton D, Kim J, Camilleri M, et al. Relationship of gastric emptying and volume changes after a solid meal in humans. Am J Physiol Gastrointest Liver Physiol 2005;289:G261–6.

58. Vasavid P, Chaiwatanarata T, Gonlachanvit S. The Reproducibility of 99mTc-pertechnetate single photon emission computed tomography (SPECT) for measurement of gastric accommodation in healthy humans: evaluation of the test results performed at the same time and different time of the day. J Neurogastroenterol Motil 2010;16(4):401–6.

59. Bouras EP, Delgado-Aros S, Camilleri M, et al. SPECT imaging of the stomach: comparison with barostat, and effects of sex, age, body mass index, and fundoplication. Single photon emission computed tomography. Gut 2002;51(6):781–6.

60. Liauy S, Camilleri M, Kim D-Y, et al. Pharmacological modulation of human gastric volumes demonstrated noninvasively using SPECT imaging. Neurogastroenterol Motil 2001;13:533–42.

61. Lacy BE, Saito YA, Camilleri M, et al. Effects of antidepressants on gastric function in patients with functional dyspepsia. Am J Gastroenterol 2018;113(2): 216–24.

62. Troncon L, Bennett R, Ahluwalia R, et al. Abnormal distribution of food during gastric emptying in functional dyspepsia patients. Gut 1994;35:327–32.

63. Piessevaux H, Tack J, Walrand S, et al. Intragastric distribution of a standardized meal in health and functional dyspepsia: correlation with specific symptoms. Neurogastroenterol Motil 2003;15:447–55.

64. Tomita T, Okugawa T, Yamasaki T, et al. Use of scintigraphy to evaluate gastric accommodation and emptying: comparison with barostat. Gastroenterol Hepatol 2013;28:106–11.

65. Maurer A, Parkman H. Towards a fuller assessment of gastric motility in patients with upper GI dyspepsia: time to accommodate! Am J Gastroenterol 2019; 114(1):16–8.

66. Orthey P, Yu D, Natta MV, et al. Intragastric meal distribution during gastric emptying scintigraphy for assessment of fundic accommodation: correlation with symptoms of gastroparesis. J Nucl Med 2018;59:691–7.

67. Orthey P, Dadparvar S, Parkman H, et al. Enhanced gastric emptying scintigraphy to assess fundic accommodation using intragastric meal distribution and antral contractility. J Nucl Med Technol 2019;47:138–43.

68. Simonian H, Maurer A, Knight L, et al. Simultaneous assessment of gastric accommodation and emptying: studies with liquid and solid meals. J Nucl Med 2004;45:1155–60.

69. Tack J, Janssen P, Tatsuhiro M, et al. Efficacy of buspirone, a fundus-relaxing drug, in patients with functional dyspepsia. Clin Gastroenterol Hepatol 2012;10: 1239–45.

70. Miwa H, Nagahara A, Tominaga K, et al. Efficacy of the 5-HT1A agonist tandospirone citrate in improving symptoms of patients with functional dyspepsia: a randomized controlled trial. Am J Physiol 2009;104:2779–87.

71. Urbain J, Vekemans M, Bouillon R, et al. Characterization of gastric antral motility disturbances in diabetes using a scintigraphic technique. J Nucl Med 1993;34:576–81.

72. Friedman M, Sarosiek I, Diaz J, et al. Scintigraphic methodology using midantrum regions of interest (ROIs) to ascertain antral contraction amplitude and peristalsis. Gastroenterology 2019;156(6 Suppl 1):796–7.

73. Diaz J, Friedman M, Makiyil J, et al. Scintigraphic methodology using midantrum regions of interest (ROIs) to ascertain antral contraction amplitude and peristalsis. Gastroenterology 2015;148(4 Suppl 1):S515–6.

74. Cogliandro R, Rizzoli G, Bellacosa L, et al. Is gastroparesis a gastric disease? Neurogastroenterol Motil 2019;31(5):e13562.

75. Barshop K, Staller K, Semler J, et al. Duodenal rather than antral motility contractile parameters correlate with symptom severity in gastroparesis patients. Neurogastroenterol Motil 2015;27:339–46.

76. Orthey P, Dadparvar S, Kamat B, et al. Using gastric emptying scintigraphy to evaluate antral contractions and duodenal bolus propagation. Am J Physiol 2020;318(1):G203–9.

77. Edelbroek M, Schuurkes J, Ridder WD, et al. Effect of cisapride on myoelectrical and motor responses of antropyloroduodenal region during intraduodenal lipid and antral tachygastria in conscious dog. Dig Dis Sci 1995;40:901–11.

78. Seidl H, Gundling F, Pfeiffer A, et al. Comparison of small-bowel motility of the human jejunum and ileum. Neurogastroenterol Motil 2012;24(8):e373–80.

79. Camilleri M, Hasler WL, Parkman HP, et al. Measurement of gastrointestinal motility in the GI laboratory. Gastroenterology 1998;115(3):747–62.

80. Maurer AH. Gastrointestinal motility, part 2: small-bowel and colon transit. J Nucl Med 2015;56(9):1395–400.

81. Antoniou A, Raja S, El-Khouli R, et al. Comprehensive radionuclide esophagogastrointestinal transit study: methodology, reference values, and initial clinical experience. J Nucl Med 2015;56(5):721–7.

82. Maqbool S, Parkman HP, Friedenberg FK. Wireless capsule motility: comparison of the SmartPill GI monitoring system with scintigraphy for measuring whole gut transit. Dig Dis Sci 2009;54(10):2167–74.

83. Prather CM, Camilleri M, Zinsmeister AR, et al. Tegaserod accelerates orocecal transit in patients with constipation-predominant irritable bowel syndrome. Gastroenterology 2000;118(3):463–8.

84. Camilleri M, Brown ML, Malagelada JR. Impaired transit of chyme in chronic intestinal pseudoobstruction. Correction by cisapride. Gastroenterology 1986;91(3):619–26.

85. Camilleri M, Zinsmeister AR, Greydanus MP, et al. Towards a less costly but accurate test of gastric emptying and small bowel transit. Dig Dis Sci 1991;36(5):609–15.

86. Bonapace ES, Maurer AH, Davidoff S, et al. Whole gut transit scintigraphy in the clinical evaluation of patients with upper and lower gastrointestinal symptoms. Am J Gastroenterol 2000;95(10):2838–47.

87. Charles F, Camilleri M, Phillips SF, et al. Scintigraphy of the whole gut: clinical evaluation of transit disorders. Mayo Clin Proc 1995;70(2):113–8.

88. Maurer AH, Krevsky B. Whole-gut transit scintigraphy in the evaluation of small-bowel and colon transit disorders. Semin Nucl Med 1995;25(4):326–38.

89. Shahid S, Ramzan Z, Maurer AH, et al. Chronic idiopathic constipation: more than a simple colonic transit disorder. J Clin Gastroenterol 2012;46(2):150–4.

90. Hasler WL, May KP, Wilson LA, et al. Relating gastric scintigraphy and symptoms to motility capsule transit and pressure findings in suspected gastroparesis. Neurogastroenterol Motil 2018;30(2). https://doi.org/10.1111/nmo.13196.

91. Read NW, Al-Janabi MN, Holgate AM, et al. Simultaneous measurement of gastric emptying, small bowel residence and colonic filling of a solid meal by the use of the gamma camera. Gut 1986;27(3):300–8. https://doi.org/10.1136/gut.27.3.300.

92. Tursi A. Gastrointestinal motility disturbances in celiac disease. J Clin Gastroenterol 2004;38(8):642–5.

93. Kamm MA, Hawley PR, Lennard-Jones JE. Outcome of colectomy for severe idiopathic constipation. Gut 1988;29(7):969–73.

94. van der Sijp JR, Kamm MA, Nightingale JM, et al. Disturbed gastric and small bowel transit in severe idiopathic constipation. Dig Dis Sci 1993;38(5):837–44.

95. Balan K, Alwis L, Sonoda LI, et al. Utility of whole gut transit scintigraphy in patients with chronic gastrointestinal symptoms. Nucl Med Commun 2010;31(4):328–33.

96. CMS. Appropriate use criteria for advanced diagnostic imaging. Secondary Appropriate use criteria for advanced diagnostic imaging. Available at: https://www.cms.gov/Outreach-and-Education/Medicare-Learning-Network-MLN/MLNProducts/Downloads/AUCDiagnosticImaging-909377.pdf.

97. Maurer A, Abell T, Bennett P, et al. Appropriate use criteria for gastrointestinal transit scintigraphy. J Nucl Med 2020;61(3):11N–7N.

# Targeting Treatment of Gastroparesis

## Use of Clinical Tests to Guide Treatments

William L. Hasler, MD

**KEYWORDS**

- Gastric emptying • Nausea and vomiting • Prokinetic treatment • Pylorospasm
- Accommodation • Gastric slow wave • Contractility • Hypersensitivity

**KEY POINTS**

- Measuring gastric emptying rates distinguishes 2 related disorders in patients with unexplained upper gut symptoms—gastroparesis and chronic unexplained nausea and vomiting (CUNV).
- There is limited evidence to suggest that rates of gastric emptying correlate with specific symptoms or can be used to reliably choose effective treatments of gastroparesis or CUNV.
- Patients with suspected gastroparesis may exhibit a diverse range of other physiologic abnormalities including pylorospasm, blunted fundic accommodation, dysrhythmic gastric slow-wave activity, altered extragastric transit or contractility, or heightened luminal sensation that can be characterized by specific test findings.
- Research is ongoing to determine if these other physiologic abnormalities relate to any specific symptom presentations and if they can be used to guide prokinetic and non-prokinetic treatment of suspected gastroparesis.

## INTRODUCTION
### Clinical Features of Gastroparesis

Gastroparesis presents with upper gastrointestinal symptoms of nausea, vomiting, early satiety, fullness, bloating, distention, and/or upper abdominal pain in association with delayed gastric emptying. In addition, gastroparesis also may lead to increased blood glucose variability including risk for early postprandial hypoglycemia due to mismatch of intestinal meal delivery with insulin given at meal time. However, between one-quarter and one-third of patients with suspected gastroparesis with characteristic symptom presentations actually exhibit gastric emptying delays.[1] Many names have been given to the large patient subset with gastroparesis symptoms but normal gastric transit including chronic unexplained nausea vomiting (CUNV) syndrome and

Division of Gastroenterology and Hepatology, University of Michigan Health System, 3912 Taubman Center, SPC 5362, Ann Arbor, MI 48109, USA
*E-mail address:* whasler@umich.edu

Gastroenterol Clin N Am 49 (2020) 519–538
https://doi.org/10.1016/j.gtc.2020.04.007
0889-8553/20/© 2020 Elsevier Inc. All rights reserved.

gastroparesis-like syndrome.[2] Gastric emptying testing is routinely used to distinguish gastroparesis from CUNV. Another approach to conferring diagnoses is to categorize patients by their symptom presentations. The Rome Foundation recently published the Rome IV criteria for gastroduodenal disorders, providing specific features for functional conditions that show overlap with gastroparesis including functional dyspepsia, chronic nausea vomiting syndrome, and cyclic vomiting syndrome.[3] One study observed that 86% of those with idiopathic gastroparesis characterized by standardized surveys satisfy Rome criteria for functional dyspepsia.[4]

Other causes of symptoms should be conducted for suspected gastroparesis should be carefully excluded. Standard work-ups typically include endoscopic and/ or radiographic testing and blood testing directed to systemic diseases that produce symptoms mimicking gastroparesis. In rare cases, unusual causes may be detected by serologic tests to evaluate for autoimmune neurologic diseases, which may have associated upper gastrointestinal manifestations.

## TREATMENTS OF GASTROPARESIS

Gastroparesis often is managed with prokinetic therapies designed to accelerate gastric emptying. Because of lack of efficacy or intolerable side effects, other medication or nonmedication treatments without prokinetic actions may be included in management regimens.

### Prokinetic Therapies

A small number of prokinetic medications are available in the United States. Metoclopramide, the only agent the Food and Drug Administration (FDA) approved for treating gastroparesis, stimulates gastric emptying by peripheral action as a dopamine $D_2$ antagonist and serotonin $5-HT_4$ agonist but also has central nervous system (CNS) antiemetic effects, which likely enhance its benefits. Use of metoclopramide is limited by significant CNS side effects (agitation, mood disorders, dystonias, sedation). Since a 2009 FDA warning for the risk of tardive dyskinesia, there has been a dramatic reduction in metoclopramide prescription over the past decade. Macrolide agents (erythromycin, azithromycin) exert intense gastric prokinetic actions serving as agonists on receptors for motilin, the endogenous stimulant of fasting upper gut motor complexes. Tolerance to chronic erythromycin use may limit its long-term prescription. Domperidone is a $D_2$ antagonist with combined antiemetic action, which acts only peripherally, thereby minimizing the CNS toxicity of metoclopramide. This agent is not available for routine prescription in the United States, but the FDA has approved its use under the Investigational New Drug approval mechanism. Domperidone has been implicated as a cause of fatal cardiac arrhythmias in patients with electrocardiographic (EKG) QTc interval prolongation. Its use should be accompanied by electrolyte and EKG surveillance. A systematic review comparing these agents concluded that erythromycin is the strongest gastric emptying stimulant, and erythromycin and domperidone both are effective for reducing gastroparesis symptoms.[5] Other drugs have some prokinetic effects and can be used to treat gastroparesis. The acetylcholinesterase inhibitor pyridostigmine increases gastrointestinal contractions and has been used to treat autoimmune upper gut dysmotility.

Research is ongoing to test new prokinetic agents for gastroparesis. Phase 3 investigations are underway for the injectable ghrelin agonist relamorelin, which was reported in earlier trials in diabetic gastroparesis to improve gastric emptying and reduce symptoms.[6] Prucalopride was recently approved by the FDA to treat chronic idiopathic constipation by acting as a serotonin $5-HT_4$ agonist. Although the drug primarily targets the colon, prucalopride was reported to accelerate gastric emptying with associated improvements in nausea/vomiting, early satiety/fullness, and bloating to greater degrees than placebo in 28 patients with idiopathic gastroparesis.[7] Velusetrag is another 5-HT$_4$ agonist with gastric prokinetic effects that improved short-term symptoms over 4 weeks in a mixed group of patients with diabetic or idiopathic gastroparesis.[8]

Endoscopic and surgical treatments for gastroparesis are offered that can accelerate gastric emptying. Case series have reported symptom and emptying benefits of endoscopic botulinum toxin injection into the pylorus in gastroparesis. In the largest series of 179 patients, higher doses of botulinum toxin (200 versus 100 units) were associated with better responses, and some patient subsets (female sex, idiopathic etiology, and age <50 years) were more likely to report benefits.[9] Another way to treat functional pyloric outlet obstruction in gastroparesis is to perform surgery. Laparoscopic pyloroplasty is the most common surgery and normalizes gastric emptying in most patients with less consistent symptom reductions. Recently, gastric per-oral myotomy (G-POEM), as an endoscopic means to cut the pylorus, has been adopted as an alternative to surgery. G-POEM performance includes an initial injection and mucosotomy to access the submucosal space, creation of a submucosal tunnel to the pylorus, followed by pyloric myotomy, and subsequent mucosal closure (**Fig. 1**). Several early studies reported improved gastric emptying and reduced symptoms. A large single-center G-POEM study noted acceleration in gastric emptying from 46% to 18% after 4-hour retention with improved overall symptoms.[10] In a second, 100-patient single-center report, 78% exhibited improved gastric emptying with normalization in 57% and a mean 4-hour retention improvement of 23.6%.[11] A meta-analysis of 7 studies with 196 patients reported success in 82% with improved symptom scores at 5 days and accelerated gastric emptying 2 to 3 months after G-POEM.[12] Another review of 291 cases in 13 studies noted technical success in

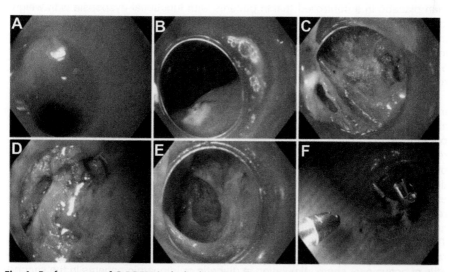

**Fig. 1.** Performance of G-POEM includes locating the procedure site proximal to the pylorus (*A*), creating a mucosotomy (*B*), tunneling in the gastric submucosa (*C*), identification of the pylorus (*D*), making the myotomy (*E*), and closing the mucosotomy site (*F*). (*From* Mekaroonkamol P, Shah R, Cai Q. Outcomes of per oral endoscopic pyloromyotomy in gastroparesis worldwide. World J Gastroenterol 2019;25:909-22.)

most patients, and 75% to 100% of patients reported improved symptoms and quality of life in most but not all reports.[13] An advantage of G-POEM over pyloroplasty is a shorter inpatient stay after the procedure. An issue with all pyloric therapies is choosing which patients are most likely to benefit from treatment. Two controlled investigations failed to observe benefits of pyloric botulinum toxin over sham injections in patients with gastroparesis.[14,15] Both studies were underpowered and one had a crossover design which precluded accurately comparing the 2 study arms. However, it is also conceivable that no benefit was seen because mixed patient groups with and without pyloric dysfunction were included in the studies. Aggressive therapy, such as completion gastrectomy, has been noted to provide benefits for patients with postsurgical gastroparesis, but this is less well accepted for other etiologies. However, some studies report short-term improvements with gastric resection in up to 60% with diabetic or idiopathic etiologies.[16]

### Antiemetic and Neuromodulator Therapies

Many antiemetic or neuromodulator treatments without prokinetic action are used in gastroparesis. Benefits in gastroparesis were reported for transdermal granisetron, a $5-HT_3$ antagonist antiemetic, in open-label studies.[17] The only antiemetic to undergo a placebo-controlled trial in patients with symptoms of gastroparesis was the neurokinin $NK_1$ antagonist aprepitant.[18] Although it did not meet its primary outcome, aprepitant was superior to placebo in improving nausea and vomiting. Tricyclic antidepressants are standard treatments for other nausea and vomiting disorders including cyclic vomiting syndrome, but nortriptyline did not improve overall symptoms compared with placebo in a 15-week randomized trial in 130 patients with idiopathic gastroparesis.[19] However, amitriptyline produced superior symptom reductions versus placebo and the serotonin reuptake inhibitor escitalopram in a large multicenter functional dyspepsia trial.[20] Likewise, the atypical antidepressant mirtazapine improved early satiety, weight gain, and quality of life more than placebo in a controlled trial in patients with functional dyspepsia with weight loss.[21] The anxiolytic agent buspirone, a $5-HT_{1A}$ agonist, reduced fullness, satiety, and bloating to greater degrees than placebo in functional dyspepsia without slowing gastric emptying.[22] In a different controlled trial in functional dyspepsia, another $5-HT_{1A}$ agonist tandospirone reduced overall symptoms and upper abdominal pain more than placebo.[23]

Gastric electrical stimulation has humanitarian device exemption for treating refractory diabetic or idiopathic gastroparesis since 2000. Case series note impressive symptom and quality of life improvements with reduced medication needs, better glycemic control, and improved nutrition. Most case studies and systematic reviews report primarily on improved nausea and vomiting, but some have also observed decreased abdominal pain. The mechanism of action of gastric stimulation likely is multifactorial, but most studies report no convincing gastric emptying stimulation. Temporary gastric stimulation has been performed by some to confirm responsiveness before permanent device implantation. Three small, blinded sham-controlled gastric stimulation trials have been conducted in the United States. There were trends to reduced vomiting in diabetics but not in idiopathic gastroparesis when the device was ON versus OFF in the first study.[24] There were no benefits of active over sham stimulation in diabetic or idiopathic patients in the second and third studies.[24–26] Some groups have coupled gastric stimulation with pyloroplasty to enhance gastric emptying. A systematic review of 38 studies reported that gastric stimulation produces less overall benefits than pyloric surgeries for gastroparesis.[27]

## GUIDING DECISIONS IN SUSPECTED GASTROPARESIS BY EMPTYING RATES

Several methods have been validated to measure gastric emptying rates to distinguish gastroparesis from CUNV. However, the relation of test findings to specific symptom presentations and responses to therapies of these 2 conditions is controversial.

### Methods of Gastric Emptying Testing

Gastric scintigraphy is the most widely used test of gastric emptying test in the United States and involves consuming a low-fat meal of egg whites labeled with $^{99m}Tc$, toast, jam, and water followed by 4-hour scanning.[28] Gastroparesis is diagnosed when greater than 60% of the radiolabel remains in the stomach at 2 hours or greater than 10% at 4 hours. Others have proposed higher fat meals to provide a more vigorous challenge for the stomach, but such methods have not achieved widespread use. Liquid-phase scintigraphy with ingestion of $[^{111}In]$DTPA has been advocated to increase the yield of solid-phase scintigraphy or for use in those who are intolerant to solid meal testing. Other test meals are used in some centers but have not been validated. Discordant diagnoses of gastroparesis have been recorded when gastric retention is measured at 2 versus 4 hours in the same test, illustrating the need to follow standardized protocols for emptying testing.

Other tests to measure gastric emptying are validated. One method involves swallowing a 2.6-cm wireless motility capsule (WMC) that measures luminal pH, contractions, and temperature. Gastric emptying is defined when the WMC passes from the acidic stomach into the more neutral pH duodenum. Three prospective investigations have validated the WMC to measure gastric emptying. In 61 patients with previously diagnosed gastroparesis and 87 healthy controls, more patients exhibited WMC delays defined by gastric emptying times of greater than 5 hours versus concurrent scintigraphy.[29] In a study of 209 patients in the NIH Gastroparesis Registry, of whom 68.8% had known gastroparesis on scintigraphy, WMC emptying delays were documented at a later date in 40.3% of patients and showed 52.8% agreement with scintigraphy.[30] The most recent prospective study of WMC performed concurrently with scintigraphy observed 75.7% agreement between the 2 tests in a nonenriched patient cohort with suspected gastroparesis, although emptying delays were more common with WMC than scintigraphy (34.6% versus 24.5%).[1] Another approved alternative, the gastric emptying breath test (GEBT), involves consuming a meal with $^{13}C$-labeled Spirulina platensis—a blue-green algae.[31] As the $^{13}C$-labeled meal is passed into the small intestine, it is digested with production of $^{13}CO_2$, which is absorbed and exhaled and quantified by mass spectrometry. GEBT showed 89% sensitivity and 80% specificity for detecting emptying delays versus concurrently performed scintigraphy. Finally, some clinicians consider visualization of retained food residue in the stomach during upper endoscopy to reflect gastric emptying delays, although other mechanical or medication (eg, opioid use) causes must be excluded.

### Correlation of Symptoms with Gastric Emptying Findings

The relation of symptoms to gastric emptying is inconsistent between different reports. In many studies, symptom severity of gastroparesis is similar in patients with and without gastric emptying delays. In one large well-characterized 425-patient cohort, scintigraphic delays did not correlate with any gastroparesis symptom.[2] Similarly, in the 209-patient WMC study, overall gastroparesis scores and all individual scores of nausea/vomiting, early satiety/fullness, bloating/distention, and pain did not relate to gastric emptying delays.[32] Delayed emptying is found in about one-third of patients with functional dyspepsia. Some studies in functional dyspepsia or using higher fat scintigraphy methods in gastroparesis have weakly correlated some symptoms (fullness, nausea, vomiting, weight loss, heartburn, regurgitation) with emptying rates. Furthermore, gastric emptying rates are not always consistent. In a recent reproducibility study of gastric scintigraphy in patients, characterization of emptying as delayed versus normal versus rapid differed between the first and second test in 30% of patients (**Fig. 2**).[33] Some have observed better correlations of gastric emptying with symptoms when standardized symptom measures are quantified during performance of emptying testing.

A recent systematic review and meta-analysis attempted to clarify this controversy by excluding studies considered to be suboptimal for measuring gastric emptying.[34] Including only scintigraphy and GEBT studies greater than 3 hours in duration, associations were noted between gastric emptying and several symptoms including nausea, vomiting, pain, early satiety, and fullness. Of note, the authors excluded the previously described well-characterized 425-patient cohort, which showed no correlation of symptoms with emptying rates because many patients were on medications known to delay gastric emptying.[2] However, their main medication class of concern was that 42% of patients who were on opioids, which were in fact discontinued at least 72 hours before gastric emptying testing. It should also be recognized that, of the studies with optimal emptying methods that were kept in the meta-analysis, approximately one-third either did not exclude or did not mention in their texts use of medications known to affect gastric emptying findings. Regardless, it is clear from the literature as a whole that there is no clinical presentation that is specific for delayed versus normal gastric emptying.

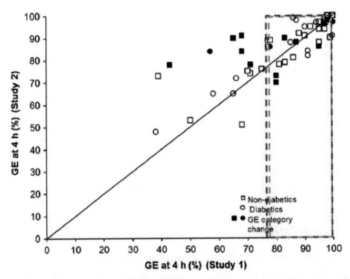

**Fig. 2.** This scatterplot shows the reproducibility of gastric scintigraphy comparing 4-hour retention values on study 2 versus study 1 in nondiabetics (*squares*) and diabetics (*circles*). The black filled markers (~30% of participants) show those subjects for whom the overall interpretation changed (eg, as normal, rapid, or delayed). (*From* Desai A, O'Connor M, Neja B, et al. Reproducibility of gastric emptying assessed with scintigraphy in patients with upper GI symptoms. Neurogastroenterol Motil 2018;30:e13365.)

### Correlation of Symptom Responses to Therapy with Gastric Emptying Findings

Studies of longitudinal outcomes in relation to gastric emptying provide varied findings. Diabetics with gastroparesis symptoms with delayed emptying reported more hospitalizations, inpatient days, and emergency department and outpatient visits even though A1c levels and other diabetic complications were similar to those with normal gastric transit.[35] Surprisingly, in a large multicenter cohort, moderate to severe emptying delays (>20% 4-hour retention) were associated with better symptom outcomes over 48 weeks versus those with milder impairments.[36] Conversely in preliminary data from another large group with gastroparesis symptoms, the 75% of patients with normal emptying reported better symptom and quality of life improvements over 6 months compared with the 25% of patients with scintigraphic emptying delays.[37]

Many clinicians use gastric emptying tests to direct treatment choices, although evidence to support this practice is weak. In a meta-analysis of 34 prokinetic trials in gastroparesis, correlations of symptom reductions with emptying acceleration were poor, which has been proposed to stem from the central sites of action of these drugs.[38] Recently, a systematic review and meta-analysis of 59 studies reported a significant reduction in symptoms with prokinetics.[39] There was no relation of accelerated gastric emptying to improved symptoms when all studies were considered. However, positive emptying associations with symptom reductions were observed when only those investigations with optimal testing methods (>3-hour studies) were included. This restriction limited analyses to only 12 studies including 5 with the 5-HT$_4$ agonist/5-HT$_3$ antagonist cisapride, 1 with domperidone, 4 with the ghrelin agonist relamorelin, and 2 with other ghrelin agonists. None of these agents is FDA approved for prescription and this analysis did not include agents prescribed in the United States for gastroparesis including metoclopramide and erythromycin, raising questions about the relevance of these findings in this country. Among newer treatments, G-POEM reduces overall and individual symptoms with associated emptying acceleration, but 43% discordance between symptom and transit improvements has been noted indicating that this correlation is incomplete.[40] In contrast, the effectiveness of some non-prokinetic therapies has been associated with normal emptying. In a placebo-controlled study of different antidepressants in functional dyspepsia, symptom benefits of amitriptyline were restricted to the patient subgroup without emptying delays.[20]

## GUIDING DECISIONS BY OTHER TESTS IN SUSPECTED GASTROPARESIS
### Rationale to Study Other Physiologic Parameters in Suspected Gastroparesis

Despite the best efforts of experts, responses to long-term management of gastroparesis and CUNV are modest because our understanding of symptom pathogenesis is incomplete. In a tertiary study, temporary nasoduodenal feedings were required for 42% of patients with gastroparesis and subsequent percutaneous endoscopic gastrostomy with jejunostomy extension was needed in 22%.[41] Although gastroparesis and CUNV are categorized as distinct disorders, evidence suggests that there is substantial overlap in their pathophysiology. Full-thickness gastric biopsies from patients with gastroparesis show decreases in interstitial cells of Cajal (ICC)—cells within the gastric wall responsible for electrical pacemaker generation and relaying neural information to gastric smooth muscle cells. Patients with CUNV exhibit qualitatively similar ICC damage as in gastroparesis but quantitatively higher ICC numbers.[42] Because of this overlap, investigators have searched for other physiologic abnormalities to better explain symptom generation in suspected gastroparesis. Emptying delays themselves may result from impaired phasic antral or spastic pyloric contractions. Other factors proposed to cause symptoms in gastroparesis and CUNV include impaired accommodation of the gastric fundus after eating, rhythm and amplitude abnormalities of gastric electrical activity, other gastric and extragastric motility abnormalities, or altered perception of gut stimulation (**Table 1**). The following sections focus on other tests of motor, myoelectric, and sensory function that can detect these abnormalities in patients with suspected gastroparesis and how findings of these tests influence care decisions.

### Pyloric Impedance Planimetry

#### Methods of testing

Early manometry studies in patients with gastroparesis showed prolonged periods of increased tonic and phasic pyloric contractility—a phenomenon termed pylorospasm.[43] Pyloric manometry is not routinely performed because catheters are difficult to secure across the pylorus and it is difficult to reliably detect tonic contractions in the absence of phasic motility. An impedance planimetry device known as the Functional Lumen Imaging Probe (EndoFLIP) is currently the test of choice to study the role of pyloric dysfunction in gastroparesis and to measure responses to endoscopic and surgical pyloric therapies. Testing usually is performed during endoscopy under

**Table 1**
**Factors other than gastric emptying proposed to cause gastroparesis symptoms**

| Physiologic Parameter | Available Testing | Test Findings |
|---|---|---|
| Pyloric motor function | Impedance planimetry (EndoFLIP) | Reduced pyloric distensibility/compliance Reduced pyloric diameter/cross-sectional area |
| Fundic accommodation | Barostat High-resolution gastric manometry Single-photon emission tomography MRI Nutrient satiety testing | Blunted accommodation |
| Gastric slow-wave activity | Single channel electrogastrography Multichannel serosal and cutaneous electrogastrography | Gastric slow-wave dysrhythmias (tachy-, bradygastria) Impaired amplitude response to meal Slow wave propagation defects |
| Extragastric transit | WMC Scintigraphy | Delayed small bowel transit Rapid small bowel transit Delayed colon transit Generalized transit delays |
| Gastrointestinal contractility | Manometry WMC Dynamic antral scintigraphy | Antral hypomotility Enteric neuropathy Enteric myopathy Rumination |
| Visceral hypersensitivity | Barostat | Hypersensitivity |

anesthesia. An EndoFLIP catheter is passed orally or through the endoscope into the stomach and visually advanced until an 8-cm deflated balloon with 16 intraballoon sensors spans the pylorus. The balloon is sequentially inflated in stages up to 50 mL while recording several pyloric parameters including diameter, cross-sectional area, pressure, and distensibility. An early EndoFLIP study found that pyloric compliance is decreased in patients with gastroparesis versus controls.[44] Other Endo-FLIP abnormalities in gastroparesis include reductions in pyloric diameter and cross-sectional area and increases in pyloric pressure.

### Correlation of symptoms with test findings
In 1 study, pyloric distensibility to EndoFLIP balloon inflation was impaired in ~40% of patients with gastroparesis, which correlated with more severe gastric emptying delays, greater early satiety and fullness, and worse quality of life.[44] Others have associated reduced distensibility with delayed emptying and symptoms.[45] Larger studies will confirm if pyloric dysfunction relates to higher symptoms in gastroparesis and may also determine if pyloric abnormalities can cause symptoms in the absence of emptying delays.

### Correlation of symptom responses to therapy with test findings
In 1 study, 19/35 (54%) patients with gastroparesis exhibited reduced pyloric distensibility with a cutoff less than 10 mm$^2$/mm Hg.[46] Those with reduced distensibility reported superior improvements in overall symptoms, fullness and bloating, gastrointestinal-specific quality of life, and GEBT emptying compared with those with normal distensibility 3 months after pyloric botulinum toxin (200 units) injection (**Fig. 3**). In a second report, higher baseline pyloric compliance correlated with greater decreases in early satiety and nausea 8 weeks after botulinum toxin injection, whereas increased pyloric distensibility after treatment correlated with better abdominal pain improvements.[45] In a third study, a threshold distensibility value of less than 9.2 mm$^2$/mm Hg on initial testing discriminated responders to G-POEM from nonresponders.[32] If confirmed on larger studies, these findings suggest that one or more EndoFLIP measures may offer potential benefits to predict responses to pyloric treatments.

### Accommodation Testing

### Methods of testing
The proximal stomach normally exhibits a nerve-mediated relaxation response to meal ingestion to maintain a stable intragastric pressure—a phenomenon termed accommodation. Several means of quantifying accommodation have been characterized. A barostat continuously records volume changes within an intragastric balloon maintained at a stable pressure and can measure accommodation to liquid nutrients. A second luminal method uses a high-resolution manometry catheter in the gastric fundus to measure gastric pressure changes after eating.[47] Accommodation can be noninvasively characterized using single-photon emission computed tomography (SPECT), in which an intravenous radiolabel that accumulates in the gastric wall is imaged after eating, or by MRI, which directly images gastric volume changes with eating. Impaired accommodation on SPECT is defined when gastric volumes are less than 428 mL after eating or if the ratio of fed to fasting volume does not reach 2.62.[48] SPECT has been validated versus barostat findings and has been subjected to testing pharmaceutical effects on gastric relaxation.[48] Gastric scintigraphy can be modified to measure separate emptying rates from the proximal and distal stomach to define intragastric meal distribution at time zero (IMD$^0$). Blunted accommodation is diagnosed when the fraction of total radioactivity in the proximal stomach immediately

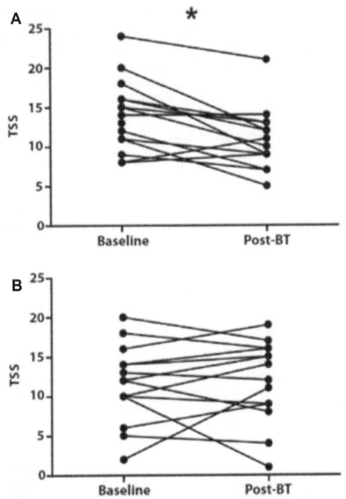

**Fig. 3.** Total symptom scores (TSS) improved in patients with gastroparesis with reduced pyloric distensibility on EndoFLIP testing (A) but not in those with normal distensibility (B). * p<0.05. (*From* Camilleri M, Chedid V, Ford AC, et al. Gastroparesis. Nat Rev Dis Primers 2018;4:41.)

after eating is less than 0.568.[49] Finally, satiety tests measure tolerance to timed ingestion of liquid nutrients. This method is claimed to provide an accurate estimate of accommodation if nutrients are consumed slowly, but results can also be influenced by luminal sensation and gastric emptying.

Accommodation defects are described for each method. Barostat studies have noted blunting of the accommodation reflex in patients with functional dyspepsia, idiopathic gastroparesis, and diabetics with upper gut symptoms. $IMD^0$ measured by regional scintigraphy was abnormally low in 14% of patients with normal overall emptying in 1 study.[49] Impaired accommodation was detected in 39% of 1 cohort using SPECT, but only 15% of the same group by $IMD^0$.[50] This disparity was postulated to possibly relate to separation of the scintigraphic radiolabel from the solid meal which then emptied faster with the liquid meal. In a large SPECT study of 1287 patients with dyspepsia, isolated accommodation defects were found in 22%, accommodation defects associated with gastric emptying delays were found in 21%, and isolated gastric emptying delays were found in 27%.[51]

### Correlation of symptoms with test findings
On barostat testing, accommodation defects correlate with early satiety, pain, and weight loss in idiopathic gastroparesis.[52] Likewise, impaired accommodation on SPECT is associated with early satiety and weight loss in functional dyspepsia.[51] However, only the prevalence of fullness and early satiety correlated with blunted accommodation using $IMD^0$.[50] Nevertheless, significant overlap in symptom presentations have been observed in those with blunted compared with normal accommodation.

### Correlation of symptom responses to therapy with test findings
Several treatments can increase accommodation in patients with functional upper gut disorders. The $5\text{-}HT_{1A}$ agonist buspirone enhanced proximal gastric relaxation and accommodation and improved symptoms (especially early satiety) in patients with functional dyspepsia in a blinded, placebo-controlled crossover trial, which were not secondary to the anxiolytic effects of this agent (**Fig. 4**).[22] A 4-week study of another $5\text{-}HT_{1A}$ agonist tandospirone in 144 patients with functional dyspepsia also showed improved epigastric pain.[23] The tricyclic agent amitriptyline similarly promotes fundic accommodation.[53] Acotiamide, an agent with antagonist actions on inhibitory muscarinic $M_1/M_2$ receptors that enhance acetylcholine release, also improved accommodation and gastric emptying and reduced symptoms in functional dyspepsia including early satiety, fullness, and bloating.[54] Patients with idiopathic gastroparesis who tolerate less than 250 mL satiety testing volumes trended to better symptom improvements on nortriptyline compared with those with normal satiety results.[19] Future investigations will determine if accommodation testing can be used to predict responses to therapies that promote proximal gastric relaxation.

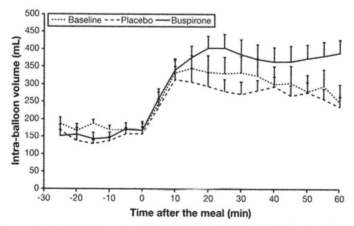

**Fig. 4.** Using gastric barostat measurements, the $5\text{-}HT_{1A}$ agonist buspirone enhanced fundic accommodation to a meal in patients with functional dyspepsia, whereas placebo did not have a significant effect. (*From* Tack J, Janssen P, Masaoka T, et al. Efficacy of buspirone, a fundus-relaxing drug, in patients with functional dyspepsia. Clin Gastroenterol Hepatol 2012;10:1239-45.)

## Electrogastrography and Related Methods

### Methods of testing

Gastric electrical activity is clinically tested using electrogastrography (EGG). EGG involves affixing cutaneous electrodes to the skin overlying the stomach with initial acquisition of fasting oscillating rhythmic gastric slow-wave signals for 15 to 60 minutes. The patient then ingests a water load or nutrient meal and postprandial slow-wave activity is recorded for another 30 to 120 minutes. Under normal conditions, the dominant slow-wave frequency ranges from 2.4 to 3.75 cycles per minute (cpm) and there is increased signal amplitude after eating. Abnormal EGG findings include bradygastria (<2.4 cpm), tachygastria (>3.75 cpm), or mixed arrhythmia greater than 30% of the recording or blunting of the amplitude increase after the meal. EGG abnormalities have been correlated with histologic abnormalities including ICC loss on full-thickness gastric biopsies from patients with gastroparesis. Unfortunately, EGG methods are highly variable from center to center in terms of recording technique, meal composition, and test interpretation, which have limited acceptance and adoption of this technique.

Gastric myoelectric recording has experienced increased activity over the past decade due to important technical advances. High-resolution recordings profiling slow-wave dysrhythmias, propagation abnormalities, and conduction blocks in patients with gastroparesis and more recently with CUNV have been obtained using 256-electrode arrays placed over the gastric serosal layer during electrical stimulator surgery.[42,55] These findings contrast with single-channel cutaneous EGGs, which cannot detect slow-wave propagation or conduction defects. Because of the need for intraoperative monitoring, these high-resolution methods are not practical for clinical testing. Early work using multichannel electrical recording arrays placed within the gastric lumen has been described, raising the possibility of future endoscopic methods to measure slow-wave dysfunction.[56] Another group recently published findings of multichannel high-resolution cutaneous EGG using a 25-electrode array placed over the stomach in 7 controls, 7 patients with functional dyspepsia, and 7 patients with gastroparesis.[57] This method characterized spatiotemporal slow-wave abnormalities in 44% of patients, including isolated reductions in propagation velocity in 5 patients, both antegrade and retrograde propagation in 6 patients, and chaotic rhythms in 3 patients, which were not detected by concurrent single-channel EGG. The investigators aim to make this technology available within 3 years.

### Correlation of symptoms with test findings

EGG disturbances are more pronounced in patients with dyspepsia than in controls in some but not all studies. In 1 report, 56% of patients with functional dyspepsia with nausea but normal gastric emptying exhibited EGG rhythm disturbances. No studies have correlated symptom severity with the degree of slow-wave disruption on 1-channel EGG, but severity of overall gastroparesis symptoms and individual symptoms of bloating/distention, fullness/early satiety, and discomfort/pain correlated with abnormal direction of slow-wave propagation in the study using high-resolution multichannel EGG (**Fig. 5**).[57] These findings should be confirmed in larger, more diverse patient populations.

### Correlation of symptom responses to therapy with test findings

In an older study, domperidone improved symptoms in 6 patients with gastroparesis with associated normalization of slow-wave dysrhythmias but not delays in gastric emptying.[58] One group reported that normal EGG dominant slow-wave frequencies in patients with gastroparesis are associated with high rates of symptom response

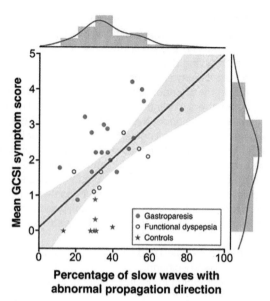

**Fig. 5.** This scatterplot shows that gastroparesis symptom severity (GCSI scores) correlated with the percentage of slow waves with abnormal propagation direction measured by high-resolution cutaneous EGG in patients with gastroparesis, functional dyspepsia, and healthy controls. (*From* Samsom M, Salet GA, Roelofs JM, et al. Compliance of the proximal stomach and dyspeptic symptoms in patients with type 1 diabetes mellitus. Dig Dis Sci 1995;40:2037-42.)

to pyloric botulinum toxin injection.[59] These findings in small single-center studies have not been evaluated in larger, multicenter cohorts.

### Testing for Gastrointestinal Contractile Abnormalities and Extragastric Transit Delays

#### Methods of testing

Observations suggest an important role for generalized gut transit and contractility abnormalities in gastroparesis and CUNV. Patients with gastroparesis more often exhibit slow transit constipation versus patients with CUNV; irritable bowel syndrome is also common in gastroparesis.[60] Other studies report prominent lower gut symptoms in CUNV as well.[30]

Manometry is performed with a fluoroscopically or endoscopically placed catheter that measures phasic contractions during fasting, after eating, and (in some cases) after prokinetic administration. However, manometry is poorly tolerated by patients and is offered in only specialized motility centers. A typical manometry study characterizes a fasting pattern, the migrating motor complex, and the increase in motor activity after eating, the fed pattern. Postprandial antral contractions on manometry are reported by some but not all investigators to inversely correlate with solid-phase gastric emptying.[61] Small intestinal abnormalities on manometry include enteric neuropathy characterized by chaotic, normal amplitude contractility with loss of normal fasting complexes and failed fed pattern conversion, and enteric myopathy characterized by low amplitude contractions with or without preservation of normal fasting and fed patterns. Reduced small intestinal activity on manometry is described in some diabetics with gastroparesis. In 88 patients with suspected gastroparesis, 70 (79.5%)

exhibited small bowel dysfunction including aberrant contractions, failed fed pattern conversion, or hypomotility.[62] GEBT emptying delays were noted in 24/70 (34.3%) patients with small bowel dysmotility, and small intestinal disturbances were found in 24/25 (96.0%) patients with emptying delays.

WMC testing defines transit delays and reduced contractility in the small bowel and colon in addition to those in the stomach. WMC measurement of fed gastric contractility includes measuring numbers of contractions greater than 10 mm Hg in amplitude and motility indices (similar to area under the pressure curve) in the hour before gastric emptying. WMC passage from the small bowel into the colon is detected when there is a characteristic greater than 1 pH unit decrease as the capsule crosses the ileocecal junction. Two prospective WMC studies reported small bowel and/or colon transit delays in greater than 40% of patients with suspected gastroparesis (Fig. 6).[1,30] Generalized WMC transit delays suggestive of global dysfunction were observed in greater than 20% of patients in the 2 studies. Numbers and motility indices of antral and small bowel contractions are lower in patients with delayed versus normal gastric emptying.[30,63]

Gastric scintigraphy can be modified to display temporal changes in antral diameter after eating. This dynamic antral scintigraphy detects contractions originating in the gastric body 11 minutes after eating in healthy subjects at a frequency similar to the slow wave (3.30 cpm).[49]

### Correlation of symptoms with test findings

Individual symptoms were similar with delayed versus normal emptying and abnormal versus normal manometry, but patients with small bowel dysmotility were more often investigator-rated as having gastric failure than with no enteric abnormalities (24% versus 5%) in 1 manometric study.[62] Reduced WMC duodenal contractions correlated with overall gastroparesis symptoms in a small study, although a larger study of well-

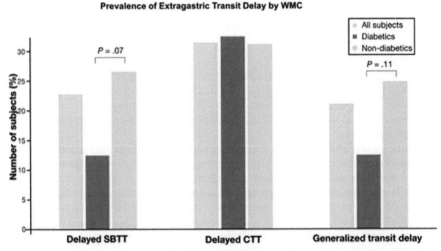

Fig. 6. The percentage of all subjects (*light blue bars*), diabetic subjects (*dark blue bars*), and nondiabetic subjects (*green bars*) exhibiting delayed small bowel transit time (SBTT), colon transit time (CTT), and generalized transit delay is shown for a prospective multicenter WMC study. (*From* Lee AA, Rao S, Nguyen LA, et al. Validation of diagnostic and performance characteristics of the wireless motility capsule in patients with suspected gastroparesis. Clin Gastroenterol Hepatol 2018 (epub ahead of print).)

characterized patients did not show relationships of small bowel contractility with either overall or individual upper gut symptoms.[30,64] At present, the relevance of contractility or extragastric transit in generating symptoms of gastroparesis or CUNV is unproved.

### Correlation of symptom responses to therapy with test findings

Retrospective reviews report that antroduodenal manometry can promote changes in treatment in less than 20% of patients with suspected dysmotility. One group of experts suggested that clinicians who perform antral and small bowel manometry in refractory patients with suspected gastroparesis use abnormal test results (including antral hypomotility) to direct treatment decisions to include initiation of jejunal feedings and placement of a gastrostomy for intermittent drainage.[65] However, in a study examining needs for long-term enteral feeding in gastroparesis, antroduodenal manometry findings were similar in those who initially required versus those who did not require jejunostomy placement.[41] WMC contractility and extragastric transit abnormalities have not been reported to correlate with symptom responses to therapies of suspected gastroparesis.

## Measurement of Sensory Perception

### Methods of testing

Heightened sensory perception of the upper gut in suspected gastroparesis is typically defined using barostat methods.[52] A highly compliant bag in the proximal stomach is inflated to predefined pressures which are maintained for set periods of time while the barostat measures volumes in the bag. During barostat bag inflation, the patient is asked to report discomfort on a standardized scale. This allows generation of both compliance curves measuring gastric wall stiffness and perceptual sensitivity to distention. Because of the uncomfortable nature of testing, clinical barostat methods to measure gastric sensation are offered in few centers worldwide. Others have documented increased chemosensitivity to capsaicin in functional dyspepsia in research settings, but clinical testing for chemical sensitivity are not routine.

### Correlation of symptoms with test findings

In 58 patients with idiopathic gastroparesis, hypersensitivity to gastric distention correlated with increased prevalence of epigastric pain, early satiety, and weight loss versus those with normal sensation.[52] In contrast, gastric emptying did not relate to symptoms in this small study. A larger barostat study in functional dyspepsia reported more prevalent hypersensitivity to distention in patients with predominant pain versus discomfort.[66] Another report in 8 patients with type 1 diabetes observed higher nausea, bloating, and epigastric pain during gastric distention compared with healthy volunteers.[67] However, all of these studies reported substantial overlap of symptoms and sensory findings.

### Correlation of symptom responses to therapy with test findings

There are no reports correlating heightened versus normal sensation to gastric distention with responses to any medication or nonmedication therapy for gastroparesis or CUNV.

## SUMMARY

Gastroparesis and CUNV present similarly with nausea, vomiting, and other upper gut symptoms, and are distinguished by the presence versus absence of delayed gastric emptying measured by one of several methods. Patients with suspected gastroparesis are managed by diverse therapies including prokinetic agents to stimulate gastric emptying and antiemetic or neuromodulator medications, which relieve symptoms by mechanisms unrelated to transit. Gastric emptying findings correlate weakly with symptoms and no specific symptom presentation reliably predicts delayed emptying, but there are emerging suggestions from the literature that emptying delays may offer prognostic information and possibly relate to responses to prokinetic treatments. Patients with gastroparesis symptoms exhibit other physiologic abnormalities including reduced phasic contractions of the stomach and small intestine, increased phasic and tonic pyloric activity, blunting of meal-induced gastric accommodation, dysrhythmias of the gastric slow wave, altered extragastric transit, and hypersensitivity to gastrointestinal stimulation. Testing can investigate each physiologic function, although some methods are infrequently used in patients with suspected gastroparesis. Early data suggest that pyloric EndoFLIP testing may offer prognostic information relating to benefits of pyloric therapies including botulinum toxin injection and G-POEM. Some accommodation tests detect abnormalities that seem to relate to slightly different symptom presentations than tests showing normal function. Nevertheless, more research is needed in large, multicenter patient cohorts before any clinical test of gastrointestinal physiology can be considered to reliably guide treatment decisions in suspected gastroparesis.

## DISCLOSURE

Dr W.L. Hasler has served as consultant for Shire Pharmaceuticals, Salix Pharmaceuticals, Nevro, Inc, and Allergan, Plc.

## REFERENCES

1. Lee AA, Rao S, Nguyen LA, et al. Validation of diagnostic and performance characteristics of the wireless motility capsule in patients with suspected gastroparesis. Clin Gastroenterol Hepatol 2019;17(9):1770–9.e2.
2. Pasricha PJ, Colvin R, Yates K, et al. Characteristics of patients with chronic unexplained nausea and vomiting and normal gastric emptying. Clin Gastroenterol Hepatol 2011;9:567–76.
3. Stanghellini V, Chan FK, Hasler WL, et al. Gastroduodenal disorders. Gastroenterology 2016;150:1380–92.
4. Parkman HP, Yates K, Hasler WL, et al. Clinical features of idiopathic gastroparesis vary with sex, body mass, symptom onset, delay in gastric emptying, and gastroparesis severity. Gastroenterology 2011;140:101–15.
5. Sturm A, Holtmann G, Goebell H, et al. Prokinetics in patients with gastroparesis: a systematic analysis. Digestion 1999;60:422–7.
6. Camilleri M, McCallum RW, Tack J, et al. Efficacy and safety of relamorelin in diabetics with symptoms of gastroparesis: a randomized, placebo-controlled study. Gastroenterology 2017;153:1240–50.
7. Carbone F, Rotondo A, Andrews CN, et al. A controlled cross-over trial shows benefit of prucalopride for symptom control and gastric emptying enhancement in idiopathic gastroparesis (abstract). Gastroenterology 2016;150:S213–4.
8. Abell T, Kuo B, Esfandyari T, et al. Velusetrag improves gastroparesis both in symptoms and gastric emptying in patients with diabetic or idiopathic gastropareis in a 12-week global phase 2B study (abstract). Gastroenterology 2019;156:S164.
9. Coleski R, Anderson MA, Hasler WL. Factors associated with symptom response to pyloric injection of botulinum toxin in a large series of gastroparesis patients. Dig Dis Sci 2009;54:2634–42.

10. Strong AT, Landreneau JP, Cline M, et al. Per-oral pyloromyotomy (POP) for medically refractory post-surgical gastroparesis. J Gastrointest Surg 2019;23: 1095–103.
11. Rodriguez J, Strong AT, Haskins IN, et al. Per-oral pyloromyotomy (POP) for medically refractory gastroparesis: short term results from the first 100 patients at a high volume center. Ann Surg 2018;268:421–30.
12. Meybodi MA, Qumseya BJ, Shakoor D, et al. Efficacy and feasibility of G-POEM in management of patients with refractory gastroparesis: a systematic review and meta-analysis. Endosc Int Open 2019;7:E322–9.
13. Mekaroonkamol P, Shah R, Cai Q. Outcomes of per oral endoscopic pyloromyotomy in gastroparesis worldwide. World J Gastroenterol 2019;25:909–22.
14. Friedenberg FK, Palit A, Parkman HP, et al. Botulinum toxin A for the treatment of delayed gastric emptying. Am J Gastroenterol 2008;103:416–23.
15. Arts J, Holvoet L, Caenepeel P, et al. Clinical trial: a randomized-controlled crossover study of intrapyloric injection of botulinum toxin in gastroparesis. Aliment Pharmacol Ther 2007;26:1251–8.
16. Zehetner J, Ravari F, Ayazi S, et al. Minimally invasive surgical approach for the treatment of gastroparesis. Surg Endosc 2013;27:61–7.
17. Simmons K, Parkman HP. Granisetron transdermal system improves refractory nausea and vomiting in gastroparesis. Dig Dis Sci 2014;59:1231–4.
18. Pasricha PJ, Yates KP, Sarosiek I, et al. Aprepitant has mixed effects on nausea and reduces other symptoms in patients with gastroparesis and related disorders. Gastroenterology 2018;154:65–76.
19. Parkman HP, Van Natta ML, Abell TL, et al. Effect of nortriptyline on symptoms of idiopathic gastroparesis: the NORIG randomized clinical trial. JAMA 2013;310: 2640–9.
20. Talley NJ, Locke GR, Saito YA, et al. Effect of amitriptyline and escitalopram on functional dyspepsia: a multicenter, randomized controlled study. Gastroenterology 2015;149:340–9.
21. Tack J, Carbone F. Functional dyspepsia and gastroparesis. Curr Opin Gastroenterol 2017;33:446–54.
22. Tack J, Janssen P, Masaoka T, et al. Efficacy of buspirone, a fundus-relaxing drug, in patients with functional dyspepsia. Clin Gastroenterol Hepatol 2012;10: 1239–45.
23. Miwa H, Nagahara A, Tominaga K, et al. Efficacy of the 5-HT$_{1A}$ agonist tandospirone citrate in improving symptoms of patients with functional dyspepsia: a randomized controlled trial. Am J Gastroenterol 2009;104:2779–87.
24. Abell T, McCallum R, Hocking M, et al. Gastric electrical stimulation for medically refractory gastroparesis. Gastroenterology 2003;125:421–8.
25. McCallum RW, Snape W, Brody F, et al. Gastric electrical stimulation with Enterra therapy improves symptoms from diabetic gastroparesis in a prospective study. Clin Gastroenterol Hepatol 2010;8:947–54.
26. McCallum RW, Sarosiek I, Parkman HP, et al. Gastric electrical stimulation with Enterra therapy improves symptoms of idiopathic gastroparesis. Neurogastroenterol Motil 2013;25. 815-e636.
27. Zoll B, Zhao H, Edwards MA, et al. Outcomes of surgical intervention for refractory gastroparesis: a systematic review. J Surg Res 2018;231:263–9.
28. Abell TL, Camilleri M, Donohoe K, et al. Consensus recommendations for gastric emptying scintigraphy: a joint report of the American Neurogastroenterology and Motility Society and the Society of Nuclear Medicine. Am J Gastroenterol 2008; 103:753–63.

29. Kuo B, McCallum RW, Koch KL, et al. Comparison of gastric emptying of a non-digestible capsule to a radio-labelled meal in healthy and gastroparetic subjects. Aliment Pharmacol Ther 2008;27:186–96.
30. Hasler WL, May KP, Wilson LA, et al. Relating gastric scintigraphy and symptoms to motility capsule transit and pressure findings in suspected gastroparesis. Neurogastroenterol Motil 2018;30:e13196.
31. Szarka LA, Camilleri M, Vella A, et al. A stable isotope breath test with a standard meal for abnormal gastric emptying of solids in the clinic and in research. Clin Gastroenterol Hepatol 2008;6:635–43.
32. Jacques J, Pagnon L, Hure F, et al. Peroral endoscopic pyloromyotomy is efficacious and safe for refractory gastroparesis: prospective trial with assessment of pyloric function. Endoscopy 2019;51:40–9.
33. Desai A, O'Connor M, Neja B, et al. Reproducibility of gastric emptying assessed with scintigraphy in patients with upper GI symptoms. Neurogastroenterol Motil 2018;30:e13365.
34. Vijayvargiya P, Jameie-Oskooei S, Camilleri M, et al. Association between delayed gastric emptying and upper gastrointestinal symptoms: a systematic review and meta-analysis. Gut 2019;68:804–13.
35. Hyett B, Martinez FJ, Gill BM, et al. Delayed radionucleotide gastric emptying studies predict morbidity in diabetics with symptoms of gastroparesis. Gastroenterology 2009;137:445–52.
36. Pasricha PJ, Yates KP, Nguyen L, et al. Outcomes and factors associated with reduced symptoms in patients with gastroparesis. Gastroenterology 2015;149:1762–74.
37. Hasler WL, Lee AA, McCallum RW, et al. Longitudinal symptom and quality of life outcomes in patients with suspected gastroparesis in relation to delays in gastric emptying and generalized gut transit: a prospective, multicenter evaluation (abstract). Gastroenterology 2018;154:S15.
38. Janssen P, Harris MS, Jones M, et al. The relation between symptom improvement and gastric emptying in the treatment of diabetic and idiopathic gastroparesis. Am J Gastroenterol 2013;108:1382–91.
39. Vijayvargiya P, Camilleri M, Chedid V, et al. Effects of promotility agents on gastric emptying and symptoms: a systematic review and meta-analysis. Gastroenterology 2019;156:1650–60.
40. Gonzalez JM, Benezech A, Vitton V, et al. G-POEM with antro-pyloromyotomy for the treatment of refractory gastroparesis: mid-term follow-up and factors predicting outcome. Aliment Pharmacol Ther 2017;46:364–70.
41. Strijbos D, Keszthelyi D, Smeets FG, et al. Therapeutic strategies in gastroparesis: results of stepwise approach with diet and prokinetics, gastric rest and PEG-J: a retrospective analysis. Neurogastroenterol Motil 2019;31:e13588.
42. Angeli TR, Cheng LK, Du P, et al. Loss of interstitial cells of Cajal and patterns of gastric dysrhythmias in patients with chronic unexplained nausea and vomiting. Gastroenterology 2015;149:56–66.
43. Mearin F, Camilleri M, Malagelada JR. Pyloric dysfunction in diabetics with recurrent nausea and vomiting. Gastroenterology 1986;90:1919–25.
44. Gourcerol G, Tissier F, Melchior C, et al. Impaired fasting pyloric compliance in gastroparesis and the therapeutic response to pyloric dilation. Aliment Pharmacol Ther 2014;41:360–7.
45. Saadi M, Yu D, Malik Z, et al. Pyloric sphincter characteristics using EndoFLIP in gastroparesis. Rev Gastroenterol Mex 2018;83:375–84.

46. Desprez C, Melchior C, Wuestenberghs F, et al. Pyloric distensibility measurement predicts symptomatic response to intrapyloric botulinum toxin injection. Gastrointest Endosc 2019;90(5):754–60.e1.

47. Janssen P, Verschueren S, Ly HG, et al. Intragastric pressure during food intake: a physiological and minimally invasive method to assess gastric accommodation. Neurogastroenterol Motil 2011;23:316–22.

48. Breen M, Camilleri M, Burton DD, et al. Performance characteristics of the measurement of gastric volume using single photon emission computed tomography. Neurogastroenterol Motil 2011;23:308–15.

49. Orthey P, Yu D, Van Natta ML, et al. Intragastric meal distribution during gastric emptying scintigraphy for assessment of fundic accommodation: correlation with symptoms of gastroparesis. J Nucl Med 2018;59:691–7.

50. Chedid V, Halawi H, Brandler J, et al. Gastric accommodation measurements by single photon emission computed tomography and two-dimensional scintigraphy in diabetic patients with upper gastrointestinal symptoms. Neurogastroenterol Motil 2019;31:e13581.

51. Park SY, Acosta A, Camilleri M, et al. Gastric motor dysfunction in patients with functional gastrointestinal symptoms. Am J Gastroenterol 2017;112:1689–99.

52. Karamanolis G, Caenepeel P, Arts J, et al. Determinants of symptom pattern in idiopathic severely delayed gastric emptying: gastric emptying rate or proximal stomach dysfunction? Gut 2007;56:29–36.

53. Lacy BE, Saito YA, Camilleri M, et al. Effects of antidepressants on gastric function in patients with functional dyspepsia. Am J Gastroenterol 2018;113:216–24.

54. Matsueda K, Hongo M, Tack J, et al. A placebo-controlled trial of acotiamide for meal-related symptoms of functional dyspepsia. Gut 2012;61:821–8.

55. O'Grady G, Angeli TR, Du P, et al. Abnormal initiation and conduction of slow-wave activity in gastroparesis, defined by high-resolution electrical mapping. Gastroenterology 2012;143:589–98.

56. Paskaranandavadivel N, Angeli TN, Manson T, et al. Multi-day, multi-sensor ambulatory monitoring of gastric electrical activity. Physiol Meas 2019;40:025011.

57. Gharibans AA, Coleman TP, Mousa H, et al. Spatial patterns from high-resolution electrogastrography correlate with severity of symptoms in patients with functional dyspepsia and gastroparesis. Clin Gastroenterol Hepatol 2019;17(13):2668–77.

58. Koch KL, Stern RM, Stewart WR, et al. Gastric emptying and gastric myoelectrical activity in patients with diabetic gastroparesis: effect of long-term domperidone treatment. Am J Gastroenterol 1989;84:1069–75.

59. Wellington J, Scott B, Kundu S, et al. Effect of endoscopic pyloric therapies for patients with nausea and vomiting and functional obstructive gastroparesis. Auton Neurosci 2017;202:56–61.

60. Zikos TA, Kamal AN, Neshatian L, et al. High prevalence of slow transit constipation in patients with gastroparesis. J Neurogastroenterol Motil 2019;25:267–75.

61. Camilleri M, Malagelada JR, Brown ML, et al. Relation between antral motility and gastric emptying of solids and liquids in humans. Am J Physiol 1985;249:G580–5.

62. Cogliandro RF, Rizzoli G, Bellacosa L, et al. Is gastroparesis a gastric disease? Neurogastroenterol Motil 2019;31:e13562.

63. Kloetzer L, Chey WD, McCallum RW, et al. Motility of the antroduodenum in healthy and gastroparetics characterized by wireless motility capsule. Neurogastroenterol Motil 2010;22:527–33.

64. Barshop K, Staller K, Semler J, et al. Duodenal rather than antral motility contractile parameters correlate with symptom severity in gastroparesis patients. Neurogastroenterol Motil 2015;27:339–46.
65. Camilleri M, Chedid V, Ford AC, et al. Gastroparesis. Nat Rev Dis Primers 2018; 4:41.
66. Karamanolis G, Caenepeel P, Arts J, et al. Association of the predominant symptom with clinical characteristics and pathophysiological mechanisms in functional dyspepsia. Gastroenterology 2006;130:296–303.
67. Samsom M, Salet GA, Roelofs JM, et al. Compliance of the proximal stomach and dyspeptic symptoms in patients with type 1 diabetes mellitus. Dig Dis Sci 1995; 40:2037–42.

# Endoscopic and Surgical Treatments for Gastroparesis
## What to Do and Whom to Treat?

Roman V. Petrov, MD[a],*, Charles T. Bakhos, MD[a],
Abbas E. Abbas, MD[a], Zubair Malik, MD[b], Henry P. Parkman, MD[b]

## KEYWORDS

- Gastroparesis • Gastric electrical stimulator • Gastric pacemaker • Pyloromyotomy
- Pyloroplasty • Gastric peroral endoscopic myotomy (GPOEM)
- Peroral pyloromyotomy (POP)

## KEY POINTS

- Failure of medical therapy for gastroparesis requires surgical or endoscopic intervention. Between multitude of treatment options available decision usually comes to gastric electrical stimulator versus pyloric intervention.
- Patients with predominant symptoms of nausea and vomiting benefit more from gastric electrical stimulation (GES) placement.
- Patient with severely delayed gastric emptying without severe nausea or vomiting proceed with pyloric intervention.
- Those with severely delayed gastric emptying and severe nausea and vomiting proceed with combined procedure—GES and pyloroplasty or pyloromyotomy.
- Endoscopic pyloric Botox injection is a temporizing intervention and enteral access tubes and gastrectomy are reserved for recalcitrant cases with failure of all previous interventions.

## INTRODUCTION

Gastroparesis is a complex chronic debilitating condition of gastric motility resulting in the delayed gastric emptying and symptoms of nausea, vomiting, early satiety, postprandial fullness, and abdominal pain, and gastroesophageal reflux disease (GERD) often leading to malnutrition and dehydration. Initial management of patients with gastroparesis focuses on the diet and lifestyle modification and medical therapy. In those

[a] Thoracic Medicine and Surgery, Lewis Katz School of Medicine at Temple University, 3401 N. Broad St, Suite C-501. Philadelphia, PA, 19140, USA; [b] Gastroenterology Medicine, Lewis Katz School of Medicine at Temple University. 3401 N. Broad St. Gi Section. Philadelphia, PA, 19140, USA
* Corresponding author.
*E-mail address:* Roman.Petrov@tuhs.temple.edu

Gastroenterol Clin N Am 49 (2020) 539–556
https://doi.org/10.1016/j.gtc.2020.04.008
0889-8553/20/© 2020 Elsevier Inc. All rights reserved.

who fail conservative management, there is no uniform way to handle further therapy. Patients with refractory gastroparesis, not responding to standard antiemetic and pro-kinetic agents or with side effects preventing their use need more complex and advanced management options. In one study of 110 patients with "refractory" gastro-paresis, 74% responded to use of another prokinetic agent and only 26% remained refractory to all prokinetic agents. These truly refractory patients underwent enteral or parenteral feedings and gastric electrical stimulation (GES) and some underwent gastrectomy. Poor responders to prokinetic agents include postgastrectomy patients, those with myopathic connective tissue disorders, type I diabetic patients with severely delayed gastric emptying, and patients with idiopathic gastroparesis with abdominal pain.[1]

An initial approach to refractory gastroparesis includes assessment of the severity of symptoms, the degree of delay of the gastric emptying, optimizing the patient's cur-rent therapy, and changing prokinetic agents.[2] Why some patients respond to one prokinetic agent and not another is uncertain. Different prokinetic agents have different mechanisms of action and the efficacy of most prokinetic agents diminishes with time. A "drug holiday," as used for L-dopa in Parkinson disease, can be used for prokinetic agents, especially erythromycin.

In patients who remain refractory to treatment, one may consider placement of a feeding jejunostomy and/or a venting gastrostomy. Other therapies might include in-jection of botulinum toxin into the pylorus, pyloromyotomy, and/or gastric electric stimulator (GES). Total parenteral nutrition (TPN), if used, should be limited and tem-porary because of the risk profile. Surgical gastrectomy should generally be discour-aged. Completion gastrectomy can be considered for selected patients with postsurgical gastroparesis.

## ENDOSCOPIC BOTOX PYLORIC THERAPY

Botulinum toxin is a potent inhibitor of neuromuscular transmission and has been used to treat spastic muscular disorders by local injection. Thus, endoscopic injection of botulinum toxin directly into the lower esophageal sphincter reduces pressure and im-proves symptoms in patients with achalasia.[3] Extrapolating success from the acha-lasia experience, several small case series of botulinum toxin injection into the pylorus demonstrated mild improvement in gastric emptying and a modest improve-ment in symptoms.[4–6] A subsequent, much larger case series of 63 patients with idio-pathic and diabetic gastroparesis demonstrated clinical response in 43% of patients with a median duration of 5 months. Notably, vomiting was associated with a lack of response to the Botox therapy.[7] In the large retrospective series of 179 patients with gastroparesis, clinical response was associated with a larger dose of the medication. Such, almost 77% of patient had a response to 200 Units of the toxin, whereas only 54% responded to 100 Units.[8] Results from placebo controlled trials have shown that although botulinum toxin injection into the pylorus may mildly improve gastric emptying, there is little difference in symptom improvement with botulinum toxin compared with placebo at 1 month.[9,10] Thus, botulinum toxin injection into the pylorus does not seem a viable long-term treatment option for patients with gastroparesis. In-surance coverage for botulinum toxin has become harder to obtain for gastroparesis, although it is often covered for achalasia and lower esophageal sphincter injection. In select patients, botulinum pyloric injections may temporize a patient for several months. It may also be used to assess response before pyloromyotomy: a positive clinical response to pyloric Botox injection may suggest better response to pyloromyotomy.[11]

## GASTRIC PERORAL ENDOSCOPIC MYOTOMY/PERORAL PYLOROMYOTOMY (GPOEM/POP)

Following the success of peroral endoscopic myotomy (POEM) for the treatment of achalasia, a similar procedure of the pyloric sphincter was introduced into clinical practice and reported in 2013 by Khashab and colleagues.[12] In the care of a 27-year-old female type I diabetic this new experimental procedure, named gastric POEM (GPOEM), was performed after failure of medical therapy and previous positive response to the pyloric stenting. Patient has responded favorably to this procedure and remained well at least 12 weeks after the intervention.[12] In a subsequent multi-center study of 30 patients with idiopathic, diabetic, and postsurgical gastroparesis the investigators observed clinical response in 86% of patients at the median follow-up of 5.5 months. Two patients had developed adverse events—capnoperitoneum and prepyloric ulcer.[13]

Because of its success (procedurally and clinically), the procedure has been enthusiastically adopted worldwide and emerging multiple reports continue to reflect positively on the outcomes. In the review article by Mekaroonkamol and colleagues[14] response rate to peroral pyloromyotomy from 12 published series ranged from 73% to 100%. A recent systematic review of 14 studies using GPOEM demonstrated pooled clinical symptom improvement rate of 88% with an intraoperative complication rate of 3%, thus demonstrating high efficacy with marginal risk.[15,16] In the investigators' experience, positive response to GPOEM procedure was more common in patients also responding to Botox injection previously.[11]

The technique of the procedure uses principles of the submucosal endoscopy, developed in the original POEM procedure (**Fig. 1**). Steps of the procedure include initial mucosal entry, submucosal tunneling, myotomy, and closure of the mucosotomy. GPOEM is technically a more challenging procedure compared with POEM due to looping of the scope in the stomach, curving of the tunnel over the pyloric muscle, field instability due to antral contraction, and difficulties in anatomic landmarking.[14] There is no consensus and standardization of the procedure regarding location, length, and depth of the myotomy. Initially procedure was more commonly performed on the anterior wall or greater curvature of the stomach. Location of the procedure on the lesser curvature was reported to have an advantage of the shorter scope length and potentially reduced looping in the stomach; shorter length of the tunnel; lesser probability of the tunnel deviation; and nondependent position with avoidance of food residue, secretions, and blood pooling.[17] Initial mucosal entry is performed after submucosal dyed saline injection and elevation of the mucosa. Depending on the planned closure type, mucosotomy is either performed longitudinally for clips closure or transversely for the OverStitch device closure.[18] After tunnel is created over the ridge of the pyloric sphincter, myotomy is performed to the subserosal layer. Although previously reported full-thickness myotomy is not routinely advocated, accidental full-thickness division is not considered a perforation and rarely requires additional attention other than a careful closure of the

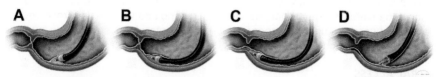

**Fig. 1.** Steps of the GPOEM procedure. (*A*) Initial mucosal entry—5 cm proximal to the pylorus on the greater curvature. (*B*) Dissection of the submucosal tunnel. (*C*) Pyloromyotomy. (*D*) Closure of the mucosotomy with the OverStitch device.

mucosotomy over the tunnel. Authors prefer closure with the suture technique for better seal of the mucosal entry.

## SURGICAL PYLOROMYOTOMY AND PYLOROPLASTY

Pyloromyotomy and pyloroplasty are well-established surgical procedures that have been applied for various indications for decades. With the minimally invasive revolution since the late 1980s, open procedures have been replaced by laparoscopic and, more recently, robotic interventions. Robotic technology provides better visualization of the stomach layers and better dexterity due to wrist motion and allows more precise dissection and preservation of the mucosal layer.[19,20] In the prospective survey of the 177 patients undergoing laparoscopic pyloroplasty as a sole treatment of the gastroparesis or in combination with antireflux surgery, 86% in total experienced improvement with 77%—complete normalization of the gastric emptying.[21] Nineteen patients (11%) required subsequent surgical interventions: gastric stimulator implantation (7%), feeding jejunostomy and/or gastrostomy tube (3%), or subtotal gastrectomy (2%). Symptom severity scores for nausea, vomiting, bloating, abdominal pain, and early satiety decreased significantly at 3 months.[21] In another report of 50 patients undergoing laparoscopic pyloroplasty for the treatment of gastroparesis, symptom improvement was observed in 82% of patients. Five patients (10%) underwent subsequent surgical interventions—gastrectomy (4%), duodenojejunostomy (4%), or gastric stimulator implantation (2%).[22] Similarly, Hibbard and colleagues in their analysis of 26 patients undergoing laparoscopic pyloroplasty for gastroparesis, reported normalization of gastric emptying in 71% with persistent significant improvement in symptoms nausea, vomiting, bloating, abdominal pain, and GERD.[23] In a systematic review of pyloric interventions, gastric stimulator implantation, and gastrectomy the investigators demonstrated overall greater response to pyloric intervention in refractory gastroparesis patients with the best outcomes in nausea and abdominal pain.[24]

Technique of laparoscopic pyloroplasty includes application of the silk stitch through the pylorus and careful division of the muscle with electrocautery hook over the stitch (**Fig. 2**). Once the fibers are divided over the stitch, the remaining fibers are carefully sought and severed until free bulging mucosa is exposed. Serosa is approximated in the transverse fashion with one silk stitch. If mucosal violation occurs, that we observe in about a half of all cases, procedure is converted to pyloroplasty with complete division of the mucosa and transverse Heineke-Mikulicz closure with running 3-0 absorbable V-Loc stitch. In these cases, closure is reinforced with omental flap to minimize the risk of leaks. In case of pyloroplasty, patient is often admitted for several days with nasogastric tube for stomach drainage to prevent stress on the closure and development of the leak. No drainage is performed in pyloromyotomy patients, and discharge is usually planned for the next day.

To facilitate dissection of the gastric wall layers, the investigators recently adopted saline injection technique from the authors' submucosal endoscopy experience. Ten milliliters of saline are injected into the area of pylorus that facilitates hydrodissection of gastric wall layers and preservation of the mucosa.

The investigators have strong preference for GPOEM as a pyloric intervention of choice in patients with gastroparesis. Surgical pyloric interventions are reserved for cases of concomitant surgical procedure in the patients with gastroparesis, such as antireflux surgery or gastric stimulator implantation or insurance denial of GPOEM.

## ENTERAL ACCESS

Enteral access in the treatment of refractory patient with severe gastroparesis serves 2 purposes—gastric venting, to alleviate nausea and vomiting and provide nutrition and

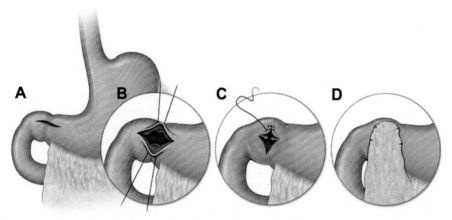

**Fig. 2.** Surgical pyloroplasty procedure. (*A*) Placement of the incisions across the pylorus. (*B*) Approximation of the defect in the transverse fashion. (*C*) Heineke-Mikulicz closure of the pyloroplasty incision. (*D*) Reinforcement of the closure with omental flap.

hydration. Placement of a gastrostomy tube for intermittent decompression by venting or suctioning may provide relief to the patient who has prominent abdominal distention. The gastrostomy tube can be opened for drainage or aspirated to decompress the stomach; this can be used when symptoms are distressing to alleviate nausea, pain, and bloating.[25] Venting gastrostomy tubes may be placed by the endoscopist, surgeon, or interventional radiologist. In an initial series, 6 of 8 patients were able to return to full-time work or school.[26] The percutaneous endoscopic gastrostomy tube can be converted to a button. Gastrostomy tubes are used much less now that refractory patients can be treated with GES; the gastrostomy tube may interfere with placement of the gastric stimulating electrodes.

Use of a gastrostomy tube for liquid feedings usually aggravates gastroparesis symptoms. For this reason, postpyloric feeding via jejunostomy is usually preferred. Transgastric dual channel gastrostomy-jejunostomy tubes can be used, allowing both feeding via jejunostomy and venting via gastrostomy.[27] However, the jejunostomy limb frequently regurgitates back into the stomach. To prevent this, the tip of the jejunostomy tube can be secured in the postpyloric position by deploying an endoclip to the duodenal mucosa.

Alternative is a direct feeding jejunostomy tubes that are effective for providing nutrition, hydration, and medications, provided that the small intestine is functioning.[28,29] Carefully regulated nutrient enteral infusion may allow better glucose control in diabetic patients whose glycemic control is otherwise poor due to vomiting and dehydration.[29] Jejunostomy tubes are usually inserted laparoscopically or at laparotomy; in some centers they are placed endoscopically.[30,31] Usually, a trial of nasoduodenal tube for feeding is used to test the ability of patient to tolerate nutrient infusions (volume, rate of infusion, and osmolality). Careful postoperative management of specifically the jejunostomy tubes is required, as they are prone to septic complications due to leaks and erosion (**Fig. 3**).[32] When starting jejunostomy feedings, one starts at a low rate (10 mL/h) and advances slowly to goal feeding rate.

## GASTRIC ELECTRICAL STIMULATION

There are several principles for electric stimulation of the stomach. First, in gastric electrical pacing the goal is to entrain and pace the gastric slow waves with low-frequency, high-energy, long-duration pulses. Pacing at 10% higher than the basal rate has been shown to accelerate gastric emptying and improve dyspeptic symptoms.[33] Second, stimulation with high-frequency, low-energy, short-duration pulses has been shown to decrease symptoms with little effect on gastric emptying; it may affect proximal stomach function and activate sensory afferent nerves to reduce symptoms.[34,35] Third, sequential muscle stimulation using bursts of supra-high frequency stimulation to induce direct gastric muscle contractions in a peristaltic sequence has accelerated emptying in animal studies.[36] Finally, sequential gastric neurostimulation has been used to entrain gastric slow waves. Preliminary open-label studies suggest that a hand-held cervical vagal stimulator may provide improvements in symptoms of gastroparesis.[37]

Enterra gastric electrical stimulator uses high-frequency GES at 12 cycles permi-nute and has received Food and Drug Administration humanitarian approval for treatment of chronic, refractory nausea and vomiting secondary to diabetic or idiopathic gastroparesis. Wires are placed into the gastric muscle at the greater curvature during laparoscopy or laparotomy. These leads are attached to an electric stimulator ("pacemaker"), which is placed in a subcutaneous abdominal pocket. An initial study demonstrated effectiveness in 20 of 26 patients with a decrease in nausea and vomiting and improvement in gastric emptying of liquids but not solids.[34] During long-term follow-up, 3 of 24 patients underwent total gastrectomy because of unsatisfactory results, and 3 had the stimulator removed because of erosion or infection. A subsequent study reported on 33 patients with chronic gastroparesis.[35] After implantation, the electrical stimulator was turned on or off in a randomized, double-blind, crossover design. Patients felt better when the stimulator was on, although the decrease in vomiting that occurred was not statistically significant. Long-term follow-up over 1 year showed a decrease in the vomiting frequency from 25 to 6 times per week, with an improvement in quality of life and mild improvement in gastric emptying. Complications were skin erosion and pocket infection in 3 patients and gastric wall perforation by the electrode in 1 patient, requiring removal of the device. One patient required revision of the device due to its migration.[35]

An open-label study in 25 patients reported an overall improvement from "severe" to "moderate" in symptoms of nausea and vomiting of 40%.[38] There was an infection rate of 15%, requiring removal of the stimulator. Studies suggest that the patients with diabetic gastroparesis with main symptoms of nausea and vomiting and not taking regular narcotic medications are the most likely to respond to Enterra therapy.[39] Subsequent studies in both diabetic and idiopathic gastroparesis, with blinded on and off periods of stimulation, did not show significant improvements in symptoms; however, a reduction of symptoms was seen with long-term open-label stimulation over 1 year.[40,41]

In one open-label study, using the Gastroparesis Cardinal Symptom Index (GCSI) to follow symptoms of gastroparesis, 29 patients underwent GES implantation over an 18-month period, with follow-up in 28 of the patients.[39] GES resulted in clinical improvement in 50% of patients with refractory gastroparesis. The overall GCSI significantly decreased with improvement in the nausea/vomiting and the postprandial subscore but no improvement in the bloating or abdominal pain subscore. The decrease in GCSI was greater for diabetic patients than idiopathic patients. Patients with main symptom of nausea/vomiting had a greater improvement than patients with abdominal pain. Patients taking narcotic analgesics at the time of implant had a poorer response compared with patients who were not. This study found 3 clinical parameters associated with a favorable clinical response to GES: (1) diabetic rather than idiopathic gastroparesis, (2) nausea/vomiting rather than abdominal pain as the primary symptom,

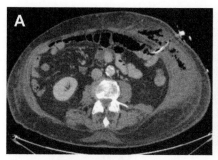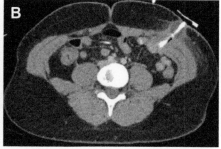

**Fig. 3.** Complication of jejunostomy tubes. (*A*) Early postoperative migration of the balloon into the abdominal wall with the leak and necrotizing fasciitis of the abdominal wall. (*B*) Late postoperative erosion of the balloon through the abdominal wall resulting in the leak and dermatitis.

and (3) independence from narcotic analgesics before stimulator implantation.[39] Knowledge of these 3 factors may allow improved patient selection for GES.

A large prospective study by Heckert and colleagues[42] details the magnitude and the pattern of improvement. Nausea, vomiting, loss of appetite, and early satiety improved significantly with stimulator use, with vomiting more improved in the diabetic cohort than idiopathic. Although GES improved symptoms in 75% of all patients, diabetic patients had a post-GES Clinical Patient Grading Assessment score statistically higher than did patients with idiopathic gastroparesis. This difference is thought to be due to the neuromolecular mechanism of diabetic gastroparesis, where blunting of the enteric nervous system may contribute to symptomatology.[42]

GES in gastroparesis was studied in a pragmatic open-label study of patients in the NIH Gastroparesis Registry.[43] In the prospectively collected database, 92 (14.5%) of patients initiated GES. Patients who underwent GES had more delayed gastric emptying at 4 hours (30.9% vs 21.8%) with worse GCSI scores (3.8 vs 3.0) before stimulator placement. After 48 weeks, GCSI scores in patients with GES improved by average of 0.9 compared with 0.3 in controls, with 43.6% showing improvement of at least 1 point compared with only 24.7% in controls. In this observational study in multiple practice settings, patients with more severe overall symptoms were more likely to improve symptomatically, primarily for nausea.[43]

A recent French study brings support for GES in a double-blind study, showing gastric stimulation leading to reduced nausea and vomiting, both in diabetic and nondiabetic patients and in both those with delayed and normal gastric emptying.[44]

### Surgical Technique

Implantation of GES procedure requires high level of precision for the best surgical outcomes (**Fig. 4**). Procedure includes implantation of 2 covered metal wires 1 cm apart into the muscular layer of the gastric wall 10 cm proximal to the pylorus on the greater curvature of the stomach. Wires are tunneled through the abdominal wall and connected to the pulse generator, placed in the subcutaneous pocket. The procedure can be performed via laparotomy, laparoscopy, and lately with robotic assistance. There is no consensus on the preferred technique of implantation of the generator. In the analysis of the 36 patients undergoing GES implantation postoperative LOS was 6.4 days for the laparotomy group and only 1.1 day for laparoscopy.[45] Long-term outcomes between 2 groups were comparable, although laparotomy group had higher vomiting scores and number of previous abdominal surgeries, suggesting

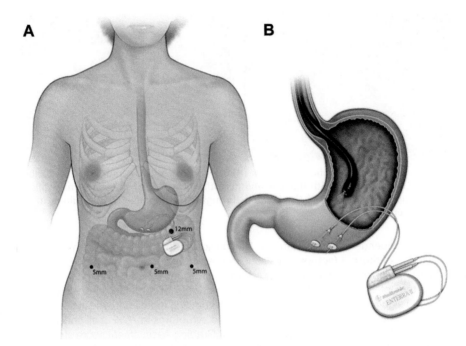

**Fig. 4.** Gastric electrical stimulator implantation procedure. (*A*) Placement of the stimulator in the subcutaneous pocket in the left subcostal area. (*B*) Intramural placement of the electrodes with direct visual control with intraoperative endoscopy.

higher preoperative morbidity as a group in whole. In another study, mini laparotomy (n = 128) had a shorter operative time (84.5 vs 137 min) and LOS (2.0 vs 3.0 days) over traditional 3-port laparoscopy (n = 37).[46] Robotic application for the implantation of the device has been recently reported.[47,48]

Likewise, there is no consensus on the location of the subcutaneous pocket for the positioning of the device generator. Technically, with the length of the leads of 35 cm, device can be located virtually in any aspect of the abdominal wall. The investigators' strong preference is to locate the device in left subcostal area, right over the site of implantation at the greater curvature of the stomach(**Fig. 5**). This location allows to maximally pull the wires out of the abdominal cavity, minimizing intrabdominal course of the leads and decreasing the risk of wire-associated complications.[49]

### Complications of Gastric Electrical Stimulation

Bielefeldt reported on 1587 adverse events related to the gastric electrical stimulator from Manufacturer and User Device Experience databank from January 2001 to October 2015.[50]

### Skin erosion, wound dehiscence

This is one of the most common reported complications. Skin erosion and wound dehiscence may be related to superficial placement or inadequate securing of the device to the fascia ( **Fig. 6**A). Abscess can develop as a seeding of the hematoma or seroma postoperatively or may be a sign of lead erosion into the lumen, tracking along the leads into subcutaneous tissue. Direct contamination of the device can occur by insulin injection or glucose-monitoring device needles. Infected device cannot be

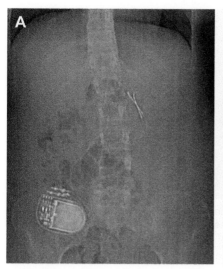
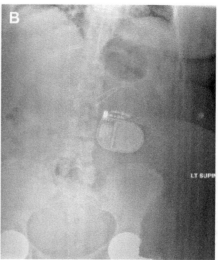

**Fig. 5.** Different location of the device in the abdominal wall. (*A*) Right lower quadrant location with long intraabdominal course of the leads. (*B*) Left subcostal area location with very short intraabdominal length of the wires with the majority coiled over the fascia under the device. (*Reprinted with permission* from Frontline Medical Communications Inc., publisher of the Journal of Clinical Outcomes Management; 2019; 26(1):31–32. All rights reserved.)

salvaged and requires explantation. Another implantation of a new device can be attempted once all wound issues resolve.

### Device migration, flipping, and twiddler syndrome

Malposition of the device likely occurs due to inadequate device fixation to the underlying fascia or erosion of the sutures. Occasionally, this may be a result of patients constantly picking and manipulating the device a condition known as Twiddler's syndrome. (**Fig. 7**).[51] Unless symptomatic, device migration can be observed. In case of flipping, there might be difficulties in communicating with the device, requiring its repositioning. Twiddler syndrome can lead to twisting, bradding, and fracture of the wires and requires repositioning. Although approved only for cardiac pacemakers,

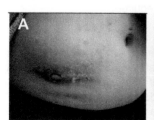
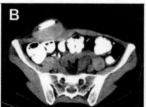
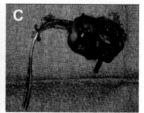

**Fig. 6.** Complications of the gastric electrical stimulator. (*A*) Erosion of the device through the skin. (*B*) Postoperative hematoma.(*C*) Specimen of resected segment of the gastric wall due to erosion of the GES lead component (please note silicone retention disk protruding through the mucosa). (*Reprinted with permission from* Frontline Medical Communications Inc., publisher of the Journal of Clinical Outcomes Management; 2019; 26(1):31-32. All rights reserved.)

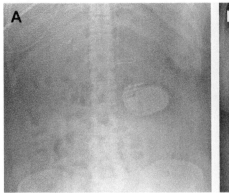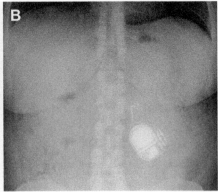

**Fig. 7.** Twiddler syndrome. (*A*) Postoperative image after implantation of the GES. (*B*) The same patient 11 month postoperatively. Patient returned with recurrence of symptoms and image reveals flipped device with braided leads.

off-label use of TYRX antibiotic envelope (**Fig. 8**) can potentially facilitate better device fixation to prevent this occurrence.

### Perforation and erosion of the leads

Very seldom leads can erode into the stomach (**Fig. 6**C). Usually it is associated with the loss of the device function. Endoscopy confirms the finding. In rare cases, infection can track along the lead and present as an infection at subcutaneous pocket. This complication requires explantation of the leads and the device with planned repeat placement after all infection resolves.

### Intestinal obstruction

Positioning the device in the left upper quadrant minimizes intraabdominal length of the leads, decreasing risk of lead-associated complications. In other locations long intraabdominal length of the leads can predispose to various complications. Although rare, the intestines can wrap around the leads of the device, causing different degree of obstruction (**Fig. 9**A, B). In case of surgical intervention for obstruction, all efforts are made to preserve the stimulator leads as damage will require re-impantation of the whole system at a later date. (**Fig. 9**C). In cases of bowel resection, lead contamination is a serious concern; however, lead explantation is not mandatory. Close postoperative monitoring for the development of lead infection is required.

### Hematoma and seroma

Postoperative hematomas can occur from inadequate hemostasis (**Fig. 6**B). Seromas frequently occur in the stimulator pocket as a reactive effusion to the trauma and a foreign body. They can be observed until full resolution if small and not complicated. In cases of large hematomas with skin compromise or dehiscence, prompt washout and drainage is required. In ideal cases, the device can be salvaged. Relocation to another site might be required if skin necrosis develops increasing risk of device contamination.

### Incisional hernia

Hernias can develop after any abdominal surgery and as such are not unique to device. Minimally invasive technique of the GES implantation minimizes this complication.

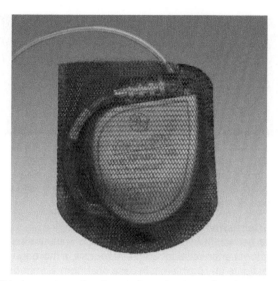

**Fig. 8.** TYRX antibiotic envelope for the cardiac stimulator. (Medtronic, Minneapolis, MN, USA.)

### Electric shock sensations

Shocks may occur from damage of the plastic lining of the device wires or from fluid buildup around the insertion of the wires into the stimulator. This can also happen from shortening of the leads to the muscles of the abdominal wall. Patients describe periodic muscle cramps with the frequency of the device impulses (every 5 seconds). The investigators successfully used omental flap coverage of the freshly implanted leads to isolate them from the abdominal wall (**Fig. 10**).[49] In patients who continue to feel shocks despite all efforts, the possibility of visceral hypersensitivity should be considered. A trial of nortriptyline for symptoms modulation and lowering of the output

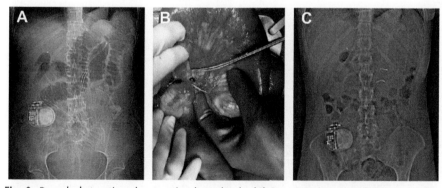

**Fig. 9.** Bowel obstruction due to stimulator leads. (*A*) Preoperative scout image revealing high-grade bowel obstruction and stimulator leads. (*B*) Intraoperative image of the same patient, demonstrating loops of bowels wrapped around the leads. Leads were preserved. (*C*) Postoperative image of another patient after laparotomy for bowel obstruction where leads were sacrificed. (*Reprinted with permission* from Frontline Medical Communications Inc., publisher of the Journal of Clinical Outcomes Management; 2019; 26(1):31–32. All rights reserved.)

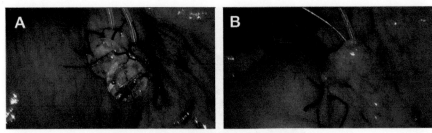

**Fig. 10.** Placement of gastric stimulator leads. (*A*) Fixation of the leads in the muscular layer of the gastric wall. (*B*) Omental flap coverage of the implanted leads.

current can be undertaken. If nothing works, the device will have to be turned off for a time period, occasionally requiring explantation.

### Lack of effect/persistent symptoms

When a patient has persistent symptoms after device implantation (no response) or recurrence of symptoms after initial favorable response, a thorough workup is undertaken aimed to investigate any problems. In case of abnormal impedance values, plain abdominal radiography can be performed to rule out leads migration or fracture (**Fig. 11**). If no abnormalities are detected, the output of the device can be turned up. After adjusting device settings, at least 1- to 3-month period is undertaken to assure any improvement. One report suggests repositioning the stimulator leads on the gastric wall in patients not responding to GES.[52]

### COMBINATION OF GASTRIC ELECTRICAL STIMULATION AND PYLOROMYOTOMY

Recently, the combination of GES with pyloric intervention procedure has been introduced in the clinical practice. Initial concerns of the device contamination have dissipated after several favorable reports. In the group of 49 patients with 26 receiving combined GES with pyloroplasty procedure, significant improvement in total

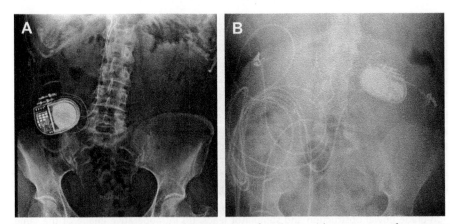

**Fig. 11.** Abdominal imaging in the investigation of patients with recurrence of symptoms and abnormal impedance values. (*A*) Fracture of the lead along the medial border of the device. (*B*) Migration of the lead. Please note wide spaced distance between the leads and lack of association of the medial lead with retention clips. (*Reprinted with permission from* Frontline Medical Communications Inc., publisher of the Journal of Clinical Outcomes Management; 2019; 26(1):31–32. All rights reserved.)

symptom score was observed. However, improved gastric emptying time was seen by 64% at 4 hours in combined procedure, whereas in GES-alone therapy only modest 7% improvement was observed.[53] In the analysis of long-term efficacy of combined GES and pyloroplasty procedure in 24 patients, 71% improvement in total symptom score at follow-up between 3 and 38 months (mean 17 months), with significant improvement in gastric emptying times and normalization in 60% of patients.[48] Patients with refractory symptoms of gastroparesis undergoing stimulator placement, pyloromyotomy, or combined stimulator with pyloromyotomy each have improvement of their gastroparesis symptoms in open-label studies.[54] Gastric stimulation and combined stimulator with pyloromyotomy improved nausea/vomiting, whereas pyloromyotomy alone tended to improve early satiety and postprandial fullness.[24]

## GASTRECTOMY

Gastrectomy is a morbid and invasive procedure regardless of the approach (open or minimally invasive) and usually regarded as a last resort intervention in the care of gastroparesis patients. The outcomes of surgical gastric resection for the treatment of idiopathic and diabetic gastroparesis has generally been disappointing.[55]

For selected patients with refractory postsurgical gastroparesis, usually due to vagotomy, in whom medical therapy has failed, subtotal gastrectomy may occasionally be considered. In the report of 40 patients (32 postvagotomy, 6 idiopathic, and 2 diabetic), a subtotal or a near-total gastrectomy with Roux-Y reconstruction was performed. Twenty-two patients (56%) had moderate response to resection with improvements in their symptoms.[56] In a series of 62 patients who underwent completion gastrectomy for severe postvagotomy gastric stasis, good symptomatic improvement in nausea, vomiting, and postprandial abdominal pain was obtained in only 43%. There was no improvement in chronic pain, diarrhea, or dumping syndrome. The combination of nausea, need for TPN, and retained food at endoscopy predicted a poor outcome.[57] In another series of 81 patients with severe postsurgical gastroparesis, near-complete gastrectomy with a 55-cm Roux-en-Y reconstruction was performed. Follow-up averaged 56 months for 52 patients; 78% reported improvement of their gastrointestinal symptoms, 7% believed that there was no change, and 15% stated that their condition had worsened. A subtotal (70%) gastrectomy with resection of the antrum and pylorus, closure of the duodenum, and restoration of GI continuity with a 60-cm Roux-en-Y jejunal loop was reported in 4 patients with insulin-dependent diabetes with intractable vomiting from gastroparesis.[58] In total, 3 of the 4 patients did well, eliminating frequent hospital admissions.

In the analysis of 35 patients (43% postoperative, 34% idiopathic, and 23% diabetic) undergoing near-total gastrectomy different symptoms improved in 70% to 89% of patients. Six patients suffered postoperative leak, requiring reintervention. There were no postoperative mortalities.[59] Landreneau and colleagues[60] reported on the 53 patients undergoing Roux-Y reconstruction for the treatment of gastroparesis with either gastrectomy (27 patients) or stomach left in situ ( similar to gastric bypass) (26 patients). Patients had similar symptom response to intervention. Gastrectomy patients required longer operative times (223 vs 155 min), longer hospital stay (7 vs 4 days), and experienced higher rate of postoperative complications (44% vs 8%). However, patients with retained stomach were more likely to require subsequent surgical interventions (23% vs 4%), suggesting that gastrectomy may be a more definitive procedure for the treatment of gastroparesis.[60] Recent report on sleeve gastrectomy in 19 gastroparesis patients suggests good response with improvement in Barium Emptying Radiography Index and Gastrointestinal Quality of Life Index.[61]

## DECISION-MAKING FOR SURGICAL TREATMENTS

With the array of the endoscopic and surgical options for the management of patients with refractory gastroparesis, it is frequently difficult to decide on the best course of action and sequence of intervention (**Fig. 12**). At the authors' institution, we offer patients each of the treatments discussed in this article. As described earlier, the authors reserve gastrectomy for the "end of the road situations" where no other intervention has proved helpful.

Botox pyloric injection is considered a temporizing intervention and the authors use it sparingly to bridge patient until more definitive intervention is performed, which is sometimes delayed by the insurance approval process. Occasionally, we use Botox injection to see if the patient is more likely to respond to surgical or endoscopic pyloromyotomy.

Enteral access is also reserved to refractory patients in whom pyloric intervention and or GES implantation has not produced the desired effect, and patient continues to lose weight, remains TPN dependent for nutritional support and hydration, or requires gastric venting for uncontrolled nausea and vomiting.

In most cases, the decision comes to either gastric stimulator or pyloromyotomy, and / or combination of both. Patients with contraindications to GES implantation (anticipated need for MRI, lack of insurance coverage, patient preference, or abdominal wall infection, precluding safe implant) are offered pyloric intervention, preferably GPOEM or surgical pyloromyotomy or pyloroplasty as a backup. In patients with severe and predominant symptoms of nausea and vomiting we proceed with GES. In patients with significantly delayed gastric emptying in the absence of severe nausea and vomiting, the authors' preferred intervention is endoscopic pyloromyotomy. If patients have significant nausea and vomiting with markedly delayed gastric emptying, patients often undergo a combined stimulator placement with surgical pyloromyotomy or pyloroplasty. Those patents who had undergone one of the procedures—either GES implantation or pyloric interventions—and remain symptomatic later can

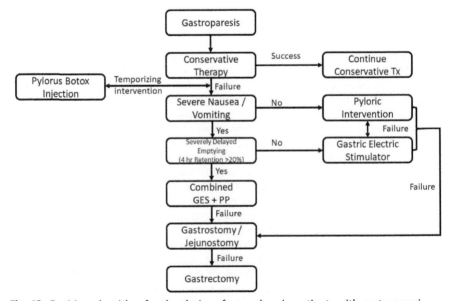

**Fig. 12.** Decision algorithm for the choice of procedure in patients with gastroparesis.

crossover and undergo the other procedure, essentially ending up with the combined intervention in the sequential fashion.

In patients who remain refractory to treatment, placement of a feeding jejunostomy or a venting gastrostomy may be considered. TPN, if used, should be limited and temporary because of the risk profile. Surgical gastrectomy should generally be discouraged and reserved for selected patients with postsurgical gastroparesis.

Studies are currently being performed to evaluate this type of patient-oriented approach—selecting between pyloric intervention and GES.

## DISCLOSURE

Funded by: NIHHYB. Grant number(s): NIH/NCI Cancer Center Support Grant P30 CA006927. NIHMS-ID: 1591505.

## REFERENCES

1. Soykan I, Sivri B, Sarosiek I, et al. Demography, clinical characteristics, psychological and abuse profiles, treatment, and long-term follow-up of patients with gastroparesis. Dig Dis Sci 1998;43(11):2398–404.
2. Rabine JC, Barnett JL. Management of the patient with gastroparesis. J Clin Gastroenterol 2001;32(1):11–8.
3. Pasricha PJ, Ravich WJ, Hendrix TR, et al. Intrasphincteric botulinum toxin for the treatment of achalasia. N Engl J Med 1995;332(12):774–8.
4. Miller LS, Szych GA, Kantor SB, et al. Treatment of idiopathic gastroparesis with injection of botulinum toxin into the pyloric sphincter muscle. Am J Gastroenterol 2002;97(7):1653–60.
5. Lacy BE, Crowell MD, Schettler-Duncan A, et al. The treatment of diabetic gastroparesis with botulinum toxin injection of the pylorus. Diabetes Care 2004;27(10): 2341–7.
6. Ezzeddine D, Jit R, Katz N, et al. Pyloric injection of botulinum toxin for treatment of diabetic gastroparesis. Gastrointest Endosc 2002;55(7):920–3.
7. Bromer MQ, Friedenberg F, Miller LS, et al. Endoscopic pyloric injection of botulinum toxin A for the treatment of refractory gastroparesis. Gastrointest Endosc 2005;61(7):833–9.
8. Coleski R, Anderson MA, Hasler WL. Factors associated with symptom response to pyloric injection of botulinum toxin in a large series of gastroparesis patients. Dig Dis Sci 2009;54(12):2634–42.
9. Arts J, Holvoet L, Caenepeel P, et al. Clinical trial: a randomized-controlled crossover study of intrapyloric injection of botulinum toxin in gastroparesis. Aliment Pharmacol Ther 2007;26(9):1251–8.
10. Friedenberg FK, Palit A, Parkman HP, et al. Botulinum toxin A for the treatment of delayed gastric emptying. Am J Gastroenterol 2008;103(2):416–23.
11. Malik Z, Kataria R, Modayil R, et al. Gastric per oral endoscopic myotomy (G-POEM) for the treatment of refractory gastroparesis: early experience. Dig Dis Sci 2018;63(9):2405–12.
12. Khashab MA, Stein E, Clarke JO, et al. Gastric peroral endoscopic myotomy for refractory gastroparesis: first human endoscopic pyloromyotomy (with video). Gastrointest Endosc 2013;78(5):764–8.
13. Khashab MA, Ngamruengphong S, Carr-Locke D, et al. Gastric per-oral endoscopic myotomy for refractory gastroparesis: results from the first multicenter study on endoscopic pyloromyotomy (with video). Gastrointest Endosc 2017; 85(1):123–8.

14. Mekaroonkamol P, Shah R, Cai Q. Outcomes of per oral endoscopic pyloromyotomy in gastroparesis worldwide. World J Gastroenterol 2019;25(8):909–22.

15. Spadaccini M, Maselli R, Chandrasekar VT, et al. Gastric peroral endoscopic pyloromyotomy for refractory gastroparesis: a systematic review of early outcomes with pooled analysis. Gastrointest Endosc 2019;91(4):746–52.e5.

16. Mohan BP, Chandan S, Jha LK, et al. Clinical efficacy of gastric per-oral endoscopic myotomy (G-POEM) in the treatment of refractory gastroparesis and predictors of outcomes: a systematic review and meta-analysis using surgical pyloroplasty as a comparator group. Surg Endosc 2019. https://doi.org/10.1007/s00464-019-07135-9.

17. Allemang MT, Strong AT, Haskins IN, et al. How I Do It: Per-Oral Pyloromyotomy (POP). J Gastrointest Surg 2017;21(11):1963–8.

18. Chung H, Khashab MA. Gastric peroral endoscopic myotomy. Clin Endosc 2018; 51(1):28–32.

19. Petrov R, Bakhos C, Abbas A. Robotic esophagectomy. In: Tsuda S, Kudsi OY, editors. Robotic-assisted minimally invasive surgery. Switzerland: Springer Nature; 2019. p. 277–93.

20. Petrov RV, Bakhos CT, Abbas AE. Robotic substernal esophageal bypass and reconstruction with gastric conduit-frequently overlooked minimally invasive option. J Vis Surg 2019;5. https://doi.org/10.21037/jovs.2019.04.02.

21. Shada AL, Dunst CM, Pescarus R, et al. Laparoscopic pyloroplasty is a safe and effective first-line surgical therapy for refractory gastroparesis. Surg Endosc 2016;30(4):1326–32.

22. Toro JP, Lytle NW, Patel AD, et al. Efficacy of laparoscopic pyloroplasty for the treatment of gastroparesis. J Am Coll Surg 2014;218(4):652–60.

23. Hibbard ML, Dunst CM, Swanstrom LL. Laparoscopic and endoscopic pyloroplasty for gastroparesis results in sustained symptom improvement. J Gastrointest Surg 2011;15(9):1513–9.

24. Zoll B, Zhao H, Edwards MA, et al. Outcomes of surgical intervention for refractory gastroparesis: a systematic review. J Surg Res 2018;231:263–9.

25. Borrazzo EC. Surgical management of gastroparesis: gastrostomy/jejunostomy tubes, gastrectomy, pyloroplasty, gastric electrical stimulation. J Gastrointest Surg 2013;17(9):1559–61.

26. Kim CH, Nelson DK. Venting percutaneous gastrostomy in the treatment of refractory idiopathic gastroparesis. Gastrointest Endosc 1998;47(1):67–70.

27. Toh Yoon EW, Yoneda K, Nakamura S, et al. Percutaneous endoscopic transgastric jejunostomy (PEG-J): a retrospective analysis on its utility in maintaining enteral nutrition after unsuccessful gastric feeding. BMJ Open Gastroenterol 2016;3(1):e000098.

28. Fontana RJ, Barnett JL. Jejunostomy tube placement in refractory diabetic gastroparesis: a retrospective review. Am J Gastroenterol 1996;91(10):2174–8.

29. Jacober SJ, Narayan A, Strodel WE, et al. Jejunostomy feeding in the management of gastroparesis diabeticorum. Diabetes Care 1986;9(2):217–9.

30. Hotokezaka M, Adams RB, Miller AD, et al. Laparoscopic percutaneous jejunostomy for long term enteral access. Surg Endosc 1996;10(10):1008–11.

31. Bakhos C, Patel S, Petrov R, et al. Jejunostomy-technique and controversies. J Vis Surg 2019;5. https://doi.org/10.21037/jovs.2019.03.15.

32. Choi AH, O'Leary MP, Merchant SJ, et al. Complications of Feeding Jejunostomy Tubes in Patients with Gastroesophageal Cancer. J Gastrointest Surg 2017;21(2): 259–65.

33. McCallum RW, Chen JD, Lin Z, et al. Gastric pacing improves emptying and symptoms in patients with gastroparesis. Gastroenterology 1998;114(3):456–61.
34. Abell TL, Van Cutsem E, Abrahamsson H, et al. Gastric electrical stimulation in intractable symptomatic gastroparesis. Digestion 2002;66(4):204–12.
35. Abell T, McCallum R, Hocking M, et al. Gastric electrical stimulation for medically refractory gastroparesis. Gastroenterology 2003;125(2):421–8.
36. Mintchev MP, Sanmiguel CP, Amaris M, et al. Microprocessor-controlled movement of solid gastric content using sequential neural electrical stimulation. Gastroenterology 2000;118(2):258–63.
37. Gottfried-Blackmore A, Adler EP, Fernandez-Becker N, et al. Open-label pilot study: Non-invasive vagal nerve stimulation improves symptoms and gastric emptying in patients with idiopathic gastroparesis. Neurogastroenterol Motil 2020;32(4):e13769.
38. Forster J, Sarosiek I, Delcore R, et al. Gastric pacing is a new surgical treatment for gastroparesis. Am J Surg 2001;182(6):676–81.
39. Maranki JL, Lytes V, Meilahn JE, et al. Predictive factors for clinical improvement with Enterra gastric electric stimulation treatment for refractory gastroparesis. Dig Dis Sci 2008;53(8):2072–8.
40. McCallum RW, Snape W, Brody F, et al. Gastric electrical stimulation with Enterra therapy improves symptoms from diabetic gastroparesis in a prospective study. Clin Gastroenterol Hepatol 2010;8(11):947–54 [quiz: e116].
41. McCallum RW, Sarosiek I, Parkman HP, et al. Gastric electrical stimulation with Enterra therapy improves symptoms of idiopathic gastroparesis. Neurogastroenterol Motil 2013;25(10). 815-e636.
42. Heckert J, Sankineni A, Hughes WB, et al. Gastric electric stimulation for refractory gastroparesis: a prospective analysis of 151 patients at a single center. Dig Dis Sci 2016;61(1):168–75.
43. Abell TL, Yamada G, McCallum RW, et al. Effectiveness of gastric electrical stimulation in gastroparesis: Results from a large prospectively collected database of national gastroparesis registries. Neurogastroenterol Motil 2019;31(12):e13714.
44. Ducrotte P, Coffin B, Bonaz B, et al. Gastric electrical stimulation reduces refractory vomiting in a randomized crossover trial. Gastroenterology 2020;158(3):506–14.e2.
45. Al-Juburi A, Granger S, Barnes J, et al. Laparoscopy shortens length of stay in patients with gastric electrical stimulators. JSLS 2005;9(3):305–10.
46. Smith A, Cacchione R, Miller E, et al. Mini-laparotomy with adjunctive care versus laparoscopy for placement of gastric electrical stimulation. Am Surg 2016;82(4):337–42.
47. Mowzoon M, Macedo FIB, Kaur J, et al. Effectiveness and feasibility of robotic gastric neurostimulator placement in patients with refractory gastroparesis. J Robot Surg 2018;12(2):303–10.
48. Davis BR, Sarosiek I, Bashashati M, et al. The long-term efficacy and safety of pyloroplasty combined with gastric electrical stimulation therapy in gastroparesis. J Gastrointest Surg 2017;21(2):222–7.
49. Zoll B, Jehangir A, Malik Z, et al. Gastric electric stimulation for refractory gastroparesis. J Clin Outcomes Manag 2019;26(1):27–38.
50. Bielefeldt K. Adverse events of gastric electrical stimulators recorded in the Manufacturer and User Device Experience (MAUDE) Registry. Auton Neurosci 2017;202:40–4.
51. Higuchi S, Shoda M, Satomi N, et al. Unique abdominal twiddler syndrome. J Arrhythm 2019;35(1):142–4.

52. Harrison NS, Williams PA, Walker MR, et al. Evaluation and treatment of gastric stimulator failure in patients with gastroparesis. Surg Innov 2014;21(3):244–9.

53. Sarosiek I, Forster J, Lin Z, et al. The addition of pyloroplasty as a new surgical approach to enhance effectiveness of gastric electrical stimulation therapy in patients with gastroparesis. Neurogastroenterol Motil 2013;25(2). 134-e80.

54. Zoll B, Jehangir A, Edwards MA, et al. Surgical treatment for refractory gastroparesis: stimulator, pyloric surgery, or both? J Gastrointest Surg 2019. https://doi.org/10.1007/s11605-019-04391-x.

55. Quigley EM, Hasler WL, Parkman HP. AGA technical review on nausea and vomiting. Gastroenterology 2001;120(1):263–86.

56. Karlstrom L, Kelly KA. Roux-Y gastrectomy for chronic gastric atony. Am J Surg 1989;157(1):44–9.

57. Forstner-Barthell AW, Murr MM, Nitecki S, et al. Near-total completion gastrectomy for severe postvagotomy gastric stasis: analysis of early and long-term results in 62 patients. J Gastrointest Surg 1999;3(1):15–21 [discussion: 21–3].

58. Ejskjaer NT, Bradley JL, Buxton-Thomas MS, et al. Novel surgical treatment and gastric pathology in diabetic gastroparesis. Diabet Med 1999;16(6):488–95.

59. Bhayani NH, Sharata AM, Dunst CM, et al. End of the road for a dysfunctional end organ: laparoscopic gastrectomy for refractory gastroparesis. J Gastrointest Surg 2015;19(3):411–7.

60. Landreneau JP, Strong AT, El-Hayek K, et al. Gastrectomy versus stomach left in situ with Roux-en-Y reconstruction for the treatment of gastroparesis. Surg Endosc 2019;34(4):1847–55.

61. Lee AM, Fuchs KH, Varga G, et al. Sleeve gastrectomy for treatment of delayed gastric emptying-indications, technique, and results. Langenbecks Arch Surg 2020;405(1):107–16.

# Gastric Biopsies in Gastroparesis

## Insights into Gastric Neuromuscular Disorders to Aid Treatment

Lakshmikanth L. Chikkamenahalli, PhD[a,b],
Pankaj J. Pasricha, MBBS, MD[c], Gianrico Farrugia, MD[a,b],
Madhusudan Grover, MBBS[a,b,*]

### KEYWORDS

• Gastric emptying • Immune cells • Enteric nervous system • Diabetes

### KEY POINTS

- Insulinopenic hyperglycemic animal models have provided significant insight into the pathophysiology of diabetic gastroparesis. Interstitial cells of Cajal (ICC) loss or damage is the key cellular abnormality leading to delay in gastric emptying in gastroparesis.
- A macrophage-based immune dysregulation leading to injury to ICC and other components of ENS is emerging as an important precursor step in the pathophysiology of gastroparesis.
- Full-thickness gastric biopsies obtained from patients in the NIDDK Gastroparesis Clinical Research Consortium (GpCRC) have been instrumental in delineating disease mechanisms and corroborating hypotheses generated in preclinical models.
- Future strategies using minimally invasive methodologies for tissue procurement and use of systems biology approaches will help in identifying targets for diagnosis, prognosis, and treatment of diseases associated with abnormal gastric function.

## INTRODUCTION

Gastroparesis is a chronic disorder of the upper gastrointestinal (GI) tract characterized by delayed gastric emptying of solids and/or liquids in the absence of mechanical obstruction of the gastric outlet.[1,2] The signs and symptoms include nausea, vomiting,

[a] Enteric NeuroScience Program, Division of Gastroenterology and Hepatology, Mayo Clinic, 200 1st Street Southwest, Rochester, MN 55905, USA; [b] Division of Physiology and Biomedical Engineering, Mayo Clinic, 200 1st Street Southwest, Rochester, MN 55905, USA; [c] Division of Gastroenterology and Hepatology, Center for Neurogastroenterology, Johns Hopkins School of Medicine, Ross 958, 720 Rutland Avenue, Baltimore, MD 21205, USA
* Corresponding author. Enteric NeuroScience Program, Division of Gastroenterology and Hepatology, Mayo Clinic, 200 1st Street Southwest, Rochester, MN 55905, USA.
E-mail address: grover.madhusudan@mayo.edu

Gastroenterol Clin N Am 49 (2020) 557–570
https://doi.org/10.1016/j.gtc.2020.04.009
0889-8553/20/© 2020 Elsevier Inc. All rights reserved.

abdominal pain, early satiety, and postprandial fullness,[3] which result in significant impairment of quality of life and high health care expenditures.[4]

In 1 study, diabetic gastroparesis (DG) accounted for 29% patients, and gastroparesis acquired after a surgery (postsurgical gastroparesis) accounted for 13% of the cases.[3] An unknown primary cause or idiopathic gastroparesis (IG) accounts for greater than 50% of patients.[3,5] Other etiologies include connective tissue disorders, end-stage renal disease, Parkinson disease, or medication-induced.[3,6] An epidemiologic survey by Jung and colleagues[6] shows the incidence of definite gastroparesis ranging from 6.3 to 17.2 cases per 100,000 persons in an age- and gender-adjusted population, and a 4-fold higher prevalence of gastroparesis was observed in women when compared with men, although other estimates suggest a considerably higher prevalence.

Gastric emptying is considered to be abnormal/delayed when greater than 60% of administered contents are retained at 2 hours and/or greater than 10% at 4 hours on a solid meal gastric scintigraphy.[7] Ongoing research in gastroparesis using human gastric biopsy specimens has provided deeper insights into pathologic alterations associated with this disease. In this review, we highlight the recent advancements in our understanding of gastroparesis using data from human gastric biopsy specimens and also from complementary animal model studies. In addition, we propose future directions for clinical utility of human biopsies and strategies for tissue procurement that are minimally invasive and can be applied more broadly.

## CELLULAR CONTROL OF NORMAL GASTRIC FUNCTION

Following the completion of the gastric phase, partially digested food (chyme) present in the stomach is emptied into the duodenum by coordinated gastric motility. Gastric emptying is a complex physiologic process that involves the coordinated interactions of extrinsic nerves, the enteric nervous system (ENS), smooth muscle cells (SMCs), and the ICC within the muscularis and myenteric layers of the stomach, as well as coordination between different parts of the stomach and feedback loops between the small intestine and stomach. A characteristic feature of the GI tract is the presence of its own intrinsic neuroglial circuits (the ENS). Nerve fibers innervate the muscular layers of the stomach.[8] The myenteric plexus situated between the circular and longitudinal muscle layers is known to regulate contraction and relaxation of smooth muscles.[9] Inhibitory and the excitatory neurons are categorized based on the expression pattern of neurotransmitters. For example, excitatory neurons predominantly express choline acetyltransferase (ChAT),[10] substance P (SP), and neurokinins (NKA, NKB, and neuropeptide Y [NPY]),[11] whereas inhibitory neurons express vasoactive intestinal polypeptide (VIP)[12] and neuronal nitric oxide synthase (nNOS), which generates nitric oxide (NO).[13]

Smooth muscle of GI tract is required to mix and churn intraluminal contents, enabling breakdown of ingested food. This is followed by propulsion of chyme into the duodenum, primarily by the contraction of SMCs present in the muscularis externa. This process of gastric emptying is accomplished by phasic contractions of SMCs.[14] The SMCs are linked to the neighboring pacemaker cells via gap junctions creating a syncytium,[15] which drives coordinated contractions and relaxation of SMCs.[16]

ICCs are the pacemaker cells that create the bioelectrical slow wave potential in the GI tract.[17] The syncytial network of ICCs generates electrical slow waves in a spatiotemporal manner driving rhythmic contraction of SMCs.[18,19] ICCs are also involved in integrating and mediating sequential excitatory and inhibitory neurotransmissions and in mechanotransduction—the critical components of normal GI motility.[20] Variants in Ano-1 transcripts, a protein specifically expressed in ICC, have been associated with symptoms in DG.[21]

Macrophages are increasingly recognized as key regulators of tissue homeostasis. Resident macrophages are highly heterogeneous and can acquire distinct phenotypes in response to changes in the tissue microenvironment. They display variable gene expression profiles.[22] Indeed, macrophage gene expression varies from mucosa, submucosa, muscularis, and serosa in mouse.[23] Mouse muscularis macrophages predominantly express CX3CR1 (hi), MHCII (hi), and CD11c (lo), differentiating themselves from lamina propria macrophages, which express CD11c (hi).[24] Similarly, human muscularis macrophages express high levels of CD11b and CD14, whereas low levels of CD11b and CD14 are expressed by mucosal macrophages.[25] Variability also persists in the expression pattern of well-established macrophage markers between mouse and humans[26,27]; for example, inducible NOS (iNOS), Arginase-1, and Ym1 are predominantly expressed by mouse macrophages but not by human macrophages.[28,29] Phenotypically, circular and longitudinal muscle muscularis macrophages are bipolar in shape, whereas, myenteric macrophages are stellate shaped.[23]

Muscularis macrophages live in symbiosis with the ENS, wherein macrophages produce bone morphogenetic protein-2 (BMP-2)—a secreted protein belonging to transforming growth factor β (TGF-β) superfamily.[24] BMP-2 directly acts on enteric neurons expressing BMP receptor (BMPR), leading to oligomerization of type I and type II serine kinases followed by phosphorylation and nuclear translocation of SMAD proteins.[24] Activation of BMPR promotes nitrergic enteric neuronal differentiation[30] and helps in regulating GI motility.[24] In turn, enteric neurons produce colony-stimulating fator-1 (CSF-1)—a growth factor crucial for the differentiation and maintenance of muscularis macrophages,[24] evident from the osteopetrotic (op/op) mice, which lack muscularis macrophages due to a mutation in their CSF-1 gene[31] and show a disorganized ENS architecture.[24] Recently, Avetisyan and colleagues,[32] have reported ICCs as a nonneuronal source of CSF-1, which helps in macrophage homeostasis in RetKO mice that lack enteric neurons. In this way, crosstalk between immune cells and the cells of ENS plays essential role in the maintenance of gastric physiologic processes.

## CELLULAR ABNORMALITIES ASSOCIATED WITH THE PATHOGENESIS OF GASTROPARESIS

Decades of research aiming to identify the physiologic and pathologic changes associated with the pathogenesis of gastroparesis has resulted in identifying several key abnormalities both at cellular (**Fig. 1**) and molecular levels. In the subsequent sections we will describe some of the important findings that have impacted our understanding of the pathologic basis of gastroparesis.

### Enteric Nervous System Changes Associated with Gastroparesis

In an initial case report by Kassander,[33] asymptomatic gastric retention of meal was observed on radiographic studies In patients with diabetes. This putative disturbance of gastric motor function was attributed to peripheral neuropathy involving the vagus nerve, as the radiography results resembled those of patients with gastric hypotonia after vagotomy.[33] However, in an observation made almost 2 decades later, delayed gastric emptying was noted even in the absence of extrinsic diabetic neuropathy.[34] Around the same time, a report described "intermittent gastric atony" in 5 nondiabetic patients experiencing the symptoms of gastroparesis,[35] which gave rise to the entity

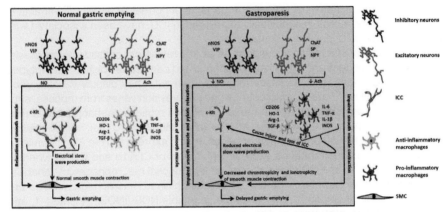

**Fig. 1.** Cellular and molecular changes associated with gastroparesis. Under normal circumstances (*left panel*), the network of ICCs (c-Kit) produces electrical slow waves leading to the membrane depolarization of smooth muscle cells (SMCs) followed by emptying of gastric contents. There is a balance of macrophages in the muscle layer and myenteric plexus with the majority expressing anti-inflammatory proteins, such as CD206, HO-1, Arg-1, or TGF-β. Neurotransmitters, such as nitric oxide (NO) and acetylcholine (Ach) released respectively by inhibitory (nNOS, VIP) and excitatory (ChAT, SP, NPY) neurons control the relaxation and contraction of smooth muscles. In gastroparesis (*right panel*), loss of ICCs results in impaired electrical slow wave production leading to reduced chronotropicity and ionotropicity of smooth muscle contraction. The changes occurring in the tissue microenvironment polarize the macrophages to acquire proinflammatory phenotype, which predominantly expresses IL-6, TNF-α, IL-1β, and iNOS, and these macrophages cause injury and loss of ICCs. In addition, defect/loss of enteric nerves and neurons leads to impaired contraction and relaxation of SMC as well as impaired pyloric relaxation. These cellular abnormalities collectively lead to delayed gastric emptying.

of IG.[36,37] A study by Yoshida and colleagues,[38] involving 16 long-term diabetic patients, of whom 5 exhibiting gastroparesis failed to show any changes in neuronal numbers or vagal morphologic abnormalities.[38] However, this study was limited by the use of only conventional histologic markers available for testing.

Although most of the initial studies focused on the extrinsic nervous system, subsequent work using animal models of DG displayed defects in the intrinsic nervous system. A report by Belai and colleagues,[39] involving a streptozotocin (STZ)-induced rat model of diabetes (without delayed gastric emptying) showed an increase in VIP-like immunoreactivity in nerve fibers, and intensely stained cell bodies in the myenteric plexus and circular muscle layer of both ileum and proximal colon ($P<.001$), but no changes in the SP innervation.[39] STZ-induced diabetic rats developing delayed gastric emptying also displayed increased VIP-like immunoreactivity.[40] These changes resolved with insulin administration in an in vitro setting, suggesting that insulin replacement may restore the defects occurring during early stages of diabetes.[41] Similar results were observed in nonobese diabetic (NOD) mice.[42] Treating these mice either with insulin or with phosphodiesterase inhibitor (Sildenafil) increased the levels of NO and also restored gastric emptying.[42] Interestingly, deletion of gene encoding nNOS in mice resulted in delayed gastric emptying of solids and liquids[43] suggesting the importance of nNOS and NO signaling in pyloric dysfunction associated with a subset of patients with gastroparesis. In a study by Chandrasekharan and colleagues,[44] enhanced apoptosis and loss of peripherin, nNOS, NPY, and ChAT neurons were observed in the colons of patients with diabetes and this neuronal loss was associated with significant decrease in ganglion size.[44] In a study on chronic estrogen deficiency using follicle-stimulating hormone receptor knockout female mice, Ravella and colleagues,[45] have reported the chronic deficiency of estrogen negatively affecting the function of tetrahydrobiopterin (BH4, a cofactor for nNOS dimerization and enzyme activity) and nNOS thereby, contributing to the development of gastroparesis.[45] This may relate to the finding that the gastroparesis is more common in females than in males with diabetes mellitus.[46] Meanwhile, in a NOD mouse model of DG, Choi and colleagues,[47] have reported the restoration of delayed gastric emptying on exogenous administration of interleukin-10 (IL-10) independent of nNOS activity. Further research aiming to understand the pathways that are involved in regulating nNOS expression would help to determine its usefulness as a molecular target to treat gastroparesis.

Studies using human tissues from patients with gastroparesis have also revealed alterations in nNOS expression. A full-thickness jejunal biopsy from a 38-year-old patient with type 1 DM showed a substantial decrease in nerve fiber content (PGP9.5) in the circular muscle when compared with the tissues from 6 control subjects ($P<.05$),[48] and the inhibitory innervation (nNOS, VIP, and PACAP) was also found to be decreased.[48] Similar findings were observed in a case report of a 32-year-old patient with severe IG where the stomach corpus sections displayed loss of nerve cell bodies (PGP9.5) by 69%.[49] A study on type 2 DM male patients with gastric cancer showed significant reduction in the expression of nNOS ($P<.01$) and SP ($P<.01$) in their antrum when compared with patients with gastric cancer without type 2 DM, suggesting the association of expression levels of nNOS and SP in the pathogenesis of DG.[50] In a case report of 2 patients with gastroparesis with type 1 DM,[51] histologic examination of a full-thickness gastric biopsy from 1 patient with long-standing, poorly controlled diabetes displayed reduced nNOS, nerve fibers, and myenteric neurons (PGP9.5). Despite this, both patients had severe refractory symptoms with malnutrition; however, the patient with short duration of diabetes that was well controlled had no significant abnormalities compared with the controls. These observations suggest an association of poor diabetic control with histopathological alterations in the ENS.[51] In another study with 28 full-thickness antral biopsies obtained from patients with refractory gastroparesis (14 each of type 1 DM and IG), a significant reduction in the numbers of ganglia, NOS$^+$, and NOS$^-$ nerve cells was seen compared with controls.[52] On the contrary, in the largest study to date carried out by the NIDDK GpCRC-defined cellular changes using gastric biopsies obtained from controls, and patients with DG and IG (20 patients in each group). There was only a 14% to 18% decrease in the expression of PGP9.5 in gastroparesis as compared with the controls.[53] These biopsies were obtained from the gastric body in contrast to the antrum in the previous study. nNOS was found to be decreased in 20% of patients with DG and 40% of patients with IG. Nonetheless, overall quantification of nNOS did not yield a significant difference between any of the groups.[53] Likewise, 20% of patients with DG and 15% of patients with IG displayed a reduction in the expression of VIP immunolabeling, but no statistically significant difference was found between the 3 groups.[53] Immunolabeling for SP was found to be increased in 1 of 20 patients with DG, whereas it was decreased in 4 of 20 patients with DG and in 2 of 20 patients with IG. No statistically significant difference in SP expression between the groups was observed.[53] These results suggest that alterations in the number of enteric nerves and neurons may be only present in a subset of gastroparesis patients and may depend on the etiology of the gastroparesis, disease duration, and site of assessment in the stomach.

An ultrastructural examination of full-thickness gastric biopsies from patients with gastroparesis conducted by Faussone-Pellegrini and colleagues[54] showed evidence for cellular damage to the nerves, even in patients with no apparent histologic changes on light microscopy. These include a loss of synaptic vesicles, thickened basal lamina, and fibrosis around nerves. Patients with IG showed a more severe damage compared with those with DG.[54]

## Smooth Muscle Changes Associated with Gastroparesis

In a report by Xue and Suzuki,[55] smooth muscles of STZ-induced diabetic rats showed antral muscle inactivity, reduced norepinephrine sensitivity, decreased Na-K pump activity, and increased sensitivity to acetylcholine without any change in their resting membrane potential. In a recent report by Herring and colleagues,[56] ablating the fork-head transcription factors—FOXF1 and FOXF2—in adult SMCs of mice resulted in impaired gastric emptying. In parallel, the authors have also observed a reduced expression of FOXF1 and FOXF2 in full-thickness gastric biopsies obtained from patients with gastroparesis, suggesting the possible importance of FOXF1 and FOXF2 in normal gastric function.[56] Interestingly, forkhead transcription factors are well known for their involvement in smooth muscle proliferation, migration, and apoptosis.[57] These results suggested that, in addition to neuropathy, diabetes can also induce multiple alterations in gastric smooth muscles, which can contribute to delayed gastric emptying.[55]

In a study by Ejskjaer and colleagues,[58] gastric histopathology of 4 patients with type 1 DM with gastroparesis showed smooth muscle degeneration and fibrosis, with eosinophilic inclusion bodies. In a study of 2 patients with DG,[51] histologic examination of full-thickness gastric biopsy from a patient with poorly controlled, long-standing diabetes showed substantial increase in fibrosis in both circular and longitudinal muscle layers and also around the myenteric plexus, whereas the same was not observed in another patient with well-controlled diabetes over a short duration. This indicates that the clinical course of diabetes may influence the smooth muscle changes.[51] However, no significant fibrosis in the gastric wall was observed in the full-thickness gastric body biopsy specimens obtained from patients with DG or IG enrolled in the NIDDK GpCRC.[53] Immunolabeling for smoothelin-A—a specific marker for SMCs—showed a reduced expression in 23% of patients. However, the electron microscopy study failed to show any marked abnormalities in SMCs in both DG and IG.[53]

## Interstitial Cells of Cajal Changes Associated with Gastroparesis

An initial study in an animal model of diabetes (NOD/LtJ mice) conducted by Ordog and colleagues,[59] indicated a significant delay in gastric emptying of the meal (Control, 96% $\pm$ 1%; Diabetic, 45% $\pm$ 16%; $P<.02$). The delay in gastric emptying was associated with reduced ICC content ($\sim$50% reduction; $P<.05$) in the antral muscles as indicated by decreased Kit-immunoreactivity, and a lack of association between ICC and enteric nerve terminals was also observed.[59] The study suggested loss of pacemaker ICCs being the basis of DG. A study using STZ-induced rat model of diabetes showed reduced density of ICC in antrum and this effect was also associated with loss of synaptic connections and decreased gastric emptying.[60]

Similar results depicting the reduction in ICC content in human biopsy specimens of jejunum,[48,61] muscle layer of colon,[62,63] and antrum[64] were reported in patients with gastroparesis with or without diabetes. The diabetes-induced loss of ICCs was not due to hyperglycemia; instead, the effect was due to reduced insulin and insulin-like growth factor 1 (IGF-1) signaling.[65] This indicates that ICCs require insulin or IGF-1 for their maintenance. There are several reports depicting reduced Kit expression, indicating partial or total loss of ICCs in gastric biopsy specimens as one of the most common abnormality in patients with gastroparesis. In a study by the NIDDK GpCRC,[53] 50% of patients with either DG or IG had more than 25% reduction in Kit expression. Patients with DG or IG exhibited similar loss with a mean ICC count of ~50% compared with controls. A well-defined myenteric plexus of ICC was not seen in the human stomach in contrast to the mouse stomach. On ultrastructure, all patients with DG or IG showed signs of ICC damage. These include apoptotic features, intracytoplasmatic vacuoles, swollen mitochondria, and extended rough endoplasmic reticulum. Compared with controls, a physical separation of ICC from other ICC and nerves was seen. Both intramuscular and myenteric ICC had similar changes.[54] In a report by Lin and colleagues,[66] analysis of antral biopsies from 41 patients with refractory gastroparesis (34 diabetic, 5 idiopathic, and 2 postsurgical) showed severe loss of ICCs in 36% of patients, and the rest of the patients had no visible ICCs identified.[66] Similarly, patients enrolled in the GpCRC had greater than 60% loss of ICC, more prominent than the loss seen in the gastric body.[67] These studies from the GpCRC and others suggest that ICC loss is a hallmark feature of gastroparesis in humans.

### Changes in Macrophage Population Associated with Gastroparesis

Recently, macrophage dysregulation has been found to be a key factor in the pathogenesis of gastroparesis. Various stimuli and cytokines present in the tissue microenvironment are known to polarize macrophages into a spectrum that has been dichotomized as M1 (proinflammatory) or M2 (anti-inflammatory).[68] Many disease states have been associated with an alteration in the macrophage milieu.[69,70] Expression of various surface markers has been used to differentiate the M1 and M2 spectrum of macrophages. For instance, M1 macrophages express tumor necrosis factor alpha (TNF-$\alpha$), IL-1$\beta$, and iNOS, whereas, M2 macrophages predominantly express the mannose receptor or CD206, Arginase-1 (mouse only), and TGF-$\beta$.[71] In the context of gastroparesis, there is a reduction in the number of anti-inflammatory CD206+ macrophages in the muscularis layers.[72] CD206+ macrophages are well known to express heme oxygenase 1 (HO-1), and induction of the enzyme HO-1 is a cellular defense mechanism against oxidative stress.[73] In the NOD mouse model, gastric macrophages (CD206+) displayed upregulated expression of HO-1 during early diabetes and the levels were consistently maintained in the animals that were resistant to develop delayed gastric emptying.[73] However, in mice developing delayed gastric emptying, there was loss of CD206+ macrophages expressing HO-1 in addition to the loss of Kit (ICC).[73] Also, loss of HO-1 expression increased oxidative stress in mice,[73] and treating these mice with hemin[73] or IL-10[47] resulted in HO-1 induction and restoration of Kit expression, indicating that CD206+ macrophages expressing HO-1 are crucial for the prevention of DG.

Mice lacking macrophages (CSF1$^{op/op}$ mice) do not develop delayed gastric emptying despite severe diabetes.[74] Supplementing CSF1$^{op/op}$ mice with an intraperitoneal injection of CSF1 restores the muscularis macrophages and makes them susceptible to developing gastroparesis on induction of diabetes.[75] In an in vitro study, treating cultured ICCs with conditioned media from M1 macrophages led to a reduction in ICC numbers by 41%, whereas no change in ICC was observed when treated with conditioned medium from M2 macrophages.[76] Of the 40 markers tested by immunoblot, M1 macrophage-conditioned medium was found to have increased amounts of 12 proinflammatory cytokines and chemokines when compared with the M2-conditioned medium.[76] These results suggest that the presence of macrophages and their phenotype plays a central role in the onset and progression of gastroparesis. M2 macrophages protect ICC, whereas M1 macrophages are required to damage ICC and result in delayed gastric emptying. The molecular mechanisms that are mediated by macrophages in orchestrating ENS and other cellular abnormalities still need to be understood.

An initial study focusing on changes in immune cell population in full-thickness gastric body biopsies obtained from patients with gastroparesis showed a mild lymphocytic infiltrate in the myenteric plexus as determined by H&E staining. Most of these infiltrated cells were positive for CD45 and CD3.[52] Further reports by the NIDDK GpCRC on full-thickness gastric biopsies of the antrum[67] but not body[77] from patients with DG or IG showed a significant reduction in the total number of CD206+ macrophages. The total population of immune cells (CD45+) was unchanged.[67] Remarkably, the reduction in the number of CD206+ macrophages correlated significantly with the loss of ICCs in the circular muscle of the gastric body and antrum tissues,[67,77] suggesting an interaction between CD206+ macrophages and maintenance of ICC.

## DEEP MOLECULAR PROFILING IN GASTROPARESIS

Reports describing molecular changes associated with the pathogenesis of human gastroparesis are scarce. A recent study by the NIDDK GpCRC describes the differentially expressing genes ($log_2$fold difference $|\geq 2|$, false discovery rate $< 5\%$) in DG and IG by deep transcriptomic profiling of full-thickness muscle from the gastric body.[78] Wherein, 111 genes in DG and 181 genes in IG were observed to be differentially expressed. Sixty-five of these genes were common in DG and IG. Ingenuity Pathway Analysis showed most of the differentially expressing genes to be listed in the top 5 canonical pathways associated with immune signaling.[78] Immune profile analysis using CIBERSORT revealed that genes associated with M1 (proinflammatory) macrophages were enriched in tissues from IG tissues compared with controls. A recent report by Herring and colleagues,[79] describes the increased expression of MYH11, MYLK1, and ACTA2—mRNAs encoding contractile proteins, in smooth muscle tissues obtained from patients with IG compared with lean controls. The authors also observed a decrease in platelet-derived growth factor receptor alpha (PDGFRα) and its ligand, PDGFB, mRNA expression. An interaction with body mass index (BMI) was observed in this study and the lean BMI group had more males, whereas the IG group was predominantly female. In our work on the gastric body, the numbers or distribution of PDGFRα-expressing fibroblast-like cells was not altered in gastroparesis.[80]

Recently, we have performed quantitative proteomic analysis of full-thickness gastric antrum biopsies from patients with DG or IG using aptamer-based SomaLogic tissue scan that quantitatively identifies 1300 human proteins.[81] We have found 73 proteins differentially expressing in DG, 133 proteins differentially expressing in IG, and 40 differentially expressing proteins were common between both DG and IG. The study also complements the results of a deep transcriptomic profiling study,[78] wherein "Role of Macrophages, Fibroblasts and Endothelial Cells" is the most statistically significant altered pathway. In summary, RNA- and protein-based molecular signatures complement histologic studies in suggesting an immune-based dysregulation and injury to the ENS in gastroparesis.

## CORRELATION WITH CLINICAL SYMPTOMS AND GASTRIC EMPTYING

A large study showed ICC loss to positively correlate with gastric retention of solids in patients with DG.[82] Another study showed delayed gastric emptying to be associated with ICC counts in the myenteric plexus.[83] In a study by Forster and colleagues,[64] patients with gastroparesis exhibiting no or depleted ICCs (ICC− group) had significantly higher tachygastria when compared with patients with some or adequate number of ICCs (ICC+ group). Tachygastria in the ICC− group was also associated with reduced postprandial rhythmic function. Along with these, the total symptom score in patients who were ICC− was significantly higher when compared with the ICC+ group at baseline and also after 3 months of using gastric electrical stimulator.[64] This was subsequently shown again in a larger study by the same group.[66] The study from the GpCRC also found a correlation between nausea and overall symptom severity and abundance of myenteric immune cells.[82] Overall the correlation between symptoms and cellular defect is low, suggesting that, once established, symptoms may persist independently of the original cause. Use of next-generation sequencing complemented by targeted validation can help identify molecules that can serve as biomarkers and allow target discovery for treatment of gastroparesis.

## FUTURE DIRECTIONS

Animal models have played a major role in providing us valuable information on the pathogenesis of delayed gastric emptying. Understanding of human gastroparesis is driven by work on full-thickness gastric biopsies, which has found several similarities between DG and IG. An important shift in paradigm has been the understanding of the innate immune system in driving injury to the ENS and ICC. A challenge to approaching immune-ENS interactions is the lack of an atlas for either of these cell types in the gastric muscle layers. There are differences in the expression pattern of genotypic markers in mouse and human immune cells.[84] Future studies will need to generate cellular and molecular atlases from healthy subjects that can be then used to compare patients with gastroparesis. From a diagnostic standpoint, we need to further develop minimally invasive methods for procuring gastric full-thickness tissue. In a recent study by Rajan and colleagues,[85] a no-hole gastric body biopsy using an over-the-scope clip was technically successful and provided adequate tissue (~1 cm) for ENS assessment. Endoscopic ultrasound-based approaches have also been tried but the yield for full-thickness assessment of the ENS is low.[86] From a therapeutic standpoint, strategies to influence macrophage polarization or regenerate gastroparesis may act as disease-modifying treatments of gastroparesis. Paradigms that include identification of patients with gastroparesis with changes in ENS and immune cell phenotypes followed by targeted therapies can be particularly helpful in altering the natural history as compared with current therapy, which is focused solely on alleviation of symptoms.

## DISCLOSURE

MG and GF are supported by NIH DK068055 and DK74008. MG is also supported by NIH K23 DK 103911 and R03 DK 120745. GF is also supported by NIH DK057061.

## REFERENCES

1. Matolo NM, Stadalnik RC. Assessment of gastric motility using meal labeled with technetium-99m sulfur colloid. Am J Surg 1983;146(6):823–6.

2. Abell TL, Van Cutsem E, Abrahamsson H, et al. Gastric electrical stimulation in intractable symptomatic gastroparesis. Digestion 2002;66(4):204–12.

3. Soykan I, Sivri B, Sarosiek I, et al. Demography, clinical characteristics, psychological and abuse profiles, treatment, and long-term follow-up of patients with gastroparesis. Dig Dis Sci 1998;43(11):2398–404.

4. Lacy BE, Crowell MD, Mathis C, et al. Gastroparesis: quality of life and health care utilization. J Clin Gastroenterol 2018;52(1):20–4.

5. Parkman HP, Yates K, Hasler WL, et al. Clinical features of idiopathic gastroparesis vary with sex, body mass, symptom onset, delay in gastric emptying, and gastroparesis severity. Gastroenterology 2011;140(1):101–15.

6. Jung HK, Choung RS, Locke GR 3rd, et al. The incidence, prevalence, and outcomes of patients with gastroparesis in Olmsted County, Minnesota, from 1996 to 2006. Gastroenterology 2009;136(4):1225–33.

7. Tougas G, Eaker EY, Abell TL, et al. Assessment of gastric emptying using a low fat meal: establishment of international control values. Am J Gastroenterol 2000; 95(6):1456–62.

8. Kyosola K, Rechardt L, Veijola L, et al. Innervation of the human gastric wall. J Anat 1980;131(Pt 3):453–70.

9. Yokoyama S, Ozaki T. Effects of gut distension on Auerbach's plexus and intestinal muscle. Jpn J Physiol 1980;30(2):143–60.

10. Hao MM, Bornstein JC, Young HM. Development of myenteric cholinergic neurons in ChAT-Cre;R26R-YFP mice. J Comp Neurol 2013;521(14):3358–70.

11. Jansen I, Alafaci C, McCulloch J, et al. Tachykinins (substance P, neurokinin A, neuropeptide K, and neurokinin B) in the cerebral circulation: vasomotor responses in vitro and in situ. J Cereb Blood Flow Metab 1991;11(4):567–75.

12. Mesik L, Ma WP, Li LY, et al. Functional response properties of VIP-expressing inhibitory neurons in mouse visual and auditory cortex. Front Neural Circuits 2015;9:22.

13. Sanders KM, Ward SM. Nitric oxide as a mediator of nonadrenergic noncholinergic neurotransmission. Am J Physiol 1992;262(3 Pt 1):G379–92.

14. Sanders KM. Spontaneous electrical activity and rhythmicity in gastrointestinal smooth muscles. Adv Exp Med Biol 2019;1124:3–46.

15. Berezin I, Huizinga JD, Daniel EE. Structural characterization of interstitial cells of Cajal in myenteric plexus and muscle layers of canine colon. Can J Physiol Pharmacol 1990;68(11):1419–31.

16. Preiksaitis HG, Diamant NE. Phasic contractions of the muscular components of human esophagus and gastroesophageal junction in vitro. Can J Physiol Pharmacol 1995;73(3):356–63.

17. Hennig GW, Spencer NJ, Jokela-Willis S, et al. ICC-MY coordinate smooth muscle electrical and mechanical activity in the murine small intestine. Neurogastroenterol Motil 2010;22(5):e138–51.

18. Ordog T, Ward SM, Sanders KM. Interstitial cells of Cajal generate electrical slow waves in the murine stomach. J Physiol 1999;518(Pt 1):257–69.

19. Smith TK, Reed JB, Sanders KM. Interaction of two electrical pacemakers in muscularis of canine proximal colon. Am J Physiol 1987;252(3 Pt 1):C290–9.

20. Klein S, Seidler B, Kettenberger A, et al. Interstitial cells of Cajal integrate excitatory and inhibitory neurotransmission with intestinal slow-wave activity. Nat Commun 2013;4:1630.

21. Mazzone A, Bernard CE, Strege PR, et al. Altered expression of Ano1 variants in human diabetic gastroparesis. J Biol Chem 2011;286(15):13393–403.

22. Gosselin D, Link VM, Romanoski CE, et al. Environment drives selection and function of enhancers controlling tissue-specific macrophage identities. Cell 2014; 159(6):1327–40.

23. Gabanyi I, Muller PA, Feighery L, et al. Neuro-immune interactions drive tissue programming in intestinal macrophages. Cell 2016;164(3):378–91.

24. Muller PA, Koscso B, Rajani GM, et al. Crosstalk between muscularis macrophages and enteric neurons regulates gastrointestinal motility. Cell 2014; 158(2):300–13.
25. Bujko A, Atlasy N, Landsverk OJB, et al. Transcriptional and functional profiling defines human small intestinal macrophage subsets. J Exp Med 2018;215(2): 441–58.
26. Martinez FO, Helming L, Milde R, et al. Genetic programs expressed in resting and IL-4 alternatively activated mouse and human macrophages: similarities and differences. Blood 2013;121(9):e57–69.
27. Spiller KL, Wrona EA, Romero-Torres S, et al. Differential gene expression in human, murine, and cell line-derived macrophages upon polarization. Exp Cell Res 2016;347(1):1–13.
28. Raes G, Van den Bergh R, De Baetselier P, et al. Arginase-1 and Ym1 are markers for murine, but not human, alternatively activated myeloid cells. J Immunol 2005; 174(11):6561 [author reply: 6561–2].
29. Gross TJ, Kremens K, Powers LS, et al. Epigenetic silencing of the human NOS2 gene: rethinking the role of nitric oxide in human macrophage inflammatory responses. J Immunol 2014;192(5):2326–38.
30. Liu X, Liu S, Xu Y, et al. Bone morphogenetic protein 2 regulates the differentiation of nitrergic enteric neurons by modulating Smad1 signaling in slow transit constipation. Mol Med Rep 2015;12(5):6547–54.
31. Mikkelsen HB, Thuneberg L. Op/op mice defective in production of functional colony-stimulating factor-1 lack macrophages in muscularis externa of the small intestine. Cell Tissue Res 1999;295(3):485–93.
32. Avetisyan M, Rood JE, Huerta Lopez S, et al. Muscularis macrophage development in the absence of an enteric nervous system. Proc Natl Acad Sci U S A 2018;115(18):4696–701.
33. Kassander P. Asymptomatic gastric retention in diabetics (gastroparesis diabeticorum). Ann Intern Med 1958;48(4):797–812.
34. Soler NG. Diabetic gastroparesis without autonomic neuropathy. Diabetes Care 1980;3(1):200–1.
35. Shellito PC, Warshaw AL. Idiopathic intermittent gastroparesis and its surgical alleviation. Am J Surg 1984;148(3):408–12.
36. Narducci F, Bassotti G, Granata MT, et al. Functional dyspepsia and chronic idiopathic gastric stasis. Role of endogenous opiates. Arch Intern Med 1986;146(4): 716–20.
37. Wengrower D, Zaltzman S, Karmeli F, et al. Idiopathic gastroparesis in patients with unexplained nausea and vomiting. Dig Dis Sci 1991;36(9):1255–8.
38. Yoshida MM, Schuffler MD, Sumi SM. There are no morphologic abnormalities of the gastric wall or abdominal vagus in patients with diabetic gastroparesis. Gastroenterology 1988;94(4):907–14.
39. Belai A, Lincoln J, Milner P, et al. Enteric nerves in diabetic rats: increase in vasoactive intestinal polypeptide but not substance P. Gastroenterology 1985;89(5): 967–76.
40. Kishimoto S, Kunita S, Kambara A, et al. VIPergic innervation in the gastrointestinal tract of diabetic rats. Hiroshima J Med Sci 1983;32(4):469–78.
41. Burnstock G, Mirsky R, Belai A. Reversal of nerve damage in streptozotocin-diabetic rats by acute application of insulin in vitro. Clin Sci (Lond) 1988;75(6): 629–35.

42. Watkins CC, Sawa A, Jaffrey S, et al. Insulin restores neuronal nitric oxide synthase expression and function that is lost in diabetic gastropathy. J Clin Invest 2000;106(3):373–84.
43. Mashimo H, Kjellin A, Goyal RK. Gastric stasis in neuronal nitric oxide synthase-deficient knockout mice. Gastroenterology 2000;119(3):766–73.
44. Chandrasekharan B, Anitha M, Blatt R, et al. Colonic motor dysfunction in human diabetes is associated with enteric neuronal loss and increased oxidative stress. Neurogastroenterol Motil 2011;23(2):131–8, e26.
45. Ravella K, Al-Hendy A, Sharan C, et al. Chronic estrogen deficiency causes gastroparesis by altering neuronal nitric oxide synthase function. Dig Dis Sci 2013; 58(6):1507–15.
46. Dickman R, Wainstein J, Glezerman M, et al. Gender aspects suggestive of gastroparesis in patients with diabetes mellitus: a cross-sectional survey. BMC Gastroenterol 2014;14:34.
47. Choi KM, Gibbons SJ, Sha L, et al. Interleukin 10 restores gastric emptying, electrical activity, and interstitial cells of Cajal networks in diabetic mice. Cell Mol Gastroenterol Hepatol 2016;2(4):454–67.
48. He CL, Soffer EE, Ferris CD, et al. Loss of interstitial cells of cajal and inhibitory innervation in insulin-dependent diabetes. Gastroenterology 2001;121(2):427–34.
49. Zarate N, Mearin F, Wang XY, et al. Severe idiopathic gastroparesis due to neuronal and interstitial cells of Cajal degeneration: pathological findings and management. Gut 2003;52(7):966–70.
50. Iwasaki H, Kajimura M, Osawa S, et al. A deficiency of gastric interstitial cells of Cajal accompanied by decreased expression of neuronal nitric oxide synthase and substance P in patients with type 2 diabetes mellitus. J Gastroenterol 2006;41(11):1076–87.
51. Pasricha PJ, Pehlivanov ND, Gomez G, et al. Changes in the gastric enteric nervous system and muscle: a case report on two patients with diabetic gastroparesis. BMC Gastroenterol 2008;8:21.
52. Harberson J, Thomas RM, Harbison SP, et al. Gastric neuromuscular pathology in gastroparesis: analysis of full-thickness antral biopsies. Dig Dis Sci 2010;55(2): 359–70.
53. Grover M, Farrugia G, Lurken MS, et al. Cellular changes in diabetic and idiopathic gastroparesis. Gastroenterology 2011;140(5):1575–15785.e8.
54. Faussone-Pellegrini MS, Grover M, Pasricha PJ, et al. Ultrastructural differences between diabetic and idiopathic gastroparesis. J Cell Mol Med 2012;16(7): 1573–81.
55. Xue L, Suzuki H. Electrical responses of gastric smooth muscles in streptozotocin-induced diabetic rats. Am J Physiol 1997;272(1 Pt 1):G77–83.
56. Herring BP, Hoggatt AM, Gupta A, et al. Gastroparesis is associated with decreased FOXF1 and FOXF2 in humans, and loss of FOXF1 and FOXF2 results in gastroparesis in mice. Neurogastroenterol Motil 2019;31(3):e13528.
57. Brunet A, Bonni A, Zigmond MJ, et al. Akt promotes cell survival by phosphorylating and inhibiting a Forkhead transcription factor. Cell 1999;96(6):857–68.
58. Ejskjaer NT, Bradley JL, Buxton-Thomas MS, et al. Novel surgical treatment and gastric pathology in diabetic gastroparesis. Diabet Med 1999;16(6):488–95.
59. Ordog T, Takayama I, Cheung WK, et al. Remodeling of networks of interstitial cells of Cajal in a murine model of diabetic gastroparesis. Diabetes 2000; 49(10):1731–9.
60. Wang XY, Huizinga JD, Diamond J, et al. Loss of intramuscular and submuscular interstitial cells of Cajal and associated enteric nerves is related to decreased

gastric emptying in streptozotocin-induced diabetes. Neurogastroenterol Motil 2009;21(10). 1095-e92.

61. Pardi DS, Miller SM, Miller DL, et al. Paraneoplastic dysmotility: loss of interstitial cells of Cajal. Am J Gastroenterol 2002;97(7):1828–33.
62. Nakahara M, Isozaki K, Hirota S, et al. Deficiency of KIT-positive cells in the colon of patients with diabetes mellitus. J Gastroenterol Hepatol 2002;17(6):666–70.
63. Feldstein AE, Miller SM, El-Youssef M, et al. Chronic intestinal pseudoobstruction associated with altered interstitial cells of cajal networks. J Pediatr Gastroenterol Nutr 2003;36(4):492–7.
64. Forster J, Damjanov I, Lin Z, et al. Absence of the interstitial cells of Cajal in patients with gastroparesis and correlation with clinical findings. J Gastrointest Surg 2005;9(1):102–8.
65. Horvath VJ, Vittal H, Ordog T. Reduced insulin and IGF-I signaling, not hyperglycemia, underlies the diabetes-associated depletion of interstitial cells of Cajal in the murine stomach. Diabetes 2005;54(5):1528–33.
66. Lin Z, Sarosiek I, Forster J, et al. Association of the status of interstitial cells of Cajal and electrogastrogram parameters, gastric emptying and symptoms in patients with gastroparesis. Neurogastroenterol Motil 2010;22(1):56–61, e10.
67. Grover M, Bernard CE, Pasricha PJ, et al. Diabetic and idiopathic gastroparesis is associated with loss of CD206-positive macrophages in the gastric antrum. Neurogastroenterol Motil 2017;29(6). https://doi.org/10.1111/nmo.13018.
68. Tarique AA, Logan J, Thomas E, et al. Phenotypic, functional, and plasticity features of classical and alternatively activated human macrophages. Am J Respir Cell Mol Biol 2015;53(5):676–88.
69. Satoh N, Shimatsu A, Himeno A, et al. Unbalanced M1/M2 phenotype of peripheral blood monocytes in obese diabetic patients: effect of pioglitazone. Diabetes Care 2010;33(1):e7.
70. Dionne S, Duchatelier CF, Seidman EG. The influence of vitamin D on M1 and M2 macrophages in patients with Crohn's disease. Innate Immun 2017;23(6):557–65.
71. Stoger JL, Gijbels MJ, van der Velden S, et al. Distribution of macrophage polarization markers in human atherosclerosis. Atherosclerosis 2012;225(2):461–8.
72. Nawaz A, Aminuddin A, Kado T, et al. CD206(+) M2-like macrophages regulate systemic glucose metabolism by inhibiting proliferation of adipocyte progenitors. Nat Commun 2017;8(1):286.
73. Choi KM, Kashyap PC, Dutta N, et al. CD206-positive M2 macrophages that express heme oxygenase-1 protect against diabetic gastroparesis in mice. Gastroenterology 2010;138(7):2399–409, 2409.e1.
74. Cipriani G, Gibbons SJ, Verhulst PJ, et al. Diabetic Csf1(op/op) mice lacking macrophages are protected against the development of delayed gastric emptying. Cell Mol Gastroenterol Hepatol 2016;2(1):40–7.
75. Cipriani G, Gibbons SJ, Miller KE, et al. Change in populations of macrophages promotes development of delayed gastric emptying in mice. Gastroenterology 2018;154(8):2122–36.e12.
76. Eisenman ST, Gibbons SJ, Verhulst PJ, et al. Tumor necrosis factor alpha derived from classically activated "M1" macrophages reduces interstitial cell of Cajal numbers. Neurogastroenterol Motil 2017;29(4). https://doi.org/10.1111/nmo.12984.
77. Bernard CE, Gibbons SJ, Mann IS, et al. Association of low numbers of CD206-positive cells with loss of ICC in the gastric body of patients with diabetic gastroparesis. Neurogastroenterol Motil 2014;26(9):1275–84.

78. Grover M, Gibbons SJ, Nair AA, et al. Transcriptomic signatures reveal immune dysregulation in human diabetic and idiopathic gastroparesis. BMC Med Genomics 2018;11(1):62.

79. Herring BP, Chen M, Mihaylov P, et al. Transcriptome profiling reveals significant changes in the gastric muscularis externa with obesity that partially overlap those that occur with idiopathic gastroparesis. BMC Med Genomics 2019;12(1):89.

80. Grover M, Bernard CE, Pasricha PJ, et al. Platelet-derived growth factor receptor alpha (PDGFRalpha)-expressing "fibroblast-like cells" in diabetic and idiopathic gastroparesis of humans. Neurogastroenterol Motil 2012;24(9):844–52.

81. Grover M, Dasari S, Bernard CE, et al. Proteomics in gastroparesis: unique and overlapping protein signatures in diabetic and idiopathic gastroparesis. Gastroenterology 2019;156(6). S-87–S-88.

82. Grover M, Bernard CE, Pasricha PJ, et al. Clinical-histological associations in gastroparesis: results from the Gastroparesis Clinical Research Consortium. Neurogastroenterol Motil 2012;24(6):531–9, e249.

83. Heckert J, Thomas RM, Parkman HP. Gastric neuromuscular histology in patients with refractory gastroparesis: relationships to etiology, gastric emptying, and response to gastric electric stimulation. Neurogastroenterol Motil 2017;29(8). https://doi.org/10.1111/nmo.13608.

84. Buscher K, Ehinger E, Gupta P, et al. Natural variation of macrophage activation as disease-relevant phenotype predictive of inflammation and cancer survival. Nat Commun 2017;8:16041.

85. Rajan E, Gostout CJ, Wong Kee Song LM, et al. Innovative gastric endoscopic muscle biopsy to identify all cell types, including myenteric neurons and interstitial cells of Cajal in patients with idiopathic gastroparesis: a feasibility study (with video). Gastrointest Endosc 2016;84(3):512–7.

86. Othman MO, Davis B, Saroseik I, et al. EUS-guided FNA biopsy of the muscularis propria of the antrum in patients with gastroparesis is feasible and safe. Gastrointest Endosc 2016;83(2):327–33.

# SMALL INTESTINE

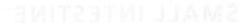
SMALL INTESTINE

# Small Intestinal Bacterial Overgrowth
## How to Diagnose and Treat (and Then Treat Again)

Brian Ginnebaugh, MD, MS[a],*, William D. Chey, MD, FACG[b],
Richard Saad, MD, MS[b]

## KEYWORDS

- SIBO • Review • Diagnosis • Pathophysiology • Treatment

## KEY POINTS

- Small intestinal bacterial overgrowth (SIBO) is a condition that can present with a wide range of nonspecific symptoms, and can be easily overlooked in the clinical setting.
- There are several diagnostic methods available to make the diagnosis of SIBO; however, each method has advantages and disadvantages, and newer diagnostic methods must be researched.
- The mainstay of treatment for SIBO is antibiotics; however, novel therapies such as prokinetics, dietary changes, and herbal therapies are on the horizon.

## INTRODUCTION

Unlike the colon, the human small intestine is typically an inhospitable environment for bacteria to grow and flourish. This is due to a variety of host factors, which include normal fasting and fed motility, secretion of gastric acid, pancreaticobiliary secretions, structural barriers such as the ileocecal valve, an intact gut immune system, and commensal bacteria. Situations that disrupt this natural environment can lead to gut dysbiosis, as well as small intestinal bacterial overgrowth (SIBO). SIBO is defined as an overgrowth of intestinal bacteria proximal to the colon that can lead to a wide variety of clinical manifestations ranging from completely asymptomatic to malabsorption, steatorrhea, and weight loss in severely affected cases.[1] Most often, patients present with nonspecific symptoms including bloating, flatulence, abdominal pain, diarrhea, and constipation.[2]

[a] Internal Medicine, University of Michigan, 3912 Taubman Center, 1500 East Medical Center Drive, Ann Arbor, MI 48109, USA; [b] University of Michigan – Michigan Medicine, 3912 Taubman Center, 1500 East Medical Center Drive, Ann Arbor, MI 48109, USA
* Corresponding author.
*E-mail address:* bginneba@med.umich.edu

Gastroenterol Clin N Am 49 (2020) 571–587
https://doi.org/10.1016/j.gtc.2020.04.010
0889-8553/20/© 2020 Elsevier Inc. All rights reserved.

In part related to the heterogeneity in clinical phenotype, SIBO can be easy for the clinician to overlook. Further complicating matters are challenges regarding diagnosing and treating SIBO. The current dogma suggests small bowel aspiration and quantitative culture is the diagnostic gold standard for SIBO; however, this method is expensive, invasive, and time-consuming. Other modalities of diagnosis include breath testing, which is noninvasive and less expensive, yet lacks the sensitivity and specificity of aspiration and culture. Empiric treatment with antibiotics is another option that is often used in clinical practice; however, with continued concerns about the development of multi-antibiotic–resistant bacteria, side effects of antibiotics, and potential for infection of noncommensal bacteria such as *Clostridium difficile,* empiric treatment does have clear limitations.[3] New diagnostic modalities, such as gas-sensing capsules, are currently being investigated. These tools aim to provide real-time information and more specific diagnosis for the physician. Although antibiotics remain the mainstay of SIBO treatment, various alternative or adjunctive therapies are available, including prokinetic agents, dietary interventions, probiotics, and herbal combinations. This review outlines the pathophysiology of SIBO, current and future diagnostic methods, and treatment options available to the clinician.

## PATHOPHYSIOLOGY
### Symptoms of Small Intestinal Bacterial Overgrowth

The human microbiome contains trillions of organisms, most of which are bacteria contained in the gastrointestinal tract. More than 70% of the gastrointestinal microbiota reside in the colon where counts reach $10^{12}$. By comparison, typical bacterial counts in the stomach and duodenum are $10^2$ to $10^3$ and counts in the jejunum are usually less than $10^4$. Distally, counts increase up to $10^9$ in the terminal ileum.[4] The intestinal microbiome is extremely diverse and contributes to the normal development and ongoing health and integrity of the visceral smooth muscle, enteric nervous system, and gut immune system by controlling pathogen overgrowth, regulating endocrine functions, conjugating bile acids, and modifying ingested toxins.[5] The microbiome is acquired in utero, and its composition matures and adapts throughout life. Disruptions in the intestinal microbiome are known to be associated with a number of diseases throughout the body, including the respiratory, neurologic, hepatic, and gastrointestinal systems. Natural human physiology maintains stable and relatively low populations of bacteria in the stomach and small intestine, when compared with the colon. These defenses that maintain this state and their associated pathophysiologic conditions are depicted in **Table 1**. When 1 or more of these defenses are compromised, bacterial counts can increase, and SIBO can develop.

### Gastric Acid Secretion

Acid-secreting oxyntic cells in the gastric fundus create an acidic milieu with a pH range of 1.5 to 3.5 in the stomach. Conditions that disrupt acid production, such as surgery, autoimmune gastritis, and medications that potently suppress acid secretion, can lead to increased intragastric pH, allowing ingested bacteria an opportunity to multiply. Although available studies have reported conflicting data,[6,7] a recent meta-analysis found an association between chronic proton pump inhibitor (PPI) use and an increased risk of SIBO.[8] The meta-analysis of Su and colleagues,[8] which included more than 7000 patients in 19 studies, showed a statistically significant odds ratio (OR) of 1.71 (confidence interval [CI] 1.2–2.4) between chronic PPI use and SIBO. In this meta-analysis, the diagnosis of SIBO was made by a variety of methods including glucose breath test, lactulose breath test, and small bowel aspiration and quantitative

**Table 1**
Protective measures against small intestinal bacterial overgrowth and common associated disorders

| Gastric Acid Secretion | Pancreaticobiliary Secretions | Intestinal Motility | Anatomic Integrity | Innate and Adaptive Immunity |
|---|---|---|---|---|
| Acid-suppressing medications<br>• Proton pump inhibitor<br>Autoimmune gastritis<br>Surgery (vagotomy) | Chronic pancreatitis<br>Exocrine pancreatic insufficiency<br>Cirrhosis | Medications (ie, opioids)<br>Autonomic Neuropathy<br>Scleroderma | Small bowel diverticulum<br>Surgical revision<br>• Roux-en-y<br>• Lack of ileocecal valve<br>Fistulae/Stricture<br>• Inflammatory bowel disease<br>• Radiation | Immunosuppressive medications<br>Combined variable immunodeficiency<br>Immunoglobulin A deficiency<br>Human immunodeficiency virus/AIDS |

culture. The meta-analysis of Lo and Chan[9] pooled 11 studies with 3134 patients, and found an OR of 2.282 (CI 1.23–4.2); however, this was only observed in subgroup analysis of small bowel aspirates, which is considered to be a more accurate test.[9]

### Pancreaticobiliary Secretions

The human pancreas performs a variety of exocrine functions, which include the secretion of proteases and lipase into the duodenum, which aides in digestion. These enzymes likely have antimicrobial properties that prevent the development of SIBO.[10] Support of this hypothesis includes studies showing that patients with chronic pancreatitis (CP) and/or exocrine pancreatic insufficiency (EPI) without previous surgery are 15% to 42% more likely to have SIBO.[10,11] Capurso and colleagues[12] showed that up to 92% of patients with CP have SIBO, regardless of whether related symptoms were present or not. Patients with CP and EPI may present with diarrhea and steatorrhea from the lack of enzyme production; however, with adequate pancreatic enzyme replacement, diarrhea and steatorrhea can often persist.[10] SIBO causes diarrhea by the de-conjugation of bile acids and likely a secondary enteritis and is the second leading cause of diarrhea among patients with CP.[11] Patients with CP have multiple etiologies of SIBO, such as prior surgery, dysmotility, PPI use, diabetes mellitus, and opioid use. Risk factors for SIBO in patients without previous surgery include more severe CP, marked by low zinc levels, opioid use, coexisting diabetes mellitus, and hypoalbuminemia. Lee and colleagues[11] also found that symptoms are often unreliable, and that the diagnosis of SIBO should be considered in any patients with CP with the previously mentioned risk factors and persistent weight loss or diarrhea.

Patients with chronic liver disease, such as cirrhosis, can develop hepatic dysfunction including decreased bile production and secretion. Bile is a detergent that also has antimicrobial properties. Not surprisingly, patients with chronic liver disease have been shown to have increased rates of SIBO compared with controls without liver disease. A 2018 meta-analysis published by Maslennikov and colleagues,[13] which investigated 21 studies (1264 patients) showed an increased prevalence of SIBO (diagnosed by either lactulose hydrogen breath test [LHBT], glucose hydrogen breath test [GHBT], or quantitative culture) in patients with cirrhosis (40.8% vs 10.7%; OR 6.83; 95% CI 4.16–11.21; $P<.001$).

### Fasting Intestinal Motility

Propulsion of food and chyme through the gastrointestinal tract sweeps bacteria toward the colon and is an important reason that bacterial counts in the proximal small intestine are normally low. Disruptions of motility, particularly the migrating motor complex (MMC) observed in the fasting state, can predispose to the development of SIBO. This was suggested in a study by Vantrappen and colleagues[14] in 1977, which showed positive correlation between patients with SIBO (defined by positive $^{14}CO_2$ bile acid breath test) and disrupted MMCs. Further supporting this theory, Huseby and colleagues[15] showed that radiation-induced injury resulted in alterations to the MMC, which promoted the development of SIBO. Medications that disrupt the MMC, including anticholinergics, opioids, and anti-diarrheal medications, have all been shown to predispose to SIBO.[3,4]

Abnormalities in small intestinal motility are more common in a number of disease states commonly encountered in clinical practice. It has long been known that type 1 diabetes mellitus can be complicated by autonomic neuropathy, which can impair normal gastric intestinal or colonic motility. Further, with the obesity epidemic, dysmotility as a consequence of autonomic neuropathy in the setting of type 2 diabetes mellitus is becoming increasingly common.[4] Patients with diabetes and autonomic neuropathy are predisposed to SIBO compared with patients with diabetes mellitus who do not have autonomic neuropathy.[16] On the contrary, prokinetic agents such as itopride, cisapride, or levosulpiride, have been shown to decrease the prevalence of SIBO.[17]

### Structural/Anatomic Abnormalities

When congenital, acquired, or iatrogenic structural/anatomic abnormalities of the small intestines arise, SIBO can develop.[18] These include diverticulae, fistulae, strictures, and/or surgical alterations, particularly those that affect the integrity of the ileocecal valve.[4]

Small bowel diverticulae are typically asymptomatic, as they are encountered in 1% to 5% of patients[19]; however, these benign outpouchings of the small bowel can lead to stasis of intestinal contents, which can predispose to the development of SIBO.[20]

Patients with inflammatory bowel disease (IBD) are also predisposed to the development of SIBO by underlying gut dysbiosis, as well as structural abnormalities from strictures, fistulizing disease, or previous surgery.[21] Treatment with immunosuppressive medications may also contribute to the development of SIBO. Shah and colleagues[21] performed a meta-analysis using hydrogen breath testing to determine the prevalence of SIBO in IBD. SIBO was significantly higher in patients with Crohn's disease (25.4%, 95% CI 22.48–28.34; OR 10.86, 95% CI 2.76–42.69). What was surprising was that patients with ulcerative colitis were also significantly more likely than controls to have SIBO (14.3%, 95% CI 10.52–18.08; OR 7.99, CI 1.66–38.35). This was attributed to the underlying dysbiosis in patients with IBD, although further research to address this issue are clearly warranted.[21] Last, patients with surgical abnormalities, particularly the lack of an intact ileocecal valve or blind loop (ie, Roux-en-Y) anatomy are much more likely to develop SIBO.[22] This is worthy of note in a day and age when bariatric surgery is increasingly common in westernized countries like the United States.

### Gut Immune System

The immune system of the intestine demonstrates an important relationship between innate (mucus) and adaptive (secretory immunoglobulin [Ig]A) immunity, which protects against SIBO. Overlying the small intestinal endothelium is a layer of mucin that is produced by goblet cells. This semi-permeable layer allows nutrients to be absorbed; however, along with permeability, bacteria are also able to penetrate. To protect against bacterial translocation, Paneth cells located at the bottom of crypts secrete IgA designed to encapsulate bacteria and prevent their ability to reach enterocytes.[23] Patients with humoral immunodeficiency such as combined variable immunodeficiency, IgA deficiency, and acquired immunodeficiency syndrome (AIDS) have higher rates of SIBO.[24] Along with permeability, these systems provide the last level of defense against the ravages of SIBO in the small bowel.

## DIAGNOSIS

There a several ways to evaluate for SIBO; each method has strengths and limitations. Current methods include aspiration of small intestinal fluid for quantitative culture, various forms of breath testing, and novel diagnostic platforms in development, such as gas, fluid, or tissue sampling capsules.

### Small Intestinal Fluid Aspiration for Quantitative Culture

As mentioned previously, when juice is aspirated from the small intestine, bacterial counts are normally less than $10^3$ in the stomach and duodenum, and less than $10^4$

in the jejunum. The microbiome transitions from aerobic bacteria proximally to anaerobic bacteria in the distal small intestine and colon.[25] This physiologic principle is the basis for small intestinal fluid aspiration for quantitative culture. Successfully performing such testing requires training, appropriate infrastructure, is expensive, and not without risk.

In the original studies that defined SIBO, it was determined that a concentration of greater than $10^5$ colony-forming units per milliliter (CFUs/mL) of aspirate was abnormal.[25] These cutoffs have been called into question, as a systematic review pointed out that the studies that suggested this cutoff almost exclusively included those with Roux-en-Y or "blind loop" anatomy. Furthermore, most healthy controls in the review had bacterial counts less than $10^3$, suggesting that a lower cutoff for diagnosis of SIBO might be appropriate.[25]

From a practical standpoint, to use the greater than $10^5$ CFU/mL cutoff for SIBO, patients must undergo enteroscopy with intubation and aspiration from the jejunum. These procedures are time-consuming and in the absence of monitored anesthesia support, can be uncomfortable for the patient. In clinical practice, it is much more common for aspiration of the proximal duodenum to assess for SIBO to be performed during routine esophagogastroduodenoscopy (EGD). Recent work has determined that the threshold for abnormal for the proximal duodenum is lower (>$10^3$ CFU/mL) than for the jejunum.[26] .

To acquire fluid samples, there are 2 main methods of collection: enteral tube placement, and endoscopy (standard EGD or enteroscopy). In the first method, a nasojejunal or orojejunal tube can be inserted with radiographic guidance such as fluoroscopy. Using endoscopy, the endoscopist intubates the esophagus and passes the scope directly into the second/third portion of the duodenum or jejunum with minimal air insufflation and no fluid aspiration. At this point a sterile catheter is placed into the endoscope, and 3 to 5 mL of fluid is aspirated.

In either method, once fluid is collected, the sample is placed into a sterile container and immediately transported to the microbiology laboratory to undergo quantitative culture.

Some investigators favor *qualitative* culture along with quantitative culture to define 2 types of SIBO: the first type is defined by gram-positive, aerobic organisms that are typically found in the upper gastrointestinal tract. In the second type, the bacterial overgrowth is dominated by gram-negative anaerobes similar to those found in the colon.[1]

Regardless of how an aspirate is obtained, there is a significant risk of contamination, sampling error, or sample mishandling. There is also the possibility that the small bowel will not contain a sufficient quantity of fluid for collection, leaving the patient to assume the risk of the procedure without the benefit of gaining a diagnosis. Although small intestinal fluid aspiration provides a direct assessment of bacterial overgrowth and is still considered the diagnostic "gold standard,"[1] its many limitations have contributed to the rising popularity of breath testing as a more practical diagnostic test for SIBO.

### Breath Testing

Unlike intestinal fluid sampling, breath testing is noninvasive, simple, less expensive, and more widely available than small bowel aspiration for quantitative culture. Breath testing relies on the principle that an orally ingested sugar or other substrate will be fermented by bacteria located in the small intestine. Currently, the most commonly used substrates are glucose and lactulose.[1,3] Fermentation of these substrates leads to the production of various gases (**Fig. 1**). Some gases are unique to bacterial

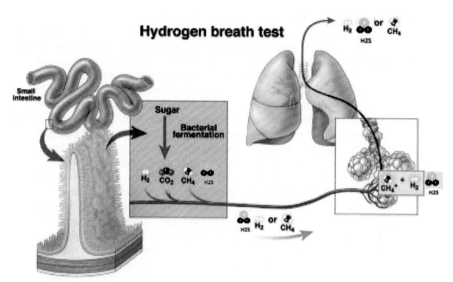

**Fig. 1.** Breath testing for SIBO.

production, whereas others can come from ingested food, diffusion from the blood stream, and chemical reactions that do not require bacteria taking place in the gut. These gases, once produced, can be expelled via the mouth or anus, or are absorbed into the systemic circulation, and then expired from the lungs in breath.[3] Gases that reflect bacterial fermentation of commonly used sugar substrates include hydrogen, methane, and hydrogen sulfide.

Because of significant heterogeneity in testing preparation, collection methods, and interpretation, groups of international experts published clinical consensus documents in 2009 [1] and 2005.[27] In 2017, Rezaie and colleagues[3] published a consensus guideline that summarized the opinions of 10 experts in neurogastroenterology from the United States, Canada, and Mexico on breath testing in North America. This document provides recommendations on breath testing indications, preparation, methodology, and interpretation.

The hydrogen breath test currently uses 1 of 2 substrates for testing, glucose (GHBT), or lactulose (LHBT). Glucose is a monosaccharide that is avidly absorbed in the proximal small bowel. In patients with normal absorptive capacity and intestinal transit, orally ingested glucose is fully absorbed in the duodenum and jejunum with little to no substrate reaching the ileum or colon.[3] Thus, a rise in breath hydrogen (or methane) excretion following oral ingestion of glucose should represent fermentation occurring somewhere in the stomach or proximal small intestine. In contrast, lactulose is a synthetic disaccharide that is nondigestible and nonabsorbable by the normal human small intestine. Thus, relevant to SIBO, lactulose "samples" the entire small intestine and on reaching the colon, is fermented by colonic bacteria. This, at least theoretically, offers the possibility of improved sensitivity but possibly reduced specificity relative to glucose breath testing.

For these reasons, the older Rome consensus document suggested that the GHBT was preferred to the LHBT regardless of differences in testing methods such as dose of substrate or duration of testing. Though different studies used 50 g to 100 g, these experts recommended a dose of 50 g[1] Although there are no studies comparing doses of glucose, the World Health Organization recommended a 75-g dose for glucose tolerance testing.[28] Because the 75-g dose of glucose is widely commercially available, the North American consensus group recommended a 75-g dose when testing for SIBO. For lactulose breath testing, both groups recommended a 10-g dose and acknowledged that higher doses might increase colonic transit times.[3]

For the hydrogen breath test, a rise of 20 ppm or greater is required for a diagnosis of SIBO; this threshold is higher than prior guidelines,[1] and results in sensitivity of 77%, and specificity or 66%.[2] Last, some have suggested that lactulose can lead to "2 peaks," one early, which represents fermentation by small intestinal bacteria, and one late, which corresponds to colonic fermentation. Unfortunately, this finding is neither sensitive or specific and thus, is not required for the diagnosis of SIBO.[3]

The main human methanogen is *Methanobrevibacter smithii*, and is one of the first inhabitants of the human gut microbiome, likely acquired from the mother's microbiota.[29] Approximately 35% of healthy humans host methanogens, and several studies have shown a positive association between constipation and elevated methane levels on breath testing.[30,31] The opposite is true for those with elevated hydrogen or hydrogen sulfide levels who appear more likely to report diarrhea.[32,33] The pathophysiology of constipation in methane-predominant SIBO is incompletely understood, however, translational studies have demonstrated that the presence of methane production is correlated with altered intestinal motility and slow intestinal transit.[34,35]

Diagnosis of methane-associated SIBO may be important therapeutically, as *M smithii* is resistant to many antibiotics, and treatment recommendations differ from hydrogen-predominant SIBO. Thus, breath testing for SIBO should at a minimum include the measurement of both hydrogen and methane levels.3 Unlike hydrogen, a rise of only 10 ppm is needed for a positive test result. Indeed, studies suggest that this threshold demonstrates a specificity of up to 100%.[3] Recent studies suggest that measurement of hydrogen sulfide might also be of value though this remains to be adequately validated in human trials.[33]

### Future Diagnostics

Given the clear limitations of quantitative culture and breath testing; a number of alternative diagnostic platforms are in development for SIBO. For example, gas-sensing capsules that will provide real-time measurements of luminal gases are in development.[36] In 2018, Berean and colleagues[37] published an investigation of the diagnostic safety and accuracy of such a gas-sensing capsule compared with hydrogen breath testing in 12 subjects. This novel capsule collected gas measurements every 5 minutes and transmitted the information wirelessly to a cell phone device held by the subject. No adverse events were reported and the capsule demonstrated high sensitivity and reliability.[37] Although larger studies are clearly needed, this pilot study provides proof of concept that a gas-sensing capsule could be developed that could detect SIBO. Another novel capsule technology that is, in development allows assessment of jejunal fluid for unique bacterial fluorescence profiles and algorithms derived from machine learning enables quantitation of the bacteria.[38]

## TREATMENT OF SMALL INTESTINAL BACTERIAL OVERGROWTH

The goals of treatment for SIBO include small intestinal decontamination and/or the prevention of recurrence. Antibiotics therefore represent an obvious choice for the initial decontamination of the small bowel. A second facet of therapy involves treatment of the underlying cause and pathogenesis for recurrent bacterial overgrowth.

Proposed therapies for this have included the use of probiotics, prokinetics and various dietary interventions.

## Antibiotics

Given the growing risk of bacterial resistance, opportunistic infections, such as *Clostridium difficile*, and other adverse effects of antibiotics, it is prudent to recommended that SIBO be diagnosed by objective testing before the pursuit of antibiotic therapy (**Table 2**). With that said, the evidence for the use of antibiotics in SIBO is largely limited to small clinical trials of low quality. A limited number of antibiotics have been evaluated in the treatment of SIBO including amoxicillin-clavulanic acid, ciprofloxacin, doxycycline, metronidazole, neomycin, norfloxacin, rifaximin, tetracycline, and trimethoprim-sulfamethoxazole.

Of the available antibiotics, rifaximin has been the most robustly evaluated as a treatment for SIBO (**Table 3**). A meta-analysis of 32 clinical trials involving more than 1300 participants assessed the safety and efficacy of rifaximin in the treatment of SIBO.[39] The overall success of therapy by intention to treat was 70% with adverse reaction occurring in 4.6%. There was great heterogeneity in the included studies and thus, many questions remain regarding the specifics of treatment. For example, the dosing of rifaximin ranged from 600 to 1600 mg a day and duration of therapy ranged from 5 to 28 days in the clinical trials. Two subsequent clinical trials have been performed assessing rifaximin for SIBO. In a trial of 18 patients with SIBO by glucose breath test following surgical resection for colorectal cancer,[40] the response rate to 10 days of rifaximin at a total daily dose of 1200 mg with a 33% based on a repeat glucose breath test following antibiotic therapy. The second trial assessed 17 cirrhotic patients with SIBO demonstrating a 76% response rate based on repeat glucose breath testing following a 7 day course of rifaximin at a total daily dose of 1200 mg.[41] Based on the aggregate data and acknowledging that only a 550 mg dose of rifaximin is commercially available, a 14-day course of therapy at 550 mg 3 times daily appears to maximize treatment efficacy (see **Table 2**). However, this dose appears to have a higher risk of adverse events compared with 550 mg taken twice daily.

Aside from rifaximin, quinolones are the next most studied group of antibiotics for SIBO. There have been 3 clinical trials assessing ciprofloxacin in the treatment of SIBO. The first study compared 10 days of ciprofloxacin 500 mg twice daily with

**Table 2**
**Summary of results for rifaximin clinical trials**

|  | Treatment Efficacy, % | Adverse Events, % |
| --- | --- | --- |
| Total daily dosage, mg |  |  |
| 600 | 16.7 | 10 |
| 800 | 50–100 | 3–13 |
| 1200 | 34–87 | 2–8 |
| 1600 | 80 | 15 |
| Duration of therapy, d |  |  |
| 5 | 66.7 | Not reported |
| 7 | 16–80 | 8.8–13.0 |
| 10 | 33–100 | 3.5 |
| 14 | 87 | 2–4.7 |
| 28 | 34 | 3.6–9.0 |

**Table 3**
**Antibiotic regimens to consider in the treatment of small intestinal bacterial overgrowth**

| Antibiotic | Dosage | Duration of Therapy, d |
|---|---|---|
| Amoxicillin-clavulanic acid | 875 mg BID | 10–14 |
| Ciprofloxacin | 500 mg BID | 10–14 |
| Doxycycline | 100 mg BID | 10–14 |
| Metronidazole | 250 mg TID | 10–14 |
| Neomycin[a] | 500 mg BID | 10–14 |
| Norfloxacin | 400 mg BID | 10–14 |
| Rifaximin | 550 mg TID | 14 |
| Tetracycline | 250 mg QID | 10–14 |
| Trimethoprim-sulfamethoxazole | 1 double strength tablet BID | 10–14 |

*Abbreviations:* BID, twice a day; QID, 4 times a day; TID, 3 times a day.
[a] Consider adding to a second antibiotic when breath test positive by methane.

metronidazole 250 mg 3 times daily in 29 patients with Crohn's disease and SIBO based on glucose breath testing.[42] In this study, all 14 adults treated with ciprofloxacin responded compared with 13 (86%) of the 15 of those receiving metronidazole based on repeat breath testing. The second trial assessed 7 patients with nonalcoholic steatohepatitis with SIBO based on glucose breath testing. Those treated with 5 days of ciprofloxacin 500 mg bid yielded a treatment response of 71% based on repeat breath testing.[43] A third trial assessed 10 patients with cystic fibrosis and SIBO based on glucose breath testing. Each pediatric patient received ciprofloxacin at a dose of 35 to 50 mg per kg per day for an unspecified duration, yielding a response rate of 90% based on repeat breath testing.[44] There has also been a randomized, placebo-controlled trial assessing norfloxacin at a dose of 400 mg twice daily for 10 days in 15 patients with irritable bowel syndrome (IBS) and SIBO based on culture of small bowel aspirate (4 also positive by breath testing as well as culture).[45] All 4 of those consenting to retesting (2 consented to repeat small bowel aspirate and breath testing, 2 consented only to repeat breath testing) for SIBO were cured compared with none of the 7 receiving placebo.

Other antibiotics have been less well studied. For example, amoxicillin-clavulanic acid has only been evaluated in a single crossover trial of 10 patients with SIBO based on glucose breath testing.[46] In this study, amoxicillin-clavulanic acid given 875 mg twice daily or norfloxacin 400 mg twice daily were given for 7 days. Amoxicillin-clavulanic acid or norfloxacin achieved normalization of breath testing results in 50% versus 30%, respectively.

Trimethoprim-sulfamethoxazole has been assessed in combination with metronidazole in an open trial of 20 Brazilian children with SIBO based on lactulose breath testing yielding a response rate of 95% based on repeat lactulose breath testing.[47]

There have been 2 clinical trials assessing the efficacy of neomycin in the treatment of SIBO. The first was a placebo-controlled trial assessing neomycin in 111 IBS patients with SIBO based on lactulose breath testing.[48] In this trial, 10 days of neomycin at a dose of 500 mg of twice daily provided a 35% response (based on a composite score for severity of abdominal pain, diarrhea and constipation) compared to 11% for placebo. Of the 84 participants with an abnormal baseline lactose breath test (>3 parts per million (ppm) of methane), this normalized on repeat breath testing in 20% of those receiving neomycin compared with 1% of those receiving placebo. The second study was a retrospective chart review of 74 patients with methane-predominant SIBO based on a lactulose breath test (>3 ppm of methane).[49] In this study, response rates to 10 days of neomycin 500 mg twice daily or 10 days of rifaximin 400 mg 3 times daily or both agents for 10 days were compared. The investigators reported normalization of methane on repeat breath testing in 33% with neomycin alone, 28% with the rifaximin alone, and 87% when receiving both antibiotics.

Cases of SIBO characterized by excessive methane gas production are largely due to the presence of the archaeon, M smithii, a prokaryote lacking a cell and demonstrating resistance to multiple antibiotics including ampicillin, streptomycin, gentamicin, rifampicin, ofloxacin, tetracycline, and amphotericin B.[50] There is limited evidence to suggest that the addition of neomycin to an antibiotic regimen may improve treatment efficacy in this cohort of SIBO. In addition to the previously noted retrospective study by Pimentel and colleagues,[51] a prospective randomized controlled trial was performed on 31 adults with IBS-C based on Rome 3 criteria and methane levels greater than 3 ppm on lactulose breath testing. Methane levels fell below 3 ppm in 66.7% in the 15 participants receiving 14 days of neomycin 500 mg bid and rifaximin 550 mg tid and in 68% of those receiving 14 days of neomycin 500 mg bid. The HMG-CoA reductase inhibitor, lovastatin, has been shown to prevent methanogenous in a variety of methanobrevibacter species including M smithii.[52] Although no clinical trials have been performed in SIBO, there is emerging evidence that lovastatin may augment a treatment response in variety of functional bowel disorders promoted by methanogenesis possibly including SIBO.[53]

A single study assessed the response of 7 days of tetracycline at a total daily dose of 1 g given to 24 adults with jejunal cultures positive for Escherichia coli. Following therapy 21 of the 24 (87.5%) demonstrated negative jejunal cultures.[54] In a single study assessing elderly nursing home residents, 9 of 62 residents were positive for SIBO by glucose breath testing[55] Those testing positive received 10 days of doxycycline,100 mg a day, for 4 consecutive months. No follow-up breath testing was performed, but those with an initial positive breath demonstrated weight gain and increased body mass index (BMI) at the end of 4 months, as opposed to those with a negative breath who demonstrated a decrease in weight and BMI.

The widely accepted practice of antibiotic retreatment following SIBO recurrence is solely based on anecdotal evidence and expert opinion. Consequently, there are no universally accepted treatment approaches. There is 1 published study assessing the frequency of SIBO recurrence in 80 adults following a course of antibiotic therapy demonstrating a recurrence rate of 12.6% at 3 months, 27.5% at 6 months, and 43.7% at 9 months.[56] Another study evaluated the use of repeated antibiotics to treat SIBO and prevent recurrence in 51 patients with systemic sclerosis.[57] In this study, 7 days of norfloxacin 400 mg twice daily was alternated once monthly with 7 days of metronidazole 250 mg 3 times daily for 3 consecutive months yielding a response rate of 52% in preventing SIBO recurrence. The investigators offer the following suggestions. The frequency of retreatment should be based on the timing and characteristics of symptom recurrence so as to minimize the repeated use of antibiotics. In situations when retreatment is necessary within a short time frame (we arbitrarily say a period of <3 months), and alternative antibiotic regimen to the previous treatment should be used to reduce the development of antibiotic resistance.

## *Probiotics*

The concept of using probiotics to treat a condition with excessive bacteria may seem counterintuitive. There are currently inconclusive data to support a role for probiotics in the treatment of SIBO. A recently published, small study examined the open-label use of a proprietary probiotic cocktail on subjects with IBS with or without SIBO.[58] In this study, the 5 IBS/SIBO subjects demonstrated a 71% improvement in the IBS severity scoring system score compared with 10.6% improvement in the score for those IBS subjects without SIBO.

A recent meta-analysis and systematic review examined the existing trials of probiotics in SIBO through May of 2016.[59] Fourteen full-text trials and 8 abstracts were included in the analysis. All included studies were small in size and of overall low quality. There was no significant difference in SIBO incidence between the probiotic and nonprobiotic arms with a relative risk of 0.54 (95% CI 0.19–1.52; $P = .24$). In a separate analysis, there was a greater SIBO decontamination rate in those on probiotics with a relative risk of 1.61 (95% CI 1.19–2.17, $P < .05$).

### Prokinetics

Although it is widely believed that the restoration of normal gastrointestinal motility can reduce the risk of SIBO, the published data to support this hypothesis are scant. A small, prospective study of 5 patients with scleroderma with documented SIBO treated with 50 μg of subcutaneous octreotide each evening for 3 weeks demonstrated normalization of breath testing for SIBO and improvements in the mean daily symptoms scores for nausea, vomiting, bloating, and abdominal pain for the group collectively.[60] In another small study, 12 patients with cirrhosis treated with daily cisapride for 6 months were shown to have improvement in small bowel transit time, fasting motility, and amplitude of contractions based on small bowel manometry as well as decreased occurrence of SIBO based on hydrogen breath testing compared with placebo.[61] A chart review of 64 patients found the daily nocturnal use of a small dose of tegaserod to be superior to no therapy in preventing the recurrence of SIBO symptoms in IBS.[62]

### Diet

Given the frequent association between eating a meal and gastrointestinal symptoms, it stands to reason that dietary modification may be of benefit to patients with SIBO. Proposed dietary strategies have included the avoidance of short chain, carbohydrates, particularly Fermentable Oligosaccharide Disaccharide Monosaccharide And Polyols (FODMAPs), avoidance of sugar substitutes such as sorbitol, aspartame, and saccharine or pursuit of an elemental diet. However, published data regarding dietary therapy for SIBO is slim to nonexistent and largely extrapolated from studies in patients with IBS.

A single-center study of 93 patients with IBS with a positive lactulose breath test found a 2-week trial of an elemental diet to improve bowel symptoms (66% reduction in symptom severity) and to normalize repeat breath testing (80% following 2 weeks of therapy and 85% following 3 weeks of therapy). However, the use of an elemental diet may be logistically difficult for a multitude of reasons.[63] Perhaps a more practical dietary intervention for the management of SIBO might be the low FODMAP diet. Though there are now multiple studies that have evaluated the efficacy of the low FODMAP diet in patients with IBS,[64] there are presently no published clinical trials assessing the low FODMAP diet as a treatment for SIBO. There are data to support that a low FODMAP diet is associated with reduced fermentation and secondary gas production based on breath testing.[65] A similar finding of lower breath hydrogen was seen in a study by McIntosh and colleagues.[66] Future studies assessing the effects of a low FODMAP diet in patients with SIBO are needed. In the meantime, the low FODMAP diet is logistically feasible and increasingly used in clinical practice and thus, may provide adjunctive management strategy in patients with repetitive episodes of SIBO.

## Herbal Therapy

There is accumulating evidence demonstrating the antimicrobial properties of a growing number of herbs including garlic, black cumin, cloves, cinnamon, thyme, all-spices, bay leaves, mustard, and rosemary.[67] This has prompted an interest in herbal therapy for the treatment of SIBO. A prospective trial was performed on 104 adults with SIBO based on a lactulose breath test comparing the efficacy of rifaximin to 1 of 2 commercially available herbal products.[68] Participants received either rifaximin 400 mg 3 times daily or 1 of 2 herbal products twice daily including either Dysbiocide and FC Cidal (Biotics Research Laboratories, Rosenberg, TX) or Candibactin-AR and Candibactin-BR (Metagenics, Inc, Aliso Viejo, CA) for 4 consecutive weeks. Based on repeat lactulose breath testing there was a 46% response with the herbal therapy versus a 34% response with the rifaximin, $P = .24$.

## SUMMARY

On many levels, SIBO remains an enigma. It is critically important for clinicians to understand the associations and issues that predispose to the development of SIBO (see **Fig. 1**). That said, although SIBO is increasingly recognized as an important cause of gastrointestinal symptoms and disease, providers remain challenged by the lack of a scientifically validated diagnostic gold standard. Further, though there are many treatment options, few can make the claim of being truly evidence-based. Thus, when confronted with a patient in whom SIBO is a concern, a provider is faced with a difficult choice: ordering an imperfect test or empirically recommending a course of treatment that offers marginal efficacy.

Clearly, more research is needed to expand our thinking beyond SIBO as merely a disorder of too much bacteria in the wrong place. For example, it might be possible that the composition of the bacterial communities and their metabolic consequences are just as important as the quantity of bacteria in the small intestine. Recent work suggests that deep sequencing of the small intestinal microbiome of patients with SIBO differs dramatically from healthy volunteers.[26] Also, what role, if any, might viruses or fungi play in these patients? Furthering our understanding of the basic mechanisms by which SIBO occurs will hopefully allow the identification of targets for biomarkers and more effective treatments. This might allow us to evolve from the current model of choosing between imperfect diagnostic tests and poorly validated antibiotic treatments to more of a precision medicine model.

## DISCLOSURE

Ginnebaugh - nothing to disclose, Saad, nothing to Disclose. Chey - Biomerica, Phathom, Redhill, Takeda – consultant, Biomerica – research grant.

## REFERENCES

1. Gasbarrini A, Corazza GR, Gasbarrini G, et al. Methodology and indications of H2-breath testing in gastrointestinal diseases: the Rome Consensus Conference. Aliment Pharmacol Ther 2009;29(Suppl 1):1–49.
2. Erdogan A, Rao SS, Gulley D, et al. Small intestinal bacterial overgrowth: duodenal aspiration vs glucose breath test. Neurogastroenterol Motil 2015; 27(4):481–9.
3. Rezaie A, Buresi M, Lembo A, et al. Hydrogen and methane-based breath testing in gastrointestinal disorders: the North American Consensus. Am J Gastroenterol 2017;112(5):775–84.

4. Bures J, Cyrany J, Kohoutova D, et al. Small intestinal bacterial overgrowth syndrome. World J Gastroenterol 2010;16(24):2978–90.

5. Lynch SV, Pedersen O. The human intestinal microbiome in health and disease. N Engl J Med 2016;375(24):2369–79.

6. Lombardo L, Foti M, Ruggia O, et al. Increased incidence of small intestinal bacterial overgrowth during proton pump inhibitor therapy. Clin Gastroenterol Hepatol 2010;8(6):504–8.

7. Ratuapli SK, Ellington TG, O'Neill MT, et al. Proton pump inhibitor therapy use does not predispose to small intestinal bacterial overgrowth. Am J Gastroenterol 2012;107(5):730–5.

8. Su T, Lai S, Lee A, et al. Meta-analysis: proton pump inhibitors moderately increase the risk of small intestinal bacterial overgrowth. J Gastroenterol 2018; 53(1):27–36.

9. Lo WK, Chan WW. Proton pump inhibitor use and the risk of small intestinal bacterial overgrowth: a meta-analysis. Clin Gastroenterol Hepatol 2013;11(5):483–90.

10. Ni Chonchubhair HM, Bashir Y, Dobson M, et al. The prevalence of small intestinal bacterial overgrowth in non-surgical patients with chronic pancreatitis and pancreatic exocrine insufficiency (PEI). Pancreatology 2018;18(4):379–85.

11. Lee AA, Baker JR, Wamsteker EJ, et al. Small intestinal bacterial overgrowth is common in chronic pancreatitis and associates with diabetes, chronic pancreatitis severity, low zinc levels, and opiate use. Am J Gastroenterol 2019;114(7): 1163–71.

12. Capurso G, Signoretti M, Archibugi L, et al. Systematic review and meta-analysis: small intestinal bacterial overgrowth in chronic pancreatitis. United European Gastroenterol J 2016;4(5):697–705.

13. Maslennikov R, Pavlov C, Ivashkin V. Small intestinal bacterial overgrowth in cirrhosis: systematic review and meta-analysis. Hepatol Int 2018;12(6):567–76.

14. Vantrappen G, Janssens J, Hellemans J, et al. The interdigestive motor complex of normal subjects and patients with bacterial overgrowth of the small intestine. J Clin Invest 1977;59(6):1158–66.

15. Husebye E, Skar V, Høverstad T, et al. Abnormal intestinal motor patterns explain enteric colonization with gram-negative bacilli in late radiation enteropathy. Gastroenterology 1995;109(4):1078–89.

16. Ojetti V, Pitocco D, Scarpellini E, et al. Small bowel bacterial overgrowth and type 1 diabetes. Eur Rev Med Pharmacol Sci 2009;13(6):419–23.

17. Revaiah PC, Kochhar R, Rana S, et al. Risk of small intestinal bacterial overgrowth in patients receiving proton pump inhibitors versus proton pump inhibitors plus prokinetics. JGH Open 2018;2(2):47–53.

18. Quigley EM. Small intestinal bacterial overgrowth: what it is and what it is not. Curr Opin Gastroenterol 2014;30(2):141–6.

19. Bach AG, Lubbert C, Behrmann C, et al. [Small bowel diverticula - diagnosis and complications]. Dtsch Med Wochenschr 2011;136(4):140–4.

20. Choung RS, Ruff KC, Malhotra A, et al. Clinical predictors of small intestinal bacterial overgrowth by duodenal aspirate culture. Aliment Pharmacol Ther 2011; 33(9):1059–67.

21. Shah A, Morrison M, Burger D, et al. Systematic review with meta-analysis: the prevalence of small intestinal bacterial overgrowth in inflammatory bowel disease. Aliment Pharmacol Ther 2019;49(6):624–35.

22. Adike A, DiBaise JK. Small intestinal bacterial overgrowth: nutritional implications, diagnosis, and management. Gastroenterol Clin North Am 2018;47(1):193–208.

23. Johansson ME, Hansson GC. Immunological aspects of intestinal mucus and mucins. Nat Rev Immunol 2016;16(10):639–49.

24. Sachdev AH, Pimentel M. Gastrointestinal bacterial overgrowth: pathogenesis and clinical significance. Ther Adv Chronic Dis 2013;4(5):223–31.

25. Khoshini R, Dai S-C, Lezcano S, et al. A systematic review of diagnostic tests for small intestinal bacterial overgrowth. Dig Dis Sci 2008;53(6):1443–54.

26. Leite G, Villanueva-Millan MJ, Celly S. et al. First Large Scale Study Defining the Characteristic Microbiome Signatures of Small intestinal Bacterial overgrowth (SIBO): Detailed analysis from the Reimagine Study, in Digestive Disease Week. 2019: San Diego, CA.

27. Keller J, Franke A, Storr M, et al. Clinically relevant breath tests in gastroenterological diagnostics–recommendations of the German Society for Neurogastroenterology and Motility as well as the German Society for Digestive and Metabolic Diseases. Z Gastroenterol 2005;43(9):1071–90 [in German].

28. Alberti KG, Zimmet PZ. Definition, diagnosis and classification of diabetes mellitus and its complications. Part 1: diagnosis and classification of diabetes mellitus provisional report of a WHO consultation. Diabet Med 1998;15(7):539–53.

29. Grine G, Boualam MA, Drancourt M. Methanobrevibacter smithii, a methanogen consistently colonising the newborn stomach. Eur J Clin Microbiol Infect Dis 2017;36(12):2449–55.

30. Pimentel M, Mayer AG, Park S, et al. Methane production during lactulose breath test is associated with gastrointestinal disease presentation. Dig Dis Sci 2003; 48(1):86–92.

31. Attaluri A, Jackson M, Valestin J, et al. Methanogenic flora is associated with altered colonic transit but not stool characteristics in constipation without IBS. Am J Gastroenterol 2010;105(6):1407–11.

32. Chatterjee S, Park S, Low K, et al. The degree of breath methane production in IBS correlates with the severity of constipation. Am J Gastroenterol 2007; 102(4):837–41.

33. Tahli Singer-Englar AR, Gupta K, Pichetshote N, et al. A Novel 4-Gas Device for Breath Testing Shows Exhaled H2S is Associated with Diarrhea and Abdominal Pain in a Large Scale Prospective Trial, in DDW 2018. 2018: Washington, DC.

34. Kunkel D, Basseri RJ, Makhani MD, et al. Methane on breath testing is associated with constipation: a systematic review and meta-analysis. Dig Dis Sci 2011;56(6): 1612–8.

35. Pimentel M, Lin HC, Enayati P, et al. Methane, a gas produced by enteric bacteria, slows intestinal transit and augments small intestinal contractile activity. Am J Physiol Gastrointest Liver Physiol 2006;290(6):G1089–95.

36. Ou JZ, Yao CK, Rotbart A, et al. Human intestinal gas measurement systems: in vitro fermentation and gas capsules. Trends Biotechnol 2015;33(4):208–13.

37. Berean KJ, Ha N, Ou JZ, et al. The safety and sensitivity of a telemetric capsule to monitor gastrointestinal hydrogen production in vivo in healthy subjects: a pilot trial comparison to concurrent breath analysis. Aliment Pharmacol Ther 2018; 48(6):646–54.

38. Singh S, AN, Wahl C, et al. Development of a Swallowable Diagnostic Capsule to Monitor Gastrointestinal Health. May 2019. 156(6):p. S-376.

39. Gatta L, Scarpignato C. Systematic review with meta-analysis: rifaximin is effective and safe for the treatment of small intestine bacterial overgrowth. Aliment Pharmacol Ther 2017;45(5):604–16.

40. Deng L, Liu Y, Zhang D, et al. Prevalence and treatment of small intestinal bacterial overgrowth in postoperative patients with colorectal cancer. Mol Clin Oncol 2016;4(5):883–7.
41. Zhang Y, Feng Y, Cao B, et al. Effects of SIBO and rifaximin therapy on MHE caused by hepatic cirrhosis. Int J Clin Exp Med 2015;8(2):2954–7.
42. Castiglione F, Rispo A, Di Girolamo E, et al. Antibiotic treatment of small bowel bacterial overgrowth in patients with Crohn's disease. Aliment Pharmacol Ther 2003;18(11–12):1107–12.
43. Sajjad A, Mottershead M, Syn WK, et al. Ciprofloxacin suppresses bacterial overgrowth, increases fasting insulin but does not correct low acylated ghrelin concentration in non-alcoholic steatohepatitis. Aliment Pharmacol Ther 2005;22(4):291–9.
44. Lisowska A, Pogorzelski A, Oracz G, et al. Oral antibiotic therapy improves fat absorption in cystic fibrosis patients with small intestine bacterial overgrowth. J Cyst Fibros 2011;10(6):418–21.
45. Ghoshal UC, Srivastava D, Misra A, et al. A proof-of-concept study showing antibiotics to be more effective in irritable bowel syndrome with than without small-intestinal bacterial overgrowth: a randomized, double-blind, placebo-controlled trial. Eur J Gastroenterol Hepatol 2016;28(3):281–9.
46. Attar A, Flourié B, Rambaud JC, et al. Antibiotic efficacy in small intestinal bacterial overgrowth-related chronic diarrhea: a crossover, randomized trial. Gastroenterology 1999;117(4):794–7.
47. Tahan S, Melli LC, Mello CS, et al. Effectiveness of trimethoprim-sulfamethoxazole and metronidazole in the treatment of small intestinal bacterial overgrowth in children living in a slum. J Pediatr Gastroenterol Nutr 2013;57(3):316–8.
48. Pimentel M, Chow EJ, Lin HC. Normalization of lactulose breath testing correlates with symptom improvement in irritable bowel syndrome. a double-blind, randomized, placebo-controlled study. Am J Gastroenterol 2003;98(2):412–9.
49. Low K, Hwang L, Hua J, et al. A combination of rifaximin and neomycin is most effective in treating irritable bowel syndrome patients with methane on lactulose breath test. J Clin Gastroenterol 2010;44(8):547–50.
50. Dridi B, Fardeau ML, Ollivier B, et al. The antimicrobial resistance pattern of cultured human methanogens reflects the unique phylogenetic position of archaea. J Antimicrob Chemother 2011;66(9):2038–44.
51. Pimentel M, Chang C, Chua KS, et al. Antibiotic treatment of constipation-predominant irritable bowel syndrome. Dig Dis Sci 2014;59(6):1278–85.
52. Gottlieb K, Wacher V, Sliman J, et al. Review article: inhibition of methanogenic archaea by statins as a targeted management strategy for constipation and related disorders. Aliment Pharmacol Ther 2016;43(2):197–212.
53. Triantafyllou K, Chang C, Pimentel M. Methanogens, methane and gastrointestinal motility. J Neurogastroenterol Motil 2014;20(1):31–40.
54. Shindo K, Machida M, Fukumura M, et al. Omeprazole induces altered bile acid metabolism. Gut 1998;42(2):266–71.
55. Lewis SJ, Potts LF, Malhotra R, et al. Small bowel bacterial overgrowth in subjects living in residential care homes. Age Ageing 1999;28(2):181–5.
56. Lauritano EC, Gabrielli M, Scarpellini E, et al. Small intestinal bacterial overgrowth recurrence after antibiotic therapy. Am J Gastroenterol 2008;103(8):2031–5.
57. Marie I, Ducrotté P, Denis P, et al. Small intestinal bacterial overgrowth in systemic sclerosis. Rheumatology (Oxford) 2009;48(10):1314–9.
58. Leventogiannis K, Gkolfakis P, Spithakis G, et al. Effect of a preparation of four probiotics on symptoms of patients with irritable bowel syndrome: association

with intestinal bacterial overgrowth. Probiotics Antimicrob Proteins 2018;11(2): 627–34.

59. Zhong C, Qu C, Wang B, et al. Probiotics for preventing and treating small intestinal bacterial overgrowth: a meta-analysis and systematic review of current evidence. J Clin Gastroenterol 2017;51(4):300–11.

60. Soudah HC, Hasler WL, Owyang C. Effect of octreotide on intestinal motility and bacterial overgrowth in scleroderma. N Engl J Med 1991;325(21):1461–7.

61. Madrid AM, Hurtado C, Venegas M, et al. Long-Term treatment with cisapride and antibiotics in liver cirrhosis: effect on small intestinal motility, bacterial overgrowth, and liver function. Am J Gastroenterol 2001;96(4):1251–5.

62. Pimentel M, Morales W, Lezcano S, et al. Low-dose nocturnal tegaserod or erythromycin delays symptom recurrence after treatment of irritable bowel syndrome based on presumed bacterial overgrowth. Gastroenterol Hepatol (N Y) 2009; 5(6):435–42.

63. Pimentel M, Constantino T, Kong Y, et al. A 14-day elemental diet is highly effective in normalizing the lactulose breath test. Dig Dis Sci 2004;49(1):73–7.

64. Dionne J, Ford AC, Yuan Y, et al. A systematic review and meta-analysis evaluating the efficacy of a gluten-free diet and a low FODMAPs diet in treating symptoms of irritable bowel syndrome. Am J Gastroenterol 2018;113(9):1290–300.

65. Ong DK, Mitchell SB, Barrett JS, et al. Manipulation of dietary short chain carbohydrates alters the pattern of gas production and genesis of symptoms in irritable bowel syndrome. J Gastroenterol Hepatol 2010;25(8):1366–73.

66. McIntosh K, Reed D, Schneider T, et al. FODMAPs alter symptoms and the metabolome of patients with IBS: a randomised controlled trial. Gut 2017;66(7): 1241–51.

67. Lai PK, Roy J. Antimicrobial and chemopreventive properties of herbs and spices. Curr Med Chem 2004;11(11):1451–60.

68. Chedid V, Dhalla S, Clarke J, et al. Herbal therapy is equivalent to rifaximin for the treatment of small intestinal bacterial overgrowth. Glob Adv Health Med 2014; 3(3):16–24.

# COLON

# Assessing Anorectal Function in Constipation and Fecal Incontinence

Alice C. Jiang, MD[a], Ami Panara, MD[b], Yun Yan, MD[c], Satish S.C. Rao, MD, PhD[d],*

## KEYWORDS

- Translumbosacral anorectal magnetic stimulation • Anorectal function
- Constipation • Fecal incontinence • Digital rectal examination

## KEY POINTS

- Assessment of anorectal function includes comprehensive history, rectal examination, and prospective stool diary or electronic App diary that accurately captures bowel symptoms, evaluation severity, and quality life measures.
- Evaluation of a suspected patient with dyssynergic constipation includes anorectal manometry, balloon expulsion test, and defecography.
- Investigation of a suspected patient with fecal incontinence includes high-resolution anorectal manometry; anal ultrasound or MR imaging; and neurophysiology tests, such as translumbosacral anorectal magnetic stimulation (TAMS) or pudendal nerve latency.

## INTRODUCTION

The evaluation of anorectal function in a patient with symptoms of constipation or fecal incontinence (FI) begins with a comprehensive history that includes assessment of quality of life and psychological stressors; disease severity; digital rectal examination (DRE); and a thoughtful plan for testing anorectal sensorimotor function, structure, and neurophysiology. In this overview, we provide our approach to the assessment of anorectal function.

[a] Division of Gastroenterology, Department of Internal Medicine, Rush University Medical Center, 600 S Paulina St, Chicago, IL 60612, USA; [b] Division of Gastroenterology, Department of Internal Medicine, University of Miami Leonard M. Miller School of Medicine, 1601 NW 12th Ave, Miami, FL, USA; [c] Division of Gastroenterology and Hepatology, Department of Internal Medicine, Augusta University, Augusta, GA, USA; [d] Division of Gastroenterology and Hepatology, Augusta University Medical Center, 1120 15th Street, AD 2226, Augusta, GA 30912, USA
* Corresponding author.
E-mail address: srao@augusta.edu

Gastroenterol Clin N Am 49 (2020) 589–606
https://doi.org/10.1016/j.gtc.2020.04.011
0889-8553/20/© 2020 Elsevier Inc. All rights reserved.

## ASSESSMENT OF SYMPTOMS

A thorough assessment of symptoms is critical for the evaluation and management of anorectal disorders. Patients have different perspectives on what defines constipation or FI. Hence, it is important to inquire about specific symptoms that can help to assist with correct diagnosis and management. In a recent cross-sectional survey across the United Kingdom, the most commonly perceived constipation symptoms reported by the general population were straining, spending a long time on the toilet without passing stool, and the need to use laxatives, whereas general practitioners and specialists described infrequent bowel movements and hard stools as the most important constipation symptoms.[1] The differences in perceived symptoms of constipation highlight the need to ask for six symptoms outlined in the Rome IV criteria for constipation[2] so that an appropriate diagnosis is made.

Important symptoms to ask in patients complaining of constipation and occurring with at least 25% of defecations are straining, lumpy or hard stools (Bristol Stool Form Scale type 1 or 2), sensation of incomplete evacuation, manual maneuvers to facilitate defecation (ie, digital evacuation, support of the pelvic floor), and fewer than three defecations per week. The presence of alarming features, such as unintentional weight loss (>10% in 3 months), rectal bleeding (in the absence of documented bleeding hemorrhoids or anal fissures), and a family history of colon cancer or familial polyposis syndromes should prompt earlier endoscopic evaluation.

Symptoms for dyssynergic defecation can vary from one patient to another and, based on one study, symptoms were not a good predictor of dyssynergic defecation.[3] The three most common symptoms based on one survey of 118 subjects with dyssynergic defecation were excessive straining (84%), feeling of incomplete evacuation (76%), and abdominal bloating (74%).[4] A study of 190 constipated patients showed that a sense of obstruction/digital evacuation was specific but not sensitive for dyssynergic defecation.[5] Other reported symptoms included the passage of hard stools (65%), a stool frequency of fewer than three bowel movements per week (62%), and digital maneuvers (35%), although this symptom is likely underreported.[4] Providers should ask patients about these symptoms directly because patients may not offer this information. Phone APPs such as FI stool diary can help.

FI is defined as the uncontrolled passage of solid or liquid stool, regardless of cause.[6] Patients should be asked about factors that cause or exacerbate incontinence, such as loose stools; use of laxatives and artificial sweeteners; or prior obstetric injury or surgical procedures, such as lateral sphincterotomy. Timing of incontinence episodes, such as during or after meals, bowel movements, exercise, or nocturnal symptoms, can help determine cause.[7] It is important to distinguish between urge and passive FI; urge incontinence is marked by having a strong sensation to defecate, but inability to reach the toilet in time, whereas passive incontinence is little to no awareness of the desire to defecate before incontinence. Patients with urge incontinence often have reduced squeeze pressures,[8] reduced rectal capacity, and increased perception of rectal balloon distention,[9] whereas patients with passive incontinence have lower resting pressures[8,10] and neuropathy.[11]

## DIGITAL RECTAL EXAMINATION

A DRE is an essential component of the physical examination in patients that present with anorectal complaints, constipation or FI. It can readily be performed in the office setting and can provide information to guide selection of any future diagnostic tests.[12] However, surveys have shown that DRE is underused.[13]

**Table 1**
**Components of the digital rectal examination, technique, expected findings, and grading of responses**

| Examination Component | Technique | Findings and Grading of Response |
|---|---|---|
| Inspection of the anus and surrounding tissue | Place patient in the left lateral position with hips flexed to 90°. Inspect perineum under good light. | Skin excoriation, skin tags, anal fissure, scars or external hemorrhoids, gaping anus, prolapsed hemorrhoids or rectum, condyloma. |
| Testing of the perineal sensation and anocutaneous reflex | Stroke the skin around the anus in a centripetal fashion (toward anus), in all four quadrants, by using a stick with a cotton bud. | Normal response is brisk contraction of the perianal skin, the anoderm, and the external anal sphincter with the cotton and wooden ends. Response only with the wooden end is an impaired response. |
| Digital palpation | Slowly advance a lubricated and gloved index finger into the rectum and feel the mucosa and surrounding muscle, bone, uterus, prostate, and pelvic structures. | Tenderness, mass, stricture, and stool and the consistency of the stool (Bristol Stool Form Scale). Assess for retroverted uterus, rectocele. |
| Assessment of resting tone | Assess resting tone with gloved index finger. | Normal, weak or increased tone. |
| Assessment of squeeze | Ask the patient to squeeze and hold as long as possible (up to 30 s). | Normal, weak or increased squeeze. |
| Push and bearing down maneuver | In addition to the finger in the rectum, place the other hand over the patients' abdomen. Ask the patient to push and bear down as if to defecate and assess changes in abdominal muscle tightening, perineal descent, and contraction or relaxation of anal sphincter and puborectalis. | i. Assess the abdominal push effort as normal, weak, or excessive. ii. Assess if the anal relaxation is normal, impaired, or if paradoxic contraction if present. iii. Assess if puborectalis relaxation is normal, impaired, or if paradoxic contraction is present. iv. Assess if perineal descent is normal, excessive, or absent. v. Assess for presence of rectal mucosal intussusception or prolapse. |

*Adapted from* Rao SS. Rectal Exam: Yes, it can and should be done in a busy practice! Am J Gastroenterol 2018;113:635–638.

The patient should be placed on the examination table in the left lateral decubitus position with hips flexed to 90°. Inspection should be performed before digital evaluation. First, look for any skin tags, anal fissures, prolapsed hemorrhoids, rashes, scars, or condylomas (**Table 1**). Next, the stick with cotton bud is used to assess the anocutaneous reflex. Gently stroke the skin around the anus in all four quadrants in a centripetal fashion (toward anus) and look for contraction of the perianal skin, the anoderm, and the external anal sphincter (EAS). Brisk contraction is normal, absent contraction with the cotton bud end is an impaired reflex and absent contraction with both ends suggests an absent reflex. Afterward, the provider's gloved index finger is lubricated and is initially placed perpendicular to the anal canal and then slowly inserted into the canal. The provider can rotate the finger to assess for masses; strictures; anal tone; stool; mucosal defects, such as rectocele; and the prostate. Pain during the examination may suggest a fissure. Next, the patient is asked to squeeze the anal sphincter and hold for up to 30 seconds. Finally, the examiner places the free hand on the patient's abdomen and asks the patient to push and bear down. The provider can assess the abdominal push effort, anal relaxation, puborectalis relaxation, perineal descent, and the presence of rectal mucosal intussusception.

## ANORECTAL MANOMETRY

Anorectal manometry (ARM) is an important diagnostic tool for the evaluation of chronic constipation and FI, because it helps to evaluate anorectal motor and sensory function. Chronic functional constipation can include one or a combination of slow transit constipation or obstructed defecation syndrome. In patients with FI, anal resting and squeeze pressures help determine the presence of internal anal sphincter (IAS) and EAS dysfunction. Measurements of anorectal function during simulated defecation can help to establish a proper diagnosis for effective management.

Conventional ARM records pressure data from single points in the anal canal using a water perfused or solid-state system, compared with high-resolution ARM (HR-ARM), which records circumferential pressure data, simultaneously, from the whole anal canal and distal rectum.[14] HR-ARM offers greater physiologic resolution and a minimization of movement artifact, and is gaining popularity as a first-line test to increase the diagnostic accuracy for patients with functional defecation disorders.[15]

Within high-resolution manometry, there are two methods of measurement. Two-dimensional (HR-ARM) records luminal pressures circumferentially from sensors on a flexible catheter and displays the data either topographically in color plots or as an average circumferential pressure at different levels of the anorectum.[14,16] Three-dimensional (3D) ARM records pressures longitudinally and radially from sensors on a rigid, solid state probe with data represented in two-dimensional and 3D form.[14,16–18]

Before starting the ARM study, DRE is performed to exclude an obstructive process in the anal canal, which would prevent advancement of the probe; bleeding; or pain in the anal canal. An enema is given to the patient 2 hours before the study. The patient is placed in the left lateral decubitus position, and the probe is positioned so that the sensors span the distal rectum to beyond the anal verge.

A protocol for standardized measurements obtained during ARM was first proposed by American Neurogastroenterology Motility Society (ANMS)[19] and recently modified

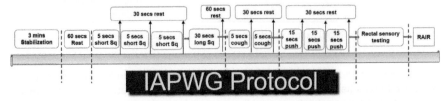

**Fig. 1.** Standardized protocol for high-resolution anorectal manometry as recommended by the IAPWG. IAPWG, international anorectal physiology working Group; RAIR, rectal anal inhibitory reflex.

by the International Anorectal Physiology Working Group (IAPWG) in 2018 (**Fig. 1**).[20] This consists of rest (basal anal pressures at rest over 60 seconds), squeeze (anal pressure during voluntary effort), long squeeze (anal pressure during sustained voluntary effort), cough (anorectal pressure changes during cough; reflux increase in rectal and anal sphincter pressure during abrupt increase in intra-abdominal pressure), push (anorectal pressure changes during simulated defecation), Rectoanal Inhibitory Reflex (reflex anal response to rectal distention), and rectal sensation (assessment of rectal sensitivity to distention).[20]

Normal values for HR-ARM have been described in several studies to date,[21–23] and for 3D-ARM in adults.[17,18,24] Clinically notable findings include sphincter hypotonia (low anal resting pressure), which has been associated with passive FI (**Fig. 2**),[8] compared with sphincter hypertonia (high anal resting pressure), which is seen in anal fissure[25] or evacuation disorder.[26] Sphincter hypocontractility (impaired ability to voluntarily contract the anal sphincter) is associated with fecal urge incontinence.[8] Lower intrarectal pressure with straining and paradoxic anal sphincter contraction during push are associated with obstructive defecation.[26]

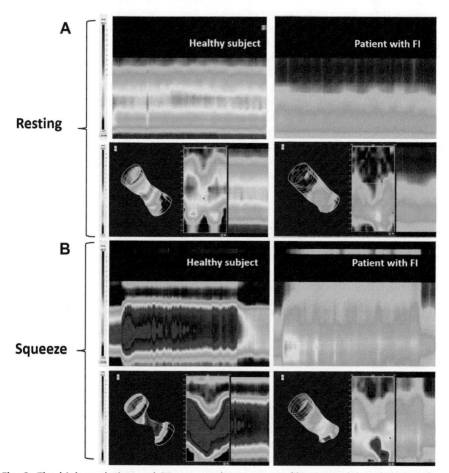

**Fig. 2.** The high-resolution and 3D anorectal pressure profile at rest (*A*) and during the squeeze (*B*) in a healthy subject (*left*) and in a patient with FI (*right*). When compared with healthy subject, the patient with FI shows significantly decreased resting and squeeze anal sphincter pressure.

Pressure defects within the anal canal found on 3D-ARM is suggestive of rectal intussusception. However, anal sphincter defects should be confirmed anatomically by endoanal ultrasound, and presence of intussusception confirmed with defecography because agreement between the studies is unreliable.[27,28]

## RECTAL SENSATION TESTING

Rectal sensation to distention is an important physiologic initiator for defecation. When sensation is either reduced (hyposensitivity) or heightened (hypersensitivity), this can result in impaired anorectal motor response. Rectal sensation is evaluated by a simple balloon distention test. An elastic balloon attached to a catheter is intermittently distended with air in the rectum. Patients are asked to report when they perceive first sensation, desire to defecate, urgency, and maximum tolerance. At each sensation, the volume of air used to distend the balloon is recorded.[29]

Rectal hyposensitivity is seen in irritable bowel syndrome with constipation, FI, chronic constipation, and patients with evacuation disorder secondary to spinal cord injury.[30] A recent study compared barostat-assisted sensory training (BAST) with syringe-assisted (standard) method of sensory testing and suggested that the BAST technique was better and preferred by the therapist.[31] Sensory retraining and biofeedback have been shown to be effective treatments for hyposensitivity associated with FI in patients with diabetes.[32] Similarly, behavioral training and sensory retraining with temporary sacral nerve stimulation has been shown to improve continence in patients with FI because of rectal hyposensitivity.[33] A recent study suggested that sensory adaptation training, a technique of desensitizing the rectum using repeated balloon distention, was better than a selective serotonin reuptake inhibitor; the latter is commonly used for treating irritable bowel syndrome with hypersensitivity. Rectal hypersensitivity is found in patients with fecal urgency and urge incontinence, such as in diarrhea-predominant irritable bowel syndrome, ulcerative colitis, and radiation proctitis.[34]

## BALLOON EXPULSION TESTING

The balloon expulsion test (BET) evaluates whether pelvic floor dyssynergia may be causing constipation.[35] It is performed by having the patient lie in the left lateral decubitus position with hips and knees flexed. A lubricated balloon attached to a catheter is inserted into the rectum and inflated with 50 mL of warm water. The patient is instructed to sit on a commode in privacy and asked to expel the balloon. An expulsion time of more than 1 minute suggests evacuation disorder.[36–38]

There is fair level of agreement between BET and ARM for dyssynergia[36] and between BET and defecography.[39] One example of the need for additional anatomic testing is in the case of rectocele or occluding intussusception for which BET by itself is insufficient. Therefore, BET should be used in conjunction with other anatomic and functional testing to confirm a diagnosis of evacuation disorder.

## DEFECOGRAPHY

Defecography provides real-time dynamic imaging of the defecatory process that is performed using barium contrast (radiograph) or MRI. Barium defecography fluoroscopically tracks the evacuation of a radiopaque barium paste as the patient is defecating in a seated position. The anorectal angulation, degree of opening of the anal canal, rectal wall morphology, perineal descent, and evacuation of rectal contents are recorded.[40,41] Barium defecography can identify anatomic features, which only become evident during the defecation process, such as rectal prolapse, rectocele, or obstructing intussusception. Additionally, MRI defecography allows visualization of all pelvic floor compartments and structures to evaluate for possible cystocele or uterovaginal prolapse.[42,43] In a prospective comparative study, evacuative proctography was found to be more sensitive in detecting rectal intussusception than MR defecography.[44]

Normative data for evacuation proctography and MRI defecography are not yet widely established, but is being actively studied.[39,45] Pathologic differences of pelvic floor descent in straining and defecation phases has been found to differentiate patients with pelvic floor dysfunction from healthy volunteers.[46,47] Some abnormal findings are repaired operatively, but the defecographic parameters do not seem to influence the clinical outcome of surgery.[48]

## ANAL ULTRASOUND

Anal ultrasonography (AUS) can aid with anatomic assessment of the sphincteric complex, including the IAS, EAS, and puborectalis muscle (**Fig. 3**A, B). If properly done, it can detect tears, scarring, and loss of muscle tissue.[49]

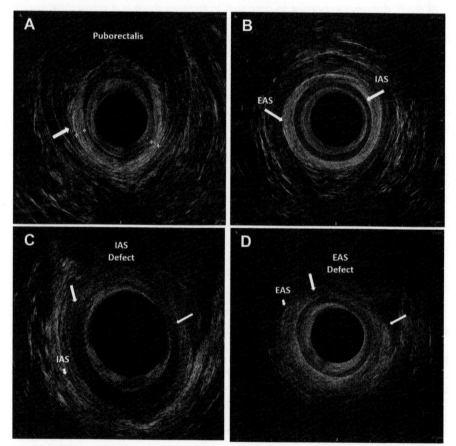

**Fig. 3.** Endoanal ultrasound views of normal subject (*A, B*) and patient with fecal incontinence (*C, D*). The puborectalis is demonstrated as a U-shaped sling (hyperechoic) surrounding the anal canal (*A*). An intact inner IAS (hypoechoic) and outer EAS (hyperechoic) are indicated by *arrows* (*B*). The scan demonstrates an IAS defect between 10 o'clock and 3 o'clock (*C*) and an EAS defect between 11 o'clock and 2 o'clock (*D*) see arrows, in a patient with FI.

Conventionally, AUS is performed with a 5 to 15 mHz rotating transducer that creates a 360° view with penetration of 2.8 to 6.2 cm.[50] Currently available 3D technology collects a series of axial images every 0.05 mm in an automated manner.[51] These images form a cube, which are analyzed in sagittal, coronal, or longitudinal cuts.[52] An experienced endosonographer should perform and interpret the test.

To prepare for the study the patient is placed in the left lateral decubitus position on the examination table. The ultrasound probe is lubricated and placed about 5 cm into the anal canal and slowly withdrawn.[53] During withdrawal, cross-sectional images of the IAS, EAS, and puborectalis are obtained and reconstructed into multiplanar 3D images that are used to calculate anal sphincter volumes.

Normally, two discrete rings of tissue are seen, the inner IAS appears hypoechoic and the outer EAS is more hyperechoic (see **Fig. 3**B).[54] The puborectalis appears U-shaped in the upper section and generally cannot be clearly distinguished from the deeper part of the EAS.[50,55] There are subtle differences between male and female anatomy in relation to thickness. One trial suggested that females have an average anterior IAS thickness of 0.12 cm, whereas the average thickness in males is 0.19 cm.[52] It is also important to note that in females there is a physiologic gap in the upper and middle part of the anterior EAS adjacent to the anovaginal septum[50] and this should not be confused for an injury.

IAS and EAS findings on AUS should be interpreted separately. IAS pathology includes muscle disruption suggesting defects; diffuse muscle thinning suggesting atrophy[34]; or increased muscle thickness and/or hypertrophy, which is seen with rectal intussusception or prolapse.[8,52,56] EAS can also have defects but have focal thinning because of atrophy or scarring.[57,58] Both IAS (**Fig. 3**C)[57,59] and EAS defects (**Fig. 3**D)[60,61] have been associated with symptoms of FI.

Although AUS is considered the gold standard for ultrasound imaging of the anal sphincters, there is paucity of data and disagreement regarding the accuracy and sensitivity of this instrument in diagnosing sphincter injuries. In their series of 51 patients, Gold and colleagues[62] found interobserver agreement in diagnosing IAS injuries, but interobserver disagreement ranging to 5 mm when assessing the EAS thickness. Sultan and colleagues[63] asked 12 patients with EAS injuries to undergo preoperative evaluation with ultrasound. AUS correctly identified the EAS injuries found on surgery, suggesting that AUS is an accurate examination for diagnosing EAS injuries.

The limited availability of AUS has led to studies evaluating the sensitivity of transvaginal ultrasound (TVUS) and transperineal ultrasound (TPUS) for the diagnosis of anal sphincter injuries. There are limited studies with conflicting findings. In their cohort of 50 patients, Stewart and Wilson[64] found TVUS findings as accurate as AUS; however, Frudinger and colleagues[65] noted less than 50% accuracy of TVUS in diagnosis of IAS and EAS injuries when compared with AUS. TPUS is limited by incomplete visualization of the EAS[66] and it showed lower accuracy than TVUS for the diagnosis of defects.[67] A more recent cross-sectional study of 250 women with obstetric anal sphincter injuries who underwent AUS, TVUS, and TPUS found TVUS and TPUS to have low positive predictive values but high negative predictive values for diagnosing anal sphincter defects, suggesting that these techniques were not reliable for identifying defects, but were good at identifying an intact sphincter.[68] Therefore, if available, AUS is a helpful tool for the diagnosis of anal sphincter defects.

## ENDOANAL AND EXTERNAL PHASED-ARRAY MRI

Endoluminal MRI is a specialized technique where coils are introduced into the anus to obtain high-resolution images of the anal sphincters and surrounding perineal structures, an advantage of this technique when compared with AUS. External phased-array MRI is a noninvasive high-resolution imaging technique.

For endoanal MRI the patient is placed in the left lateral decubitus position and a thin cylindrical coil covered with a condom and lubricant is introduced into the anus. A bowel relaxant is given to reduce artifact from peristalsis. The patient is then placed in the supine position. Imaging is done with a T2-weighted imaging sequence. The procedure takes about 30 minutes.[69]

There have been good reproduction of data suggesting that the accuracy of endoanal MRI in diagnosing EAS defects is similar to AUS,[70–74] but that it is inferior for diagnosing IAS defects.[70] Both techniques are only available at specialized centers.

For external phased-array MRI the patient is placed in the supine position and an external coil is placed anterior to the patient. As with endoanal MRI, a T2-weighted sequence is used. The procedure takes about 15 minutes to complete.[75] Terra and colleagues[75] found good correlation of findings between this technique and endoanal MRI for defects and atrophy of the EAS.[76]

AUS has also been compared with external phased-array MRI. One recent study of 40 women with obstetric injuries suggested moderate interrater reliability between the two techniques when diagnosing anal sphincter defects.[77] Therefore, in experienced centers external phased-array MRI may be a suitable and less invasive technique for evaluation of the anal sphincter in patients with FI.

## NEUROPHYSIOLOGY TESTING

Neurophysiologic tests of anorectal function can provide useful information about neuronal innervation and neuromuscular function. These tests, however, are less frequently used in clinical practice because of limited availability; adoption of less-invasive surrogate measures, such as ARM[78]; and concerns about accuracy[79,80] and/or sensitivity and specificity.[81]

## ELECTROMYOGRAPHY

Electromyography (EMG) is electrical recording of muscle activity from the anal sphincter and is performed with either a fine wire needle electrode or a surface electrode, such as an anal plug.[82–84] A disposable needle electrode is placed into the EAS to record motor unit recruitment at rest, with voluntary contraction or with reflex contraction.[20] Alternatively, surface EMG is recorded using a plug electrode.

Abnormal EMG activity, such as fibrillation potentials and high-frequency spontaneous discharges, provides evidence of chronic denervation.[82,85] Anal sphincter denervation is commonly seen in patients with FI secondary to cauda equina syndrome or pudendal nerve injury,[86] but this finding may not be specific. The number of motor units recruited during anal squeeze maneuver with needle EMG correlates with anal canal squeeze pressure,[84] therefore needle EMG is used as a complimentary test to ARM.

Needle EMG may be more accurate than surface EMG because the electrode more accurately records muscle activity and is less likely to register artifact from nearby muscles.[87] However, surface EMG is less invasive and in one study showed similar findings to needle EMG when assessing paradoxic anal sphincter response during bear down manuever[84] (for dyssynergia), but not for nerve injury.

Unfortunately, has not gained popularity among clinicians because it is cumbersome and painful and is only used in a selected few research centers.

## PUDENDAL NERVE TERMINAL MOTOR LATENCY

The pudendal nerve arises from sacral plexus nerves 2 to 4 and is responsible for innervation of the EAS and the levator ani muscles along with much of the sensory innervation of the perineum. Pudendal nerve terminal motor latency (PNTML) measures neuromuscular integrity between the terminal portion of the pudendal nerve and the EAS.

PNTML is commonly performed with a disposable fingerstall device with electrodes (St Mark's electrode, Dantec-Medtronics, Minneapolis, MN)[88] that the examiner wears on a gloved index finger. An electrode gel is placed on the electrodes mounted on the examiner's finger, which is then guided toward the ischial spine on one side.[89] Next, short electrical impulses are delivered through the electrodes.[90] Serial stimulations are performed and the values are averaged. The same process is then repeated on the opposite side.[89] A normal nerve latency is 2.0 ± 0.2 milliseconds and a longer latency suggests damage to the pudendal nerve.[91] However, only a few intact nerve fibers can give a normal result; therefore, a normal nerve latency does not rule out nerve damage.[92]

FI after obstetric injuries has been associated with pudendal nerve neuropathy,[93,94] but incontinence generally occurs many years after injury, suggesting that there could be other contributing factors.[94] PNTML is influenced by age[92,95–97] and does not correlate with manometric pressures.[98–101] Because of these methodologic and scientific concerns including assessment of only the terminal portion and not the entire nerve, an American Gastroenterological Association technical review did not recommend PNTML.[85]

## TRANSLUMBOSACRAL ANORECTAL MAGNETIC STIMULATION TEST

The measurement of translumbar and transsacral motor evoked potentials (MEP) from the anorectum has been shown to be a useful assessment of anorectal neuropathy in patients with FI[102] and spinal cord injury.[103]

The test requires three components (**Fig. 4**): a magnetic stimulator (The Magstim Company Limited, Whiteland, Wales, UK), with 70 or 90 mm magnetic coils for stimulation, and an anorectal probe with two pairs of bipolar steel ring electrodes (Gaeltec, Gaeltec Devices Ltd, Dunvegan, Scotland), and a neurophysiology recorder.

For the translumbar magnetic stimulation, the coil is applied on each side at the L3 level, about 4 cm lateral to the midline. For the transsacral magnetic stimulation the coil is applied on each side at the S3 level, about 4 cm lateral to the midline. Magnetic stimulations begin with 50% intensity and are slowly increased until an optimal and reproducible MEP response at the anal and rectal sites are obtained.[104] At least five MEP responses are recorded at each site and the data are analyzed manually using the Neuropack (Nihon Kohden, Tokyo, Japan) software.

There are two studies that have assessed the motor response of the anal sphincter with translumbosacral anorectal magnetic stimulation (TAMS) in patients with FI and compared with normal control subjects (see **Fig. 4**).[102,104] Rao and colleagues[102] showed significant and patchy neuropathy in 50% to 70% of patients with FI and the TAMS test was superior to PNTML. Xiang and colleagues[104] also found that most translumbar and transsacral MEP latencies were significantly prolonged in patients with FI versus control subjects, but that there was no difference in the corticospinal conduction time, suggesting that the neuropathy was mostly peripheral. A recent large study that examined the clinical utility of the TAMS test in 251 patients reported that anal neuropathy was more prevalent than rectal neuropathy, whereas the prevalence of lumbar and sacral neuropathy were similar.[105]

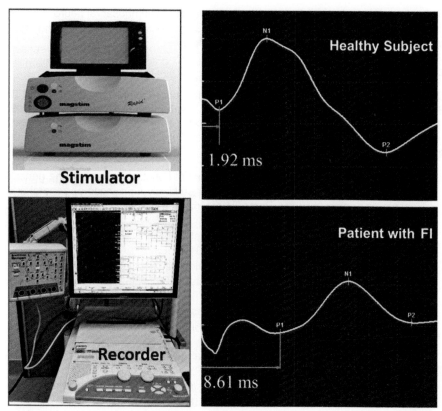

**Fig. 4.** Translumbosacral anorectal magnetic stimulation equipment (*left*) and anal MEP responses in a healthy normal subject and a patient with fecal incontinence (*right*). The latency of the MEP response in FI is significantly prolonged compared with healthy subject.

## NEWER TECHNIQUES

Newer techniques, such as Anal EndoFLIP (Medtronics, MN, USA) [106–108] and Fecobionics,[109,110] provide unique and novel perspectives of anorectal dynamics including improved characterization of anal sphincter opening and closing pressures. These techniques are promising and require further validation. Likewise, rectal barostat testing can provide useful and more accurate information regarding rectal sensation and compliance.[111] Recently, BAST has also been used as a therapeutic tool in two randomized controlled trials for improving rectal hyposensitivity[112,113] and for rectal hypersensitivity using sensory adaptation training.[114]

## SUMMARY

Constipation and FI are complaints commonly encountered complaints in the gastrointestinal clinic. Detailed assessment of symptoms together with a trustworthy patient-provider relationship and phone APP symptom diaries can help to determine possible etiologies and guide diagnostic testing. A range of tests now exist to further define the mechanisms underlying symptoms including HR-ARM, rectal sensation testing, defecography, and AUS to look for anatomic defects, and TAMS test for anorectal neuropathy. These provide a basis for recommending effective treatments including biofeedback therapy, sacral nerve stimulation, and translumbosacral neuro modulation therapy, and rarely surgery. Newer techniques, such as Anal EndoFlip and barostat sensory testing, are novel promising techniques.

## DISCLOSURE

Dr A.C. Jiang, Dr A. Panara, and Dr Y. Yan report no conflicts of interest to disclose. Dr S.S.C. Rao serves on the advisory board for Neurogut Inc (U-01- DK115572-02; R01DK104127-02).

## REFERENCES

1. Dimidi E, Cox C, Grant R, et al. Perceptions of constipation among the general public and people with constipation differ strikingly from those of general and specialist doctors and the Rome IV criteria. Am J Gastroenterol 2019;114(7): 1116–29.
2. Mearin F, Lacy BE, Chang L, et al. Bowel disorders. Gastroenterology 2016. https://doi.org/10.1053/j.gastro.2016.02.031.
3. Glia A, Lindberg G, Nilsson LH, et al. Clinical value of symptom assessment in patients with constipation. Dis Colon Rectum 1999;42(11):1401–8 [discussion: 1408–10].
4. Rao SS, Tuteja AK, Vellema T, et al. Dyssynergic defecation: demographics, symptoms, stool patterns, and quality of life. J Clin Gastroenterol 2004;38(8): 680–5.
5. Koch A, Voderholzer WA, Klauser AG, et al. Symptoms in chronic constipation. Dis Colon Rectum 1997;40(8):902–6.
6. Rao SS, Bharucha AE, Chiarioni G, et al. Functional anorectal disorders. Gastroenterology 2016. https://doi.org/10.1053/j.gastro.2016.02.009.
7. Bharucha AE, Seide BM, Zinsmeister AR, et al. Relation of bowel habits to fecal incontinence in women. Am J Gastroenterol 2008;103(6):1470–5.
8. Engel AF, Kamm MA, Bartram CI, et al. Relationship of symptoms in faecal incontinence to specific sphincter abnormalities. Int J Colorectal Dis 1995;10(3): 152–5.
9. Siproudhis L, El Abkari M, El Alaoui M, et al. Low rectal volumes in patients suffering from fecal incontinence: what does it mean? Aliment Pharmacol Ther 2005;22(10):989–96.
10. Chiarioni G, Scattolini C, Bonfante F, et al. Liquid stool incontinence with severe urgency: anorectal function and effective biofeedback treatment. Gut 1993; 34(11):1576–80.
11. Rao SS. Pathophysiology of adult fecal incontinence. Gastroenterology 2004; 126(1 Suppl 1):S14–22.
12. Rao SSC. Rectal exam: yes, it can and should be done in a busy practice! Am J Gastroenterol 2018;113(5):635–8.
13. Wong RK, Drossman DA, Bharucha AE, et al. The digital rectal examination: a multicenter survey of physicians' and students' perceptions and practice patterns. Am J Gastroenterol 2012;107(8):1157–63.
14. Dinning PG, Carrington EV, Scott SM. Colonic and anorectal motility testing in the high-resolution era. Curr Opin Gastroenterol 2016;32(1):44–8.
15. Zhao Y, Ren X, Qiao W, et al. High-resolution anorectal manometry in the diagnosis of functional defecation disorder in patients with functional constipation: a retrospective cohort study. J Neurogastroenterol Motil 2019;25(2):250–7.

16. Tetangco E, Yan Y, Rao S. Performing and analyzing high-resolution anorectal manometry. NeuroGastroLatam Rev 2018;2:1–13. https://doi.org/10.24875/NGL.19000016.
17. Coss-Adame E, Rao SS, Valestin J, et al. Accuracy and reproducibility of high-definition anorectal manometry and pressure topography analyses in healthy subjects. Clin Gastroenterol Hepatol 2015;13(6):1143–50.
18. Li Y, Yang X, Xu C, et al. Normal values and pressure morphology for three-dimensional high-resolution anorectal manometry of asymptomatic adults: a study in 110 subjects. Int J Colorectal Dis 2013;28(8):1161–8.
19. Rao SS, Azpiroz F, Diamant N, et al. Minimum standards of anorectal manometry. Neurogastroenterol Motil 2002;14(5):553–9.
20. Carrington EV, Scott SM, Bharucha A, et al. Expert consensus document: advances in the evaluation of anorectal function. Nat Rev Gastroenterol Hepatol 2018;15(5):309–23.
21. Noelting J, Ratuapli SK, Bharucha AE, et al. Normal values for high-resolution anorectal manometry in healthy women: effects of age and significance of rectoanal gradient. Am J Gastroenterol 2012;107(10):1530–6.
22. Carrington EV, Brokjaer A, Craven H, et al. Traditional measures of normal anal sphincter function using high-resolution anorectal manometry (HRAM) in 115 healthy volunteers. Neurogastroenterol Motil 2014;26(5):625–35.
23. Sauter M, Heinrich H, Fox M, et al. Toward more accurate measurements of anorectal motor and sensory function in routine clinical practice: validation of high-resolution anorectal manometry and Rapid Barostat Bag measurements of rectal function. Neurogastroenterol Motil 2014;26(5):685–95.
24. Mion F, Garros A, Brochard C, et al. 3D High-definition anorectal manometry: values obtained in asymptomatic volunteers, fecal incontinence and chronic constipation. Results of a prospective multicenter study (NOMAD). Neurogastroenterol Motil 2017;29(8):pp1–9.
25. Farouk R, Duthie GS, MacGregor AB, et al. Sustained internal sphincter hypertonia in patients with chronic anal fissure. Dis Colon Rectum 1994;37(5):424–9.
26. Rao SS, Welcher KD, Leistikow JS. Obstructive defecation: a failure of rectoanal coordination. Am J Gastroenterol 1998;93(7):1042–50.
27. Vitton V, Ben Hadj Amor W, Baumstarck K, et al. Comparison of three-dimensional high-resolution manometry and endoanal ultrasound in the diagnosis of anal sphincter defects. Colorectal Dis 2013;15(10):e607–11.
28. Benezech A, Cappiello M, Baumstarck K, et al. Rectal intussusception: can high resolution three-dimensional ano-rectal manometry compete with conventional defecography? Neurogastroenterol Motil 2017;29(4):pp1–7.
29. Scott SM, Gladman MA. Manometric, sensorimotor, and neurophysiologic evaluation of anorectal function. Gastroenterol Clin North Am 2008;37(3):511–38.
30. Gladman MA, Lunniss PJ, Scott SM, et al. Rectal hyposensitivity. Am J Gastroenterol 2006;101(5):1140–51.
31. Rao SS, Erdogan A, Coss-Adame E, et al. Rectal hyposensitivity: randomized controlled trial of barostat vs. syringe-assisted sensory training. Gastroenterology 2013;144(suppl 1):S363.
32. Wald A, Tunuguntla AK. Anorectal sensorimotor dysfunction in fecal incontinence and diabetes mellitus. Modification with biofeedback therapy. N Engl J Med 1984;310(20):1282–7.
33. Madbouly KM, Hussein AM. Temporary sacral nerve stimulation in patients with fecal incontinence owing to rectal hyposensitivity: a prospective, double-blind study. Surgery 2015;157(1):56–63.

34. Bharucha AE, Fletcher JG, Harper CM, et al. Relationship between symptoms and disordered continence mechanisms in women with idiopathic faecal incontinence. Gut 2005;54(4):546–55.

35. Minguez M, Herreros B, Sanchiz V, et al. Predictive value of the balloon expulsion test for excluding the diagnosis of pelvic floor dyssynergia in constipation. Gastroenterology 2004;126(1):57–62.

36. Chiarioni G, Kim SM, Vantini I, et al. Validation of the balloon evacuation test: reproducibility and agreement with findings from anorectal manometry and electromyography. Clin Gastroenterol Hepatol 2014;12(12):2049–54.

37. Lee YY, Erdogan A, Yu S, et al. Anorectal manometry in defecatory disorders: a comparative analysis of high-resolution pressure topography and waveform manometry. J Neurogastroenterol Motil 2018;24(3):460–8.

38. Rao SS, Mudipalli RS, Stessman M, et al. Investigation of the utility of colorectal function tests and Rome II criteria in dyssynergic defecation (Anismus). Neurogastroenterol Motil 2004;16(5):589–96.

39. Palit S, Thin N, Knowles CH, et al. Diagnostic disagreement between tests of evacuatory function: a prospective study of 100 constipated patients. Neurogastroenterol Motil 2016;28(10):1589–98.

40. Mahieu P, Pringot J, Bodart P. Defecography: I. Description of a new procedure and results in normal patients. Gastrointest Radiol 1984;9(3):247–51.

41. Chan CL, Scott SM, Knowles CH, et al. Exaggerated rectal adaptation: another cause of outlet obstruction. Colorectal Dis 2001;3(2):141–2.

42. American Gastroenterological A, Bharucha AE, Dorn SD, et al. American Gastroenterological Association medical position statement on constipation. Gastroenterology 2013;144(1):211–7.

43. Wald A, Bharucha AE, Cosman BC, et al. ACG clinical guideline: management of benign anorectal disorders. Am J Gastroenterol 2014;109(8):1141–57.

44. Zafar A, Seretis C, Feretis M, et al. Comparative study of magnetic resonance defaecography and evacuation proctography in the evaluation of obstructed defaecation. Colorectal Dis 2017;19(6):O204–9.

45. Tirumanisetty P, Prichard D, Fletcher JG, et al. Normal values for assessment of anal sphincter morphology, anorectal motion, and pelvic organ prolapse with MRI in healthy women. Neurogastroenterol Motil 2018;30(7):e13314.

46. Schawkat K, Heinrich H, Parker HL, et al. How to define pathologic pelvic floor descent in MR defecography during defecation? Abdom Radiol (NY) 2018; 43(12):3233–40.

47. Patcharatrakul T, Rao SSC. Update on the pathophysiology and management of anorectal disorders. Gut Liver 2018;12(4):375–84.

48. van Dam JH, Ginai AZ, Gosselink MJ, et al. Role of defecography in predicting clinical outcome of rectocele repair. Dis Colon Rectum 1997;40(2):201–7.

49. Savoye-Collet C, Koning E, Dacher JN. Radiologic evaluation of pelvic floor disorders. Gastroenterol Clin North Am 2008;37(3):553–67, viii.

50. Villanueva-Herrero JA, Reyes Hansen M, Alarcon-Bernes L, et al. Endoanal Ultrasound for Anorectal Disease Gastrointestinal Diseases - Publisher: SM Group Project: Dynamic Sono-Manometry for Obstructive Defecation, 2017;pp 1-23.

51. Hildebrandt U, Feifel G, Schwarz HP, et al. Endorectal ultrasound: instrumentation and clinical aspects. Int J Colorectal Dis 1986;1(4):203–7.

52. Regadas SM, Regadas FS, Rodrigues LV, et al. Importance of the tridimensional ultrasound in the anorectal evaluation. Arq Gastroenterol 2005;42(4):226–32 [in Portuguese].

53. Frudinger A, Bartram CI, Halligan S, et al. Examination techniques for endosonography of the anal canal. Abdom Imaging 1998;23(3):301–3.
54. Abdool Z, Sultan AH, Thakar R. Ultrasound imaging of the anal sphincter complex: a review. Br J Radiol 2012;85(1015):865–75.
55. Hussain SM, Stoker J, Lameris JS. Anal sphincter complex: endoanal MR imaging of normal anatomy. Radiology 1995;197(3):671–7.
56. Vaizey CJ, Kamm MA, Bartram CI. Primary degeneration of the internal anal sphincter as a cause of passive faecal incontinence. Lancet 1997;349(9052): 612–5.
57. Dvorkin LS, Chan CL, Knowles CH, et al. Anal sphincter morphology in patients with full-thickness rectal prolapse. Dis Colon Rectum 2004;47(2):198–203.
58. Marshall M, Halligan S, Fotheringham T, et al. Predictive value of internal anal sphincter thickness for diagnosis of rectal intussusception in patients with solitary rectal ulcer syndrome. Br J Surg 2002;89(10):1281–5.
59. Halligan S, Sultan A, Rottenberg G, et al. Endosonography of the anal sphincters in solitary rectal ulcer syndrome. Int J Colorectal Dis 1995;10(2):79–82.
60. Titi MA, Jenkins JT, Urie A, et al. Correlation between anal manometry and endosonography in females with faecal incontinence. Colorectal Dis 2008;10(2): 131–7.
61. Pinsk I, Brown J, Phang PT. Assessment of sonographic quality of anal sphincter muscles in patients with faecal incontinence. Colorectal Dis 2009;11(9):933–40.
62. Gold DM, Halligan S, Kmiot WA, et al. Intraobserver and interobserver agreement in anal endosonography. Br J Surg 1999;86(3):371–5.
63. Sultan AH, Kamm MA, Talbot IC, et al. Anal endosonography for identifying external sphincter defects confirmed histologically. Br J Surg 1994;81(3):463–5.
64. Stewart LK, Wilson SR. Transvaginal sonography of the anal sphincter: reliable, or not? Am J Roentgenol 1999;173(1):179–85.
65. Frudinger A, Bartram CI, Kamm MA. Transvaginal versus anal endosonography for detecting damage to the anal sphincter. Am J Roentgenol 1997;168(6): 1435–8.
66. Roche B, Deleaval J, Fransioli A, et al. Comparison of transanal and external perineal ultrasonography. Eur Radiol 2001;11(7):1165–70.
67. Lohse C, Bretones S, Boulvain M, et al. Transperineal versus endoanal ultrasound in the detection of anal sphincter defects. European Journal of Obstetrics & Gynecology and Reproductive Biology 103;2002:79-82.
68. Taithongchai A, van Gruting IMA, Volloyhaug I, et al. Comparing the diagnostic accuracy of 3 ultrasound modalities for diagnosing obstetric anal sphincter injuries. Am J Obstet Gynecol 2019;221(2):134.e1–9.
69. Stoker J. Magnetic resonance imaging in fecal incontinence. Semin Ultrasound CT MR 2008;29(6):409–13.
70. Malouf AJ, Williams AB, Halligan S, et al. Prospective assessment of accuracy of endoanal MR imaging and endosonography in patients with fecal incontinence. Am J Roentgenol 2000;175(3):741–5.
71. West RL, Dwarkasing S, Briel JW, et al. Can three-dimensional endoanal ultrasonography detect external anal sphincter atrophy? A comparison with endoanal magnetic resonance imaging. Int J Colorectal Dis 2005;20(4):328–33.
72. Cazemier M, Terra MP, Stoker J, et al. Atrophy and defects detection of the external anal sphincter: comparison between three-dimensional anal endosonography and endoanal magnetic resonance imaging. Dis Colon Rectum 2006;49(1):20–7.

73. Dobben AC, Terra MP, Slors JF, et al. External anal sphincter defects in patients with fecal incontinence: comparison of endoanal MR imaging and endoanal US. Radiology 2007;242(2):463–71.

74. Tan E, Anstee A, Koh DM, et al. Diagnostic precision of endoanal MRI in the detection of anal sphincter pathology: a meta-analysis. Int J Colorectal Dis 2008;23(6):641–51.

75. Terra MP, Beets-Tan RG, van Der Hulst VP, et al. Anal sphincter defects in patients with fecal incontinence: endoanal versus external phased-array MR imaging. Radiology 2005;236(3):886–95.

76. Terra MP, Beets-Tan RG, van der Hulst VP, et al. MRI in evaluating atrophy of the external anal sphincter in patients with fecal incontinence. Am J Roentgenol 2006;187(4):991–9.

77. Kirss J Jr, Huhtinen H, Niskanen E, et al. Comparison of 3D endoanal ultrasound and external phased array magnetic resonance imaging in the diagnosis of obstetric anal sphincter injuries. Eur Radiol 2019;29(10):5717–22.

78. Carrington EV, Heinrich H, Knowles CH, et al. Methods of anorectal manometry vary widely in clinical practice: results from an international survey. Neurogastroenterol Motil 2017;29(8):e13016.

79. Podnar S, Rodi Z, Lukanovic A, et al. Standardization of anal sphincter EMG: technique of needle examination. Muscle Nerve 1999;22(3):400–3.

80. Wiesner A, Jost WH. EMG of the external anal sphincter: needle is superior to surface electrode. Dis Colon Rectum 2000;43(1):116–8.

81. Thomas C, Lefaucheur JP, Galula G, et al. Respective value of pudendal nerve terminal motor latency and anal sphincter electromyography in neurogenic fecal incontinence. Neurophysiol Clin 2002;32(1):85–90.

82. Lefaucheur JP. Neurophysiological testing in anorectal disorders. Muscle Nerve 2006;33(3):324–33.

83. Sorensen M, Nielsen MB, Pedersen JF, et al. Electromyography of the internal anal sphincter performed under endosonographic guidance. Description of a new method. Dis Colon Rectum 1994;37(2):138–43.

84. Lopez A, Nilsson BY, Mellgren A, et al. Electromyography of the external anal sphincter: comparison between needle and surface electrodes. Dis Colon Rectum 1999;42(4):482–5.

85. Diamant NE, Kamm MA, Wald A, et al. AGA technical review on anorectal testing techniques. Gastroenterology 1999;116(3):735–60.

86. Infantino A, Melega E, Negrin P, et al. Striated anal sphincter electromyography in idiopathic fecal incontinence. Dis Colon Rectum 1995;38(1):27–31.

87. Merletti R, Bottin A, Cescon C, et al. Multichannel surface EMG for the noninvasive assessment of the anal sphincter muscle. Digestion 2004;69(2):112–22.

88. Kiff ES, Swash M. Slowed conduction in the pudendal nerves in idiopathic (neurogenic) faecal incontinence. Br J Surg 1984;71(8):614–6.

89. Van Koughnett JA, da Silva G. Anorectal physiology and testing. Gastroenterol Clin North Am 2013;42(4):713–28.

90. Saraidaridis JT, Molina G, Savit LR, et al. Pudendal nerve terminal motor latency testing does not provide useful information in guiding therapy for fecal incontinence. Int J Colorectal Dis 2018;33(3):305–10.

91. Wexner SD, Marchetti F, Salanga VD, et al. Neurophysiologic assessment of the anal sphincters. Dis Colon Rectum 1991;34(7):606–12.

92. Cheong DM, Vaccaro CA, Salanga VD, et al. Electrodiagnostic evaluation of fecal incontinence. Muscle Nerve 1995;18(6):612–9.

93. Tetzschner T, Sorensen M, Lose G, et al. Anal and urinary incontinence in women with obstetric anal sphincter rupture. Br J Obstet Gynaecol 1996; 103(10):1034–40.
94. Swash M, Snooks SJ, Henry MM. Unifying concept of pelvic floor disorders and incontinence. J R Soc Med 1985;78(11):906–11.
95. Jameson JS, Chia YW, Kamm MA, et al. Effect of age, sex and parity on anorectal function. Br J Surg 1994;81(11):1689–92.
96. Lefaucheur J, Yiou R, Thomas C. Pudendal nerve terminal motor latency: age effects and technical considerations. Clin Neurophysiol 2001;112(3):472–6.
97. Pradal-Prat D, Mares P, Peray P, et al. Pudendal nerve motor latency correlation by age and sex. Electromyogr Clin Neurophysiol 1998;38(8):491–6.
98. Vaccaro CA, Cheong DM, Wexner SD, et al. Pudendal neuropathy in evacuatory disorders. Dis Colon Rectum 1995;38(2):166–71.
99. Osterberg A, Graf W, Edebol Eeg-Olofsson K, et al. Results of neurophysiologic evaluation in fecal incontinence. Dis Colon Rectum 2000;43(9):1256–61.
100. Rasmussen OO, Christiansen J, Tetzschner T, et al. Pudendal nerve function in idiopathic fecal incontinence. Dis Colon Rectum 2000;43(5):633–6 [discussion: 636–7].
101. Suilleabhain CB, Horgan AF, McEnroe L, et al. The relationship of pudendal nerve terminal motor latency to squeeze pressure in patients with idiopathic fecal incontinence. Dis Colon Rectum 2001;44(5):666–71.
102. Rao SS, Coss-Adame E, Tantiphlachiva K, et al. Translumbar and transsacral magnetic neurostimulation for the assessment of neuropathy in fecal incontinence. Dis Colon Rectum 2014;57(5):645–52.
103. Tantiphlachiva K, Attaluri A, Valestin J, et al. Translumbar and transsacral motor-evoked potentials: a novel test for spino-anorectal neuropathy in spinal cord injury. Am J Gastroenterol 2011;106(5):907–14.
104. Xiang X, Patcharatrakul T, Sharma A, et al. Cortico-anorectal, spino-anorectal, and cortico-spinal nerve conduction and locus of neuronal injury in patients with fecal incontinence. Clin Gastroenterol Hepatol 2019;17(6):1130–7.e2.
105. Yan Y, Herekar A, Gu Q, et al. Clinical utility of translumbosacral anorectal magnetic stimulation (TAMS) test in anorectal disorders. Gastroenterology 2019; 156(6):354–5.
106. Leroi AM, Melchior C, Charpentier C, et al. The diagnostic value of the functional lumen imaging probe versus high-resolution anorectal manometry in patients with fecal incontinence. Neurogastroenterol Motil 2018;30(6):e13291.
107. Alqudah MM, Gregersen H, Drewes AM, et al. Evaluation of anal sphincter resistance and distensibility in healthy controls using EndoFLIP (c). Neurogastroenterol Motil 2012;24(12):e591–9.
108. Zifan A, Sun C, Gourcerol G, et al. Endoflip vs high-definition manometry in the assessment of fecal incontinence: a data-driven unsupervised comparison. Neurogastroenterol Motil 2018;30(12):e13462.
109. Sun D, Huang Z, Zhuang Z, et al. Fecobionics: a novel bionics device for studying defecation. Ann Biomed Eng 2019;47(2):576–89.
110. Gregersen H, Krogh K, Liao D. Fecobionics: integrating anorectal function measurements. Clin Gastroenterol Hepatol 2018;16(6):981–3.
111. Whitehead WE, Delvaux M. Standardization of barostat procedures for testing smooth muscle tone and sensory thresholds in the gastrointestinal tract. The Working Team of Glaxo-Wellcome Research, UK. Dig Dis Sci 1997;42(2): 223–41.

112. Lee YY, Erdogan A, Rao SS. How to perform and assess colonic manometry and barostat study in chronic constipation. J Neurogastroenterol Motil 2014;20(4): 547–52.
113. Patcharatrakul T, Erdogan A, Coss-Adame A, et al. Barostat-assisted sensory training (BT) is superior to syringe-assisted training (ST) for rectal hyposensitivity. Neurogastroenterol Motil 2016;28(Supplement 1):42.
114. Mohanty S, Schulze K, Stessman M, et al. Behavioral therapy for rectal hypersensitivity. Am J Gastroenterol 2001;96:A955.

# Treating Chronic Abdominal Pain in Patients with Chronic Abdominal Pain and/or Irritable Bowel Syndrome

Lauren Stemboroski, DO, Ron Schey, MD, FACG*

## KEYWORDS

- Irritable bowel syndrome • IBS • Chronic abdominal pain • Constipation • Diarrhea

## KEY POINTS

- IBS is a chronic relapsing, remitting disease comprised of abdominal pain related to defecation and changes in bowel habits occurring at least 6 months before diagnosis and present during the last 3 months.
- The treatment of IBS focuses on the patient's predominant symptom and the underlying pathophysiology.
- Current treatment methods include lifestyle and diet modification, alternative and herbal therapies, probiotics, and pharmacotherapy, which are discussed in detail.

## INTRODUCTION

Chronic abdominal pain is characterized as occurring intermittently or constantly for at least 6 months. Visceral pain is transmitted to the brain via vagal, thoracolumbar, and lumbosacral afferent nerves.[1] Nonreferred visceral pain is perceived as diffuse, dull and midline, or epigastric because the afferent nervous system to this region is supplied by bilateral splanchnic nerves.[2] Referred pain is usually aching and near the surface of the body, and accompanied by skin hyperalgesia and increased muscle tone of the abdominal wall. Referred pain presents in a dermatomal distribution, which correlates with the site of the spinal cord level of the affected visceral organ.[2]

## CLINICAL APPROACH
### History

The first step in managing chronical abdominal pain is to elicit a detailed history, including key factors, such as onset, duration, timing, location, radiation, quality,

Division of Gastroenterology/Hepatology, Department of Internal Medicine, University of Florida College of Medicine, 653 West 8th Street, Jacksonville, FL 32209, USA
* Corresponding author.
E-mail address: Ron.Schey@jax.ufl.edu

Gastroenterol Clin N Am 49 (2020) 607–621
https://doi.org/10.1016/j.gtc.2020.05.001
0889-8553/20/© 2020 Elsevier Inc. All rights reserved.

and severity. It is important to ask about relationship to meals and bowel movements. A list of medications and supplements, along with dose and frequency of pain medications and nonsteroidal anti-inflammatory drugs should be reviewed. Abdominal pain characteristics and location can offer clues to the diagnosis (**Table 1**).

Alarm features include, but are not limited to, symptom onset after the age of 50 years, severe or progressive symptoms, unexplained weight loss, nocturnal pain, recent change in bowel habits, or rectal bleeding. The presence of alarm features should raise the suspicion for structural diseases and prompt further investigation. However, many patients with structural disease do not have alarm features.[2]

### Physical Examination

A detailed physical examination including a rectal examination is necessary to elucidate the cause of chronic abdominal pain.[2] In the event of an acute episode of chronic abdominal pain it is imperative to quickly rule out the possibility of a surgical abdomen. A detailed rectal examination can offer valuable information, such as active bleeding, mass, signs of constipation, pelvic floor dysfunction, or high anal resting tone.[3]

**Table 1**
**Locations and characteristics of common causes of abdominal pain**

| Location | Cause | Characteristics/Associated Symptoms |
|---|---|---|
| RUQ pain | Gallstones | Intense, dull discomfort that may radiate to the back |
| | Acute cholecystitis | Prolonged, steady, severe RUQ pain, positive Murphy sign |
| | Acute cholangitis | Fever, jaundice, and abdominal pain |
| | Hepatitis | Fatigue, malaise, nausea, vomiting |
| Epigastric pain | Acute coronary syndrome | Associated SOB and dyspnea on exertion |
| | Pancreatitis | Pain radiating to the back |
| | Peptic ulcer disease | Upper abdominal pain or discomfort, relationship to meals, NSAID use |
| | GERD | Heartburn, regurgitation, dysphagia |
| | Gastritis (also LUQ) | Abdominal pain, heartburn, nausea/vomiting, NSAID use or alcohol |
| | Gastroparesis | Nausea, vomiting, abdominal pain, early satiety, postprandial fullness, bloating |
| LUQ pain | Splenomegaly | LUQ pain or discomfort, referred to the left shoulder |
| | Splenic infarct | Severe LUQ pain |
| | Splenic abscess | Fever, LUQ tender |
| Lower abdominal pain | Acute appendicitis | Periumbilical pain initially that radiates to the right lower quadrant |
| | Diverticulitis | Severe, persistent, lasting days, nausea/vomiting |
| | Kidney stones | Flank pain, back pain |
| | Cystitis | Dysuria, frequency, urgency |
| | Colitis | Prolonged diarrhea with abdominal pain, weight loss, and fever |
| | Pelvic inflammatory disease | Evidence of inflammation of the genital tract |
| | Endometriosis | Dysmenorrhea, pelvic pain, dyspareunia |

Abbreviations: GERD, gastroesophageal reflux disease; LUQ, left upper quadrant; NSAID, nonsteroidal anti-inflammatory drug; RUQ, right upper quadrant; SOB, shortness of breath.

## Work-up for Chronic Abdominal Pain

Laboratory studies including complete blood count with differential, complete metabolic panel, lipase, and urinalysis should be performed. Depending on the suspected diagnosis, abdominal imaging is usually ordered as part of the initial work-up; this can include ultrasound, computed tomography scan, or MRI. Imaging is usually unrevealing in cases of undiagnosed abdominal pain and should not be repeated unless the patient's presentation changes. Repeating computed tomography scans in patients with negative findings and nontraumatic abdominal pain has been shown to have a low diagnostic yield and should be avoided.[2] Once alarm signs are excluded and the history and physical examination are not supportive of an alternate diagnosis or there is a long history of negative diagnostic studies, further testing should not be pursued.

## Systemic Diseases Leading to Diffuse Abdominal Pain

Diffuse abdominal pain poses an obstacle for the physician because there is no location to start the differential-making process. It is important to review systemic causes of abdominal pain because it is vital that the underlying disorder is recognized and treated appropriately. Examples of disease that can cause diffuse abdominal pain are outlined in **Box 1**.

## Causes of Localized Abdominal Pain

Pain that is unrelated to eating or bowel movements but related to movement should raise suspicion for possible chronic abdominal wall pain. The most common cause of chronic abdominal wall pain is from anterior cutaneous nerve entrapment syndrome. It is believed to originate from the entrapment of a cutaneous nerve emanating from T7-T12, caused by direct pressure, fibrosis, or edema.[2] Successful treatment of chronic abdominal wall pain with nonnarcotic analgesics, nonsteroidal anti-inflammatory drugs, heat, or physical therapy is beneficial to the patient and confirms the diagnosis.

Musculoskeletal pain is sharp and localized to an area of less than 2 cm, which is a stark contrast to visceral abdominal pain. Carnett sign is a physical examination finding that is used with 97% accuracy to detect abdominal wall pain.[2] Pain from palpation increases with raising the head and contracting the rectus abdominus muscle when Carnett test is positive.[4] Less than 10% of patients with visceral pain have a positive Carnett test; contraction of the abdominal wall muscles serves to protect the visceral organs from palpation, therefore visceral pain usually improves with this maneuver.[2,4]

## Causes of Functional Abdominal Pain

Disorders of gut-brain interaction (DGBI), also referred to as functional gastrointestinal (GI) disorders, are the most encountered diagnoses in gastroenterology. The symptoms of DGBI are caused by one or more of the following: motility disturbance, visceral hypersensitivity, altered mucosal and immune function, altered gut microbiota, and altered central nervous system processing.[5,6] The three most common causes of DGBI include irritable bowel syndrome (IBS) (15%–20%), functional dyspepsia (10%), and centrally mediated abdominal pain syndrome (CAPS) (0.5%–2%).[2] Functional dyspepsia and IBS are thought to be caused by increased visceral pain sensitivity; these patients experience an exaggerated response to normal events.[2,5]

IBS is chronic relapsing, remitting disease made up of abdominal pain related to defecation and changes in bowel habits.[2] Rome IV defined IBS as a functional bowel disorder in which recurrent abdominal pain is associated with defecation or a change

---

**Box 1**
**Systemic disease leading to diffuse abdominal pain**

Endometriosis
- Patients may report pain with sitting or radiating to the perineum
- Found in up to 80% of women with chronic noncyclic lower abdominal pain
- Commonly perimenstrual and accompanied by dyspareunia
- Diagnosed by laparotomy and biopsy

Familial Mediterranean fever
- Most prevalent in individuals of Turkish, Armenian, North African, Jewish, and Arab descent
- Recurrent episodes of fever and serosal inflammation
- No symptoms between attacks
- Signs of peritonitis are often present

Chronic mesenteric ischemia
- Postprandial abdominal pain caused by increased demand on splanchnic blood vessels; cramping or dull pain; lasting 1 to 2 hours
- Episodic or constant hypoperfusion of the small intestine; 50% of patients have peripheral vascular disease or coronary artery disease

Sclerosing mesenteritis
- Rare, nonneoplastic inflammatory and fibrotic disease that affects the mesentery
- Abnormal responses to healing and repair of connective tissue in response to trauma
- Can cause obstruction from mass effect

Hereditary angioedema
- Affects skin or mucosa or upper respiratory or gastrointestinal tracts
- Absence of pruritus and urticaria
- Bowel wall edema can cause colic, nausea, vomiting, and diarrhea

Mast cell activation syndrome
- Can cause a slew of gastrointestinal symptoms related to histamine release

Ehlers-Danlos syndrome
- Hereditary connective tissue disorders characterized by varying degrees of skin hyperextensibility, joint hypermobility, generalized skin fragility
- 56% of patients complain of abdominal pain
- Pathophysiology is unknown but these patients are known to have increased risk of torsion and ischemia

---

in bowel habits. Symptom onset should occur at least 6 months before diagnosis and symptoms should be present during the last 3 months. The IBS diagnostic criteria are summarized in **Box 2**.

More rarely encountered is CAPS, which is a continuous or frequently relapsing abdominal pain thought to be caused by disinhibition of pains signals rather than hyperexcitability of the afferent nervous system and is rarely related to gut function.[7] Pain in CAPS tends to be diffuse, prolonged, and colicky in nature, but sometimes presents as a burning pain related to previous surgery.[2] The management of CAPS requires a strong patient-physician relationship, focus on nonpharmacologic therapies, and behavioral therapy when needed.[8] Low-dose tricyclic antidepressants (TCAs) or serotonin-reuptake inhibitors (SSRIs) are used for pharmacologic therapy for 4 to 6 weeks and titrated up in cases of incomplete response.[8]

Another cause of chronic abdominal pain is narcotic bowel syndrome, which is seen with increasing doses of opioids, most commonly present in patients requiring more than 100 mg morphine equivalent per day.[9] Narcotic bowel syndrome is seen in about 5% of patients on chronic opioid therapy.[10] Chronic narcotic use illogically activates excitatory antianalgesic pathways producing visceral hyperalgesia.[4,10] Pain is

---

**Box 2**
**IBS diagnostic criteria**

Recurrent abdominal pain (on average at least 1 d/wk) for the last 3 months, associated with two or more of the following:
   1.Related to defecation
   2.Associated with a change in the frequency of stool
   3.Associated with a change in the form (appearance) of stool

These criteria should be fulfilled for the last 3 months with symptom onset at least 6 months before diagnosis.

*Modified from* Rome IV.

---

typically diffuse, colicky, or constant, lasting more than 3 months' duration and improves with decreasing opioid use.[2,9] Opiate detoxification provides treatment in 89.7% of cases.[8]

## Physiology

The central nervous system is directly connected to the body's organs affecting the body as a unit. Strong emotions, such as anxiety, fear, and anger, can alter motility and symptom perception. Emotional or physical stress can increase colonic contractions, induce defecation, cause diarrhea, or conversely, delay gastric emptying and decrease colonic transit time.[5] Stress can alter the gut microbiome by impairing mucosal secretory and barrier functions, which can cause transmigration of bacteria leading to pain and diarrhea.[5] However, chronic irritable bowel symptoms, such as increased motility and visceral inflammation, can contribute to depression and anxiety; the brain-gut axis is a reciprocal relationship.[5]

Pain is an important and largely unmet need in the treatment of IBS.[11] There is a fine balance between sensing pain and suppressing pain, which controls the activation status of the visceral afferent nerve endings. Neurotransmitters involved in visceral sensation include 5-HT and neurokinins, making these chemicals targets for pharmacotherapy.[11] Patients with DGBI do not have the same ability to downregulate incoming neural signals.[5] The consequences of IBS are similar to those of other pain conditions, including difficulty sleeping, fatigue, altered mood, and decreased quality of life.[12]

## TREATMENT STRATEGIES

The foundation of effective management strategies is based on a strong physician-patient relationship. It has been proposed that physicians feel less capable when treating DGBI than when treating a structural diagnosis.[4] It is important for the treating physician to understand that these patients are challenging, accept these as positive diagnoses, and reduce expectations for a quick recovery.[4] It is paramount to provide support and counsel the patient to take personal responsibility for their treatment.

The treatment of IBS focuses on the patient's predominant symptom and the underlying pathophysiology. There are currently no disease-modifying therapeutic agents to treat IBS; however, there are treatments targeting the underlying mechanisms, such as increased abnormal transit time and increased colonic bile acid concentration.[1] Current treatment methods include lifestyle and diet modification, alternative and herbal therapies, probiotics, and pharmacotherapy. These are each discussed in detail.

## Exercise

Exercise is proven to be beneficial to health because it reduces the risk of cardiovascular diseases, endocrine disorders, improves bone and muscle conditioning, and decreases the levels of anxiety and depression.[13]

Walking has been shown to improve overall GI symptoms and anxiety; yoga has also been beneficial in reducing symptom severity in IBS.[1] Johannesson and colleagues[14] reported that patients who exercised 20 to 60 minutes, three to five times per week (moderate to physical aerobic activity) had significant improvement in IBS symptom scores and psychological symptoms over a 12-week period; this was confirmed with a median follow-up of 5.2 years. There is some evidence that suggests that reduced physical activity may be related to levels of pain intensity in children with chronic pain.[15]

## Dietary Modifications

Food causes symptoms in patients with IBS. There are a few hypotheses for the mechanisms behind this including (1) altered gut microbiota, (2) sensitivity to the gastrocolic reflex, (3) insoluble fiber exacerbates symptoms, and (4) antigens in the food alter the intestinal epithelial barrier.[1,5] It is not possible to cure IBS with one specific dietary approach because of the current understanding of its multifactorial pathogenesis.

### Low-fructose, oligosaccharides, disaccharides, monosaccharides, and polyols diet

Fructose, oligosaccharides, disaccharides, monosaccharides, and polyols (FODMAPs) are found in many of the fruits and legumes we eat, and are concentrated in dairy products and artificial sweeteners. Because these chemicals are poorly absorbed, they may provoke osmotic effects or fermentation, which increases distention leading to increased colonic sensitivity.[16] Reducing the intake of foods rich in these chemicals has been proven to reduce bacterial abundance.[17] The low-FODMAP diet is the most efficacious diet approach of all. Studies from around the world have shown benefit over placebo, and 50% to 87% of adult IBS sufferers respond.[18]

Although the low-FODMAP diet is the most studied, access to a dietitian across the world varies, and even if one is available, knowledge and training in a low-FODMAP diet is highly variable.[18] Currently in the United States, most gastroenterologists use educational handouts to advocate for a FODMAP diet, with only one in five referring to a dietician.[18] These lists of "allowed" and "not allowed" foods are occasionally challenging and contradictory to current recommendations.[18,19]

For maximum efficacy, this diet should be implemented by a dietician knowledgeable in this area and in three phases: (1) FODMAP restriction, (2) FODMAP reintroduction, and (3) FODMAP personalization.[20]

### Fiber

Fibers are used as first-line therapies because of the absence of serious adverse effects, although the evidence is controversial.[21] Treatment with psyllium decreases symptom severity in IBS. Its benefits are possibly caused by decreased inflammatory effects from increased production of short-chain fatty acids or alteration the intestinal microbiota.[1] A 2011 Cochrane review including 12 studies concluded that neither soluble (psyllium) nor insoluble fibers had a beneficial effect in improving the symptoms when compared with placebo.[22] However, this was contradicted by another meta-analysis that used the same trials but had a combined end point for abdominal pain and global IBS symptoms where the relative risk (95% confidence interval) was 0.76.[23]

Bijkerk and colleagues[24] randomized 275 patients with IBS to 12 weeks of treatment with soluble fiber (psyllium), insoluble bran fiber, or placebo. The reduction in severity of symptoms in the psyllium group was higher than that in the placebo group after 3 months of treatment, whereas the change in severity of symptoms in the bran group was comparable with that in the placebo group.

### Gluten-free diet

There is a subset of patients with IBS who do not have markers of celiac disease that benefit from a gluten-free diet. There is indeterminate evidence to recommend a gluten-free diet to all patients with IBS; the studies have small sample sizes and varying conclusions.

It is possible that many patients with IBS improve on a gluten-free diet because it also reduces fructan intake, a significant element of modern wheat products that are well established to provoke IBS symptoms.[25] Vazquez-Roque and colleagues[26] found that gluten alters bowel barrier functions in patients with IBS with diarrhea (IBS-D), particularly in HLA-DQ2/8-positive patients evidenced by levels of mannitol and the lactulose/mannitol ratio.

### Prebiotics, probiotics, and synbiotics

Evidence suggesting that an imbalance in the gut microbiota also contributes to IBS has prompted the use of probiotics in the management of IBS.[27] Prebiotics include food ingredients, such as fructo-oligosaccharides or inulin, that remain undigested in the human GI system and can promote the growth or activity of gut bacteria selectively used by host microorganisms, conferring a health benefit.[28]

Probiotics are live or attenuated microorganisms. Probiotic preparations have been shown to reduce IBS symptoms, such as abdominal pain/discomfort, bloating, and distention.[29,30] Probiotics also have inflammatory properties and inhibit proinflammatory cytokines.[29,31] The results of probiotics used in randomized clinical trials (RCTs) are positive but do not consistently outweigh placebo. One meta-analysis, including 33 separate RCTs, demonstrated *Streptococcus thermophiles* (LacClean Gold) and the seven-strain combination of three *Bifidobacterium*, three *Lactobacillus*, and one *Streptococcus* were associated with significant improvements in global IBS symptoms but little evidence was found for the use of prebiotics.[28]

Two RCTs of synbiotics in IBS recruited a total of 198 patients, and although both trials were individually positive, because of significant heterogeneity between studies there was no statistically significant effect of synbiotics in reducing symptoms.[32,33]

### Herbal therapies

The use of peppermint extracts has been studied in several clinical trials that evaluated the administration of enteric coated peppermint oil (PO) capsules to patients with IBS for 4 to 8 weeks and found it was associated with significant increase in quality of life while patients were taking the oil.[34] The main component of PO is menthol. Menthol prevents calcium influx into smooth muscle, prohibiting contractility.[1] PO possesses analgesic effects, antimicrobial, anti-inflammatory, antioxidant, and immunomodulating properties.[35] Cash and colleagues[36] demonstrated that a novel formulation of PO, enteric-coated (IBgard) designed to release in the small intestine, was associated with a rapid and sustained symptomatic improvement in patients with non-constipated IBS based on significant reductions in a global IBS symptom score and reduced frequency and/or intensity of individual IBS symptoms. This finding was evident at 24 hours ($P = .009$) and 4 weeks ($P = .02$).[36] PO was well tolerated and has few adverse effects. A recent meta-analysis evaluated 835 patients with IBS in 12 different studies and found the number needed to treat with PO to prevent one patient from having persistent symptoms was three for global symptoms and four for abdominal pain.[35] However, PO can worsen gastroesophageal reflux symptoms.

Iberogast (STW 5) is a combination of nine herbal plant extracts originally used for functional dyspepsia in Germany.[34] The extract containing flowers, roots, leaves, and herbs has been used for more than 30 years to treat digestive disorders.[34] In one randomized, double-blind, placebo-controlled study protocol over a 4-week period, the herbal preparation improved dyspeptic symptoms significantly better than placebo.[37] The reduction in IBS symptoms is possibly mediated through influences on serotonin, acetylcholine, and opioid receptors in the GI tract leading to antispasmodic effects.[1,34] Another study suggests Iberogast has a prosecretory functions because of its effects on chloride channels via CFTR and calcium-dependent channels, and thus may have a role in treating secretory disorders associated with IBS and constipation.[38]

## Pharmacotherapy for Irritable Bowel Syndrome

Treatment of IBS is unique to each patient and targeted at the predominant or most troublesome symptom. There is not one sole disease process or pathophysiologic explanation for symptoms; therefore, it makes sense to target symptoms, such as pain and diarrhea or pain and constipation, when understanding the natural history of the disorder.[11] The subtypes of IBS are based on the predominant stool pattern used to dictate treatment options, such as IBS predominant constipation (IBS-C), IBS-D, or mixed stool pattern.

## Antispasmodic Drugs

Antispasmodics are group of drugs that have been used in IBS therapy for decades. It is known that a subgroup of patients with IBS have altered GI transit and abnormal contractility of smooth muscle contributing to disturbances in bowel habit and pain.[11] Included are drugs with various mechanisms of action including anticholinergic agents (ie, butyl scopolamine, hyoscine, cimetropium bromide, pirenzepine), direct smooth muscle relaxants (PO, papaverine, mebeverine), and calcium channel blockers (alverine citrate, otilonium bromide, pinaverium bromide) contributing to relief of pain in IBS.[39] A systematic review and meta-analysis of 22 RCTs compared various antispasmodics with placebo in 1778 patients and found antispasmodic agents were more effective than placebo in the treatment of IBS; however, these studies had statistically significant heterogeneity detected.[23] However, this meta-analysis studied many drugs not available in the United States, including otilonium bromide and pinaverium, which had the strongest data.[11] Subgroup analyses for different types of antispasmodics found that use of cimetropium/dicyclomine, PO, pinaverium, and trimebutine presented statistically significant benefits.[22]

## Antidepressants and Psychological Treatment

Physiologic factors seem to be related to one of the pathophysiologic aspects of IBS manifestation. There have been some indications of an association between IBS and psychiatric disorders.

The TCAs and newer serotonin-norepinephrine reuptake inhibitors (duloxetine, venlafaxine) are useful in treating chronic pain syndromes because of their noradrenergic and serotoninergic effcts.[4] These drugs are also useful in patients with coexisting psychological disorders, which is not uncommon to see in IBS. Patients may not want to take these drugs initially because of the stigma that they only treat psychiatric conditions; therefore, it is imperative to explain they are used to treat pain centrally. They have independent effects on pain and are used at lower dosages than to treat depression but titrated up to full dosage if needed.[4] Patients should also be reassured these drugs are nonaddictive and stopped without major side effects if needed. If these are ineffective the patient should be referred to psychiatry for treatment with another antidepressant, such as an SSRI, bupropion, buspirone, or an atypical antipsychotic.[4] Quetiapine is an atypical antipsychotic that has been used in low dosages for chronic pain syndromes and has antianxiety and sleep properties.

It is well known that depression changes the brain's perception of pain. The mechanism behind antidepressants positive effects in IBS is not certain; however, it is postulated that there is reduced activation of pain centers in the anterior cingulate cortex.[11] TCAs and SSRIs also act on intestinal transit. TCAs prolong orocecal transit times, whereas SSRIs decrease orocecal transit time; therefore, TCAs are used in IBS-D and SSRIs are preferred in IBS-C.[1]

Cognitive behavioral therapy is implemented to improve symptoms control through adaption of perception, maladaptive thoughts, and behaviors. Hypnosis and dynamic psychotherapy have been studied in IBS.[4]

An updated systematic review and meta-analysis by Ford and colleagues[6] demonstrated that antidepressants and psychological therapies seem to be effective treatments for IBS, although there are limitations in the quality of the evidence. Antidepressants versus placebo, or psychological therapies versus control therapy or "usual management" were eligible for the study; TCAs, SSRIs, cognitive behavioral therapy, relaxation therapy, hypnotherapy, multicomponent psychological therapy, and dynamic psychotherapy were specifically evaluated. Highest adverse effects were seen with the TCAs.[6] A recent Cochrane systematic review comparing cognitive therapy versus conventional therapy did not find any difference in comparison with placebo, regarding abdominal pain, quality of life, or symptom score improvement.[40]

### Drugs Acting on Opioid Receptors

Opioids have pharmacologic effects throughout the GI tract. In the esophagus, they decrease lower esophageal sphincter tone and cause simultaneous contractions.[9] Opioids affect the gallbladder by causing increased contraction resulting in biliary pain, sphincter of Oddi spasm, and decreased gallbladder emptying. They can also cause anxiety, nausea, vomiting, and gastroparesis by decreasing gastric motility and increasing pyloric tone. In the small bowel and colon, transit time, tone, and absorption is increased, resulting in postoperative ileus, constipation, bloating, and distention. Patients may also experience decreased rectal sensation or straining constipation from internal sphincter tone contraction caused by opioids.[9]

Loperamide, a $\mu$-opioid receptor agonist (which does not cross the blood-brain barrier), is an antidiarrheal agent used in the treatment of diarrhea in patients with IBS.[9] It's efficacy is based in little evidence from RCTs.[11] There is no evidence supporting the use of loperamide for chronic pain in IBS.[9] One study included 90 patients in a prospective double-blind trial comparing loperamide with placebo over 5 weeks. This study demonstrated improved stool consistency, reduced defecation frequency, and reduced intensity of pain.[41]

Eluxadoline is a novel mixed agent $\mu$ and $\kappa$ opioid receptor agonist and $\delta$ opioid receptor antagonist used to treat diarrhea.[9] Lacy and colleagues[42] reported that eluxadoline effectively and safely treated IBS-D symptoms of abdominal pain and diarrhea in patients who self-reported either adequate or inadequate control of their symptoms with prior loperamide treatment.

### 5-HT3 Receptor Antagonists

Ninety percent of the body's total amount of serotonin (5-HT) is found in the enterochromaffin cells within the intestine.[11] Patients with IBS-D have increased postprandial levels of serotonin, whereas patients with IBS-C have decreased levels postprandially.[11] Alosetron is a selective 5-HT3-receptor antagonist approved by the Food and Drug Administration (FDA) for the treatment of women with IBS-D who have failed conventional therapy.[43] One study enrolled patients using Rome III criteria and found the overall treatment responder rate was 44.6%, demonstrating control of the two cardinal symptoms of IBS-D, abdominal pain and diarrhea, evaluated by the FDA composite end point.[43] This trial also found fecal urgency, another important symptom of IBS-D, significantly improved during this study.[43] Another network meta-analysis assessing the efficacy of licensed pharmacologic therapies (alosetron, eluxadoline, ramosetron, and rifaximin) in adults with IBS-D or IBS with mixed stool pattern found all drugs to be superior to placebo, but alosetron and ramosetron seemed to be the most effective.[44]

This class of drugs can induce constipation, which is controlled by titrating the dose.[11] Alosetron has been reported in association with ischemic colitis in about 1:800 treated persons.[11]

### Bile Acid Sequestrants

Recent studies have documented that more than 25% of patients with IBS-D have evidence of bile acid diarrhea, and have symptom improvement on bile acid sequestrants.[45,46] Bile acid diarrhea is diagnosed through testing fecal excretion of bile or fasting serum C4 (7-α-hydroxy-4-cholesten-3-one).[45] Intraluminal bile acid binders, such as colesevelam[47] and colestipol,[48] have shown benefit in bowel symptoms and global symptoms in patients with IBS-D. Use of bile acid sequestrates is limited by their poor palatability.

### Antibiotics

Rifaximin has minimal absorption in the GI tract, broad-spectrum antimicrobial with activity against gram-positive and gram-negative aerobic and anaerobic organisms. It acts by reducing the quantity of gas-producing bacteria and altering the predominant species of bacteria present.[49]

Some patients with IBS have underlying small intestinal bacterial overgrowth detected on hydrogen breath testing; however, there is a risk of false-positive testing caused by rapid small bowel transit, which is seen in this population.[11] Two phase 3 trials showed that treatment with rifaximin at a dose of 550 mg three times daily for 14 days provides better relief of global IBS symptoms in patients without constipation than placebo for up to 10 weeks after completion of therapy.[50] The safety profile of rifaximin was similar to placebo.[50] Additional investigation into optimal dosing and treatment duration is necessary. One double-blind, randomized, placebo-controlled trial performed from 2010 to 2013 at three tertiary care centers found rifaximin plus neomycin was superior than neomycin alone in improving constipation ($P = .007$), straining ($P = .017$), and bloating ($P = .020$).[51] Rifaximin is currently FDA approved to treat patients with IBS-D and allow for up to two courses of retreatment for relapse of symptoms.[11]

### Intestinal Secretagogues

In the past decade, several novel secretagogues have been FDA approved for the treatment of IBS-C; these include lubiprostone, linaclotide, and plecanatide. They are also approved for chronic idiopathic constipation. Tenapanor is pending approval for IBS-C. These drugs were examined in a systematic review and network meta-analysis, which proved their efficacy in placebo-controlled trials in IBS-C, and were more effective than placebo for reducing global symptoms.[52]

Lubiprostone is a prostaglandin derivative that activates the intestinal chloride channel type 2 on the apical membrane of small intestinal enterocytes.[52,53] Activation leads to chloride and water efflux into the lumen. Lubiprostone was evaluated at a daily dose of 16 μg (8 μg twice daily) versus placebo (twice daily) for 12 weeks in two phase 3 double-blind, randomized, placebo-controlled trials.[54] Lubiprostone led to a significantly higher number of global responders and improved individual symptoms in patients with IBS-C compared with placebo; the overall incidence of adverse events was similar to placebo.[54] Another analysis proved lubiprostone was significantly more effective than placebo in reducing abdominal pain and bloating using the FDA-recommended criteria.[55]

Linaclotide and plecanatide are minimally absorbed peptides that stimulate the guanylate cyclase-C receptor, leading to electrolyte and fluid transport into the intestinal lumen. In one large phase 3 clinical trial, patients with IBS-C were treated with 290 μg oral linaclotide once daily in a 12-week treatment period, followed by a 4-week randomized withdrawal period.[56] Linaclotide achieved statistically significant improvement in abdominal pain and constipation, compared with placebo, and there was no worsening of symptoms compared with baseline following cessation of linaclotide during the withdrawal period.[56] Adults meeting Rome III criteria for IBS-C were randomized to placebo or plecanatide (3 or 6 mg) for 12 weeks across two identical, phase 3, randomized, double-blind, placebo-controlled trials.[57] Plecanatide significantly improved stool frequency/consistency, straining, and abdominal symptoms compared with placebo, and the drug was highly tolerated with approximately 1.3% of patients discontinuing the drug because of diarrhea.[57]

Tenapanor is a first of its class small-molecule inhibitor of the GI sodium-hydrogen exchanger-3, which results in increased intraluminal sodium and water excretion.[58] In a phase 2, double-blind study by Chey and colleagues,[58] patients with IBS-C had significantly increased stool frequency and reduced abdominal symptoms after receiving tenapanor 50 mg twice daily. These benefits were sustained over the 12-week treatment period.

### γ-Aminobutyric Acid Analogues

γ-Aminobutyric acid analogues, such as pregabalin and gabapentin, are being studied for their use in IBS. Some preliminary reports show it may have a role in reducing symptoms; however, there are insufficient data to support its use.[11]

## SUMMARY

The field of IBS is lacking the presence of validated biomarkers, that is, bile acid metabolism or colon transit time, which can be objectively measured during treatment. There is still considerable unmet need for effective and safe visceral analgesics. Further high-quality studies, such as RCTs, focusing on the pathophysiologic mechanisms underlying IBS are needed.[11] The most efficacious current therapies for visceral pain are directed primarily at bowel dysfunction (eg, 5-HT3 antagonists). Such therapies as lifestyle modifications, changes in diet, and cognitive behavioral therapy should be used in conjunction with pharmacotherapy rather than pharmacotherapy alone.

## REFERENCES

1. Camilleri M. Management options for irritable bowel syndrome. Mayo Clin Proc 2018;93(12):1858–72.

2. Pichetshote N, Pimentel M. An approach to the patient with chronic undiagnosed abdominal pain. Am J Gastroenterol 2019;114(5):726–32.

3. Talley NJ. How to do and interpret a rectal examination in gastroenterology. Am J Gastroenterol 2008;103(4):820–2.

4. Drossman DA. Severe and refractory chronic abdominal pain: treatment strategies. Clin Gastroenterol Hepatol 2008;6(9):978–82.

5. Drossman DA. Functional gastrointestinal disorders: history, pathophysiology, clinical features and Rome IV. Gastroenterology 2016 May;150(6):1257–61.

6. Ford AC, Lacy BE, Harris LA, et al. Effect of antidepressants and psychological therapies in irritable bowel syndrome: an updated systematic review and meta-analysis. Am J Gastroenterol 2019;114(1):21–39.

7. Keefer L, Drossman DA, Guthrie E, et al. Centrally mediated disorders of gastrointestinal pain. Gastroenterology 2016;150(6):1408–19.

8. Tack J, Drossman DA. What's new in Rome IV? Neurogastroenterol Motil 2017;29(9).

9. Camilleri M, Lembo A, Katzka DA. Opioids in gastroenterology: treating adverse effects and creating therapeutic benefits. Clin Gastroenterol Hepatol 2017;15(9): 1338–49.

10. Kurlander JE, Drossman DA. Diagnosis and treatment of narcotic bowel syndrome. Nat Rev Gastroenterol Hepatol 2014;11(7):410–8.

11. Camilleri M, Ford AC. Pharmacotherapy for irritable bowel syndrome. J Clin Med 2017;6(11).

12. Zhou Q, Wesselmann U, Walker L, et al. AAPT diagnostic criteria for chronic abdominal, pelvic, and urogenital pain: irritable bowel syndrome. J Pain 2018; 19(3):257–63.

13. Warburton DE, Nicol CW, Bredin SS. Health benefits of physical activity: the evidence. CMAJ 2006;174(6):801–9.

14. Johannesson E, Simrén M, Strid H, et al. Physical activity improves symptoms in irritable bowel syndrome: a randomized controlled trial. Am J Gastroenterol 2011; 106(5):915–22.

15. Kichline T, Cushing CC, Ortega A, et al. Associations between physical activity and chronic pain severity in youth with chronic abdominal pain. Clin J Pain 2019;35(7):618–24.

16. Major G, Pritchard S, Murray K, et al. Colon hypersensitivity to distension, rather than excessive gas production, produces carbohydrate-related symptoms in individuals with irritable bowel syndrome. Gastroenterology 2017;152(1): 124–33.e2.

17. Halmos EP, Christophersen CT, Bird AR, et al. Diets that differ in their FODMAP content alter the colonic luminal microenvironment. Gut 2015;64(1):93–100.

18. Halmos EP, Gibson PR. Controversies and reality of the FODMAP diet for patients with irritable bowel syndrome. J Gastroenterol Hepatol 2019;34(7):1134–42.

19. McMeans AR, King KL, Chumpitazi BP. Low FODMAP dietary food lists are often discordant. Am J Gastroenterol 2017;112(4):655–6.

20. Whelan K, Martin LD, Staudacher HM, et al. The low FODMAP diet in the management of irritable bowel syndrome: an evidence-based review of FODMAP restriction, reintroduction and personalisation in clinical practice. J Hum Nutr Diet 2018; 31(2):239–55.

21. Drossman DA, Whitehead WE, Camilleri M. Irritable bowel syndrome: a technical review for practice guideline development. Gastroenterology 1997;112(6): 2120–37.

22. Ruepert L, Quartero AO, de Wit NJ, et al. Bulking agents, antispasmodics and antidepressants for the treatment of irritable bowel syndrome (review). Cochrane Database Syst Rev 2011;(8):CD003460.

23. Ford AC, Talley NJ, Spiegel BM, et al. Effect of fibre, antispasmodics, and peppermint oil in the treatment of irritable bowel syndrome: systematic review and meta-analysis. BMJ 2008;337:a2313.

24. Bijkerk CJ, de Wit NJ, Muris JW, et al. Soluble or insoluble fibre in irritable bowel syndrome in primary care? Randomised placebo controlled trial. BMJ 2009;339: b3154.

25. Werlang ME, Palmer WC, Lacy BE. Irritable bowel syndrome and dietary interventions. Gastroenterol Hepatol (N Y) 2019;15(1):16–26.

26. Vazquez-Roque MI, Camilleri M, Smyrk T, et al. A controlled trial of gluten-free diet in patients with irritable bowel syndrome-diarrhea: effects on bowel frequency and intestinal function. Gastroenterology 2013;144(5):903–11.e3.

27. Ishaque SM, Khosruzzaman SM, Ahmed DS, et al. A randomized placebo-controlled clinical trial of a multi-strain probiotic formulation (Bio-Kult®) in the management of diarrhea-predominant irritable bowel syndrome. BMC Gastroenterol 2018;18(1):71.

28. Ford AC, Harris LA, Lacy BE, et al. Systematic review with meta-analysis: the efficacy of prebiotics, probiotics, synbiotics and antibiotics in irritable bowel syndrome. Aliment Pharmacol Ther 2018;48(10):1044–60.

29. O'Mahony L, McCarthy J, Kelly P, et al. Lactobacillus and bifidobacterium in irritable bowel syndrome: symptom responses and relationship to cytokine profiles. Gastroenterology 2005;128(3):541–51.

30. Ki Cha B, Mun Jung S, Hwan Choi C, et al. The effect of a multispecies probiotic mixture on the symptoms and fecal microbiota in diarrhea-dominant irritable bowel syndrome: a randomized, double-blind, placebo-controlled trial. J Clin Gastroenterol 2012;46(3):220–7.

31. Barbara G, Zecchi L, Barbaro R, et al. Mucosal permeability and immune activation as potential therapeutic targets of probiotics in irritable bowel syndrome. J Clin Gastroenterol 2012;46(Suppl):S52–5.

32. Tsuchiya J, Barreto R, Okura R, et al. Single-blind follow-up study on the effectiveness of a symbiotic preparation in irritable bowel syndrome. Chin J Dig Dis 2004; 5(4):169–74.

33. Min YW, Park SU, Jang YS, et al. Effect of composite yogurt enriched with acacia fiber and *Bifidobacterium lactis*. World J Gastroenterol 2012;18(33):4563–9.

34. Grundmann O, Yoon SL. Complementary and alternative medicines in irritable bowel syndrome: an integrative view. World J Gastroenterol 2014;20(2):346–62.

35. Alammar N, Wang L, Saberi B, et al. The impact of peppermint oil on the irritable bowel syndrome: a meta-analysis of the pooled clinical data. BMC Complement Altern Med 2019;19(1):21.

36. Cash BD, Epstein MS, Shah SM. A novel delivery system of peppermint oil is an effective therapy for irritable bowel syndrome symptoms. Dig Dis Sci 2016;61(2): 560–71.

37. Madisch A, Holtmann G, Mayr G, et al. Treatment of functional dyspepsia with a herbal preparation. A double-blind, randomized, placebo-controlled, multicenter trial. Digestion 2004;69(1):45–52.

38. Krueger D, Gruber L, Buhner S, et al. The multi-herbal drug STW 5 (Iberogast) has prosecretory action in the human intestine. Neurogastroenterol Motil 2009; 21(11):1203-e110.

39. Annaházi A, Róka R, Rosztóczy A, et al. Role of antispasmodics in the treatment of irritable bowel syndrome. World J Gastroenterol May 2014;20(20):6031–43.

40. Pacheco RL, Roizenblatt A, Góis AFT, et al. What do Cochrane systematic reviews say about the management of irritable bowel syndrome? Sao Paulo Med J 2019;137(1):82–91.

41. Efskind PS, Bernklev T, Vatn MH. A double-blind placebo-controlled trial with loperamide in irritable bowel syndrome. Scand J Gastroenterol 1996;31(5):463–8.

42. Lacy BE, Chey WD, Cash BD, et al. Eluxadoline efficacy in IBS-D patients who report prior loperamide use. Am J Gastroenterol 2017;112(6):924–32.

43. Lacy BE, Nicandro JP, Chuang E, et al. Alosetron use in clinical practice: significant improvement in irritable bowel syndrome symptoms evaluated using the US Food and Drug Administration composite endpoint. Therap Adv Gastroenterol 2018;11. 1756284818771674.

44. Black CJ, Burr NE, Camilleri M, et al. Efficacy of pharmacological therapies in patients with IBS with diarrhoea or mixed stool pattern: systematic review and network meta-analysis. Gut 2020;69(1):74–82.

45. Wang XJ, Camilleri M. Personalized medicine in functional gastrointestinal disorders: understanding pathogenesis to increase diagnostic and treatment efficacy. World J Gastroenterol 2019;25(10):1185–96.

46. Wedlake L, A'Hern R, Russell D, et al. Systematic review: the prevalence of idiopathic bile acid malabsorption as diagnosed by SeHCAT scanning in patients with diarrhoea-predominant irritable bowel syndrome. Aliment Pharmacol Ther 2009;30(7):707–17.

47. Camilleri M, Acosta A, Busciglio I, et al. Effect of colesevelam on faecal bile acids and bowel functions in diarrhoea-predominant irritable bowel syndrome. Aliment Pharmacol Ther 2015;41(5):438–48.

48. Bajor A, Törnblom H, Rudling M, et al. Increased colonic bile acid exposure: a relevant factor for symptoms and treatment in IBS. Gut 2015;64(1):84–92.

49. Iorio N, Malik Z, Schey R. Profile of rifaximin and its potential in the treatment of irritable bowel syndrome. Clin Exp Gastroenterol 2015;8:159–67.

50. Pimentel M, Lembo A, Chey WD, et al. Rifaximin therapy for patients with irritable bowel syndrome without constipation. N Engl J Med 2011;364(1):22–32.

51. Pimentel M, Chang C, Chua KS, et al. Antibiotic treatment of constipation-predominant irritable bowel syndrome. Dig Dis Sci 2014;59(6):1278–85.

52. Black CJ, Burr NE, Quigley EMM, et al. Efficacy of secretagogues in patients with irritable bowel syndrome with constipation: systematic review and network meta-analysis. Gastroenterology 2018;155(6):1753–63.

53. Schey R, Rao SS. Lubiprostone for the treatment of adults with constipation and irritable bowel syndrome. Dig Dis Sci 2011;56(6):1619–25.

54. Drossman DA, Chey WD, Johanson JF, et al. Clinical trial: lubiprostone in patients with constipation-associated irritable bowel syndrome–results of two randomized, placebo-controlled studies. Aliment Pharmacol Ther 2009;29(3):329–41.

55. Chang L, Chey WD, Drossman D, et al. Effects of baseline abdominal pain and bloating on response to lubiprostone in patients with irritable bowel syndrome with constipation. Aliment Pharmacol Ther 2016;44(10):1114–22.

56. Rao S, Lembo AJ, Shiff SJ, et al. A 12-week, randomized, controlled trial with a 4-week randomized withdrawal period to evaluate the efficacy and safety of linaclotide in irritable bowel syndrome with constipation. Am J Gastroenterol 2012; 107(11):1714–24 [quiz p.1725].

57. Brenner DM, Fogel R, Dorn SD, et al. Efficacy, safety, and tolerability of plecanatide in patients with irritable bowel syndrome with constipation: results of two phase 3 randomized clinical trials. Am J Gastroenterol 2018;113(5):735–45.
58. Chey WD, Lembo AJ, Rosenbaum DP. Tenapanor treatment of patients with constipation-predominant irritable bowel syndrome: a phase 2, randomized, placebo-controlled efficacy and safety trial. Am J Gastroenterol 2017;112(5): 763–74.

# Refractory Constipation
## How to Evaluate and Treat

Michael Camilleri, MD*, Justin Brandler, MD

## KEYWORDS

- Dyssynergia • Evacuation disorder • Descending perineum syndrome
- Slow transit constipation • Colonic inertia

## KEY POINTS

- The key to managing refractory constipation is to diagnose the pathophysiology.
- Advances in recent years include identification of rectal evacuation disorders.
- Treatment should be individualized to the underling pathophysiology.
- Delayed colonic transit may be due to rectal evacuation disorders and rarely represents evidence of colonic inertia.
- Descending perineum syndrome requires specific diagnosis and therapy.

## INTRODUCTION

Chronic constipation is one of most prevalent conditions presenting to primary care physicians or subspecialty physicians and surgeons and is typically diagnosed by symptom criteria.[1–3] This article addresses the management of patients with refractory constipation. In clinical practice, there are many features in the history, digital rectal examination, and the commonly performed clinical tests that either present pitfalls in the identification of the cause of refractoriness or provide clues for the management of patients with what appears to be refractory constipation. Advances in recent years have led to a greater appreciation of the prevalence, diagnosis, and treatment of dyssynergic defection in patients presenting to gastroenterologists and to development of effective pharmacologic agents for treatment of chronic constipation, as illustrated in a network meta-analysis.[4]

## REFRACTORY CONSTIPATION: TERMINOLOGY

There are several terms and synonyms of those terms that are commonly used in discussions of refractory constipation; thus, **Table 1** summarizes the various conditions that are considered in the differential diagnosis of chronic refractory constipation and

Division of Gastroenterology and Hepatology, Mayo Clinic, 200 First Street Southwest, Charlton Building, Room 8-110, Rochester, MN 55905, USA
* Corresponding author.
*E-mail address:* camilleri.michael@mayo.edu

Gastroenterol Clin N Am 49 (2020) 623–642
https://doi.org/10.1016/j.gtc.2020.05.002
0889-8553/20/© 2020 Elsevier Inc. All rights reserved.

gastro.theclinics.com

**Table 1**
**Constipation terminology**

| Term | Definition | Examples/Comments |
|------|-----------|-------------------|
| Classification | | |
| Chronic idiopathic constipation (CIC) | Symptoms: ≥2 Rome IV criteria on >25% of bowel movements *without* abdominal pain/bloating as predominant symptoms[1]<br>Duration: ≥3 mo<br>Onset: ≥6 mo before diagnosis<br>*Red flags absent, common secondary causes ruled out*[a] | Functional constipation |
| Irritable bowel syndrome-constipation predominant (IBS-C) | Symptoms: ≥2 Rome IV Criteria on >25% of bowel movements *with* abdominal pain as predominant symptom[1]<br>Duration: ≥3 mo<br>Frequency: ≥1 d/wk<br>*Red flags absent, common secondary causes ruled out*[a] | IBS-Mixed includes IBS-C, as both have >25% bowel movements Bristol Stool Form Scale (BSFS) 1–2 |
| Rectal evacuation disorder (RED) | Inability to evacuate stool from the rectum<br>Due to *physiologic* and/or *structural* pathology<br>Pathology of *rectum, anus,* and/or *anorectal unit*<br>Subset of CIC or IBS-C | • Dyssynergic defecation<br>• Pelvic floor dysfunction<br>• Pelvic floor dyssynergia<br>• Obstructed defecation syndrome<br>• Rectocele/rectal prolapse<br>• Descending perineum syndrome |
| Slow transit constipation (STC) | Slow colonic transit seen objectively on validated test<br>Tests: Sitz markers, wireless motility capsule, scintigraphy<br>Can *co-occur with RED*<br>Subset of CIC or IBS-C | Colonic inertia |
| Red flag symptoms | Symptoms requiring further testing/ investigation:<br>• Hematochezia<br>• Unintentional weight loss of ≥10 pounds<br>• Family history of colon cancer or inflammatory bowel disease<br>• Anemia<br>• Positive fecal occult blood test<br>• Acute onset constipation in elderly | |

*(continued on next page)*

| Table 1 *(continued)* | | |
|---|---|---|
| **Term** | **Definition** | **Examples/Comments** |
| Clinical pathology | | |
| Refractory chronic constipation | Constipation *not responsive* to *lifestyle modifications* (increased physical activity, fluid, or soluble fiber intake) and no response to *osmotic and stimulant laxatives* | |
| Perineal descent | Caudal movement of *anal verge* during attempted defecation as measured below an imaginary line between the coccyx and pubic symphysis (pubococcygeal line) | • Normal: 2–4 cm<br>• Absent: <2 cm<br>• Excessive: >4 cm |
| Rectal prolapse | Circumferential, full-thickness, *intussusception* of *rectal* wall<br>• External: seen on examination with patient straining in seated position<br>• Internal: seen only on defecography or proctoscopy | |
| Pelvic organ prolapse | Bulging of pelvic organs *into* anterior or posterior *vaginal* wall | |
| Rectocele | Bulging of the rectum *into* posterior *vaginal* wall | |
| Cul-de-sac hernias (peritoneocele) | Bulging of peritoneum *between vagina* and *rectum* with or without abdominal visceral organs | Peritoneocele subtype contents:<br>• Enterocele: small intestine<br>• Sigmoidocele: sigmoid colon<br>• Omentocele: omentum |

ᵃ See **Table 2** for common secondary causes.

associated clinical features. A specific category is the group of conditions summarized under the term rectal evacuation disorders with the multiple synonyms used to describe the variety of manifestations of rectal evacuation disorders. These include pelvic floor dyssynergia and obstructed defecation, which represent "spastic" disorders of the pelvic floor and anal sphincter function. In contrast, conditions associated with "flaccid" or weak pelvic floor anatomy are associated with descending perineum syndrome, as well as anatomic abnormalities such as a rectocele or rectal mucosal prolapse. **Table 1** also summarizes the clinical pathology associated with refractory chronic constipation, as well as the diverse manifestations or anatomic or structural changes that can be evident in patients with refractory constipation. Some of these terms are commonly encountered in clinical practice and include perineal descent, prolapse, and rectocele; another term such as cul-de-sac hernia represents bulging of the peritoneum in the pouch of Douglas between the vagina and rectum and may include viscera such as the small intestine, sigmoid colon, or omentum.

## REFRACTORINESS OF CONSTIPATION MAY RESULT FROM UNCONTROLLED UNDERLYING DISEASE OR TREATMENT

**Table 2** summarizes different categories that result in secondary constipation, including medications; metabolic, neuromuscular, or psychiatric disorders; as well as mechanical and lifestyle factors. A classic example is the constipation occurring in patient with Parkinson disease, which can be associated with delayed colonic transit due to damaged myenteric plexus neurons from $\alpha$-synuclein deposits, pelvic floor dyssynergia, treatment with carbidopa-levodopa and anticholinergic medications, treatment with tricyclic antidepressants for associated depression, and immobility.

In clinical practice, the most commonly encountered medications resulting in secondary refractory constipation are opioids such as codeine, tramadol, morphine, and oxycodone, as well as medications used to treat hypertension, such as calcium channel blockers, antacids, particularly those containing calcium and aluminum salts, central neuromodulators, and $5HT_3$ antagonists, such as ondansetron used for the treatment of nausea, which is often a symptom experienced in patients with constipation.

A careful evaluation for metabolic and neurologic diseases includes searching for Beighton criteria for Ehlers-Danlos syndrome,[5] orthostatic hypotension, and peripheral neuropathy on physical examination, and performing screening tests such as serum potassium, calcium, magnesium, and sensitive thyroid-stimulating hormone. In patients with recent onset of refractory constipation, especially for those older than 40 years and a positive family history, it is essential to exclude mechanical obstruction from colonic neoplasm or benign strictures secondary to diverticular disease.

## CLINICAL TESTING IN PATIENTS WITH REFRACTORY CONSTIPATION

In a classic paper by Voderholzer and colleagues,[6] clinical experience showed that patients with constipation who did not respond to an adequate trial of dietary fiber (more than 20 g per day), the sources of refractoriness were typically dyssynergic defecation, slow transit constipation due to a likely motility disorder of the colon, or concomitant use of medications causing constipation.[6,7]

**Table 3** summarizes the physiologic (motor or sensory) as well as the structural tests conducted in clinical practice to evaluate patients with chronic or refractory constipation. These include balloon expulsion test, anorectal manometry, rectal sensation studies using a latex balloon during the anorectal manometry,[8–10] or, in specialized centers, an infinitely compliant balloon distended with a barostat, and measurement of colonic transit. Rectal sensation may be reduced in patients with chronic constipation and, particularly in children, this may result from an increased rectal diameter due to stool retention, especially in those with rectal evacuation disorder or with encopresis.

Experience from a review of 449 consecutive patients with rectal evacuation disorder evaluated by a single gastroenterologist[11] shows that findings on digital rectal

**Table 2**
**Etiologies of secondary constipation**

| Categories | Examples |
|---|---|
| Medications | |
|   Analgesics | Opioids/tramadol |
|   Antihypertensives | Calcium channel blockers<br>Diuretics<br>Clonidine |
|   Antinausea | 5HT$_3$ blocker<br>Promethazine |
|   Antacids | Calcium carbonate (Maalox, Tums, Caltrate)<br>Aluminum hydroxide (Maalox, Gaviscon) |
|   Antiallergy | Antihistamines |
|   Central nervous system | |
|     Antidepressants | Tricyclic antidepressants |
|     Anti-Parkinson | Carbidopa-levodopa |
|     Neuroleptics | Typical, atypical antipsychotics |
| Metabolic diseases | |
|   Endocrine | Diabetes mellitus<br>Hypothyroidism<br>Hyperparathyroidism<br>Pregnancy |
|   Electrolytes | Hyper/hypocalcemia<br>Hypokalemia<br>Hypomagnesemia |
| Neuromuscular diseases | |
|   Neuropathy | Parkinsonism<br>Multiple sclerosis<br>Spinal cord injury<br>Autonomic neuropathy<br>Amyloidosis<br>Paraneoplastic neuropathy<br>Primary megacolon/megarectum |
|   Myopathy | Systemic sclerosis<br>Ehlers-Danlos syndrome<br>Amyloidosis |
| Obstruction | |
|   Mechanical | Colorectal neoplasm<br>Diverticulitis |
|   Functional | Pseudo-obstruction (intestinal, colonic) |
| Psychiatric disease | |
|   Mood disorders | Depression |
|   Eating disorders | Anorexia, bulimia |
| Lifestyle | |
|   Diet | Dehydration<br>Low fiber intake |
|   Exercise | Immobility |

**Table 3**
Constipation clinical testing

| Test | Description | Examples/Comments |
|---|---|---|
| **Physiologic (Motor, Sensory)** | | |
| Balloon expulsion test (BET) | 4-cm balloon in rectum filled with 50 mL water, patient attempts to expel balloon<br>Previously weight based, but often no longer used | Normal expulsion: <1 min<br>Abnormal expulsion: >2 min<br>*Testing techniques, body positions, and types of balloons highly variable* |
| Anorectal manometry (ARM) | Assess resting, anal squeeze, and *defecation* states<br>Assess motor (anus, rectum, anorectal unit)<br>Assess sensory (rectum) | Conventional ARM<br>High-resolution ARM (HR-ARM)<br>3D-HR-ARM (primarily research)<br>*Wide overlap of measurements between health and disease* |
| Pelvic floor electromyography (EMG) | Assess external anal sphincter and *levator ani* muscles<br>Use needle, skin, or anal plug electrodes<br>Intraluminal electrodes felt more accurate because closer to sphincter muscle | Useful for diagnosis and treatment of defecatory disorders using *pelvic floor biofeedback*<br>*Pudendal nerve terminal motor latencies used to assess neuromuscular integrity after pelvic floor trauma but clinical utility is controversial* |

| | | |
|---|---|---|
| Simple rectal balloon distension | *Assess motor:* rectal stiffness/capacity<br>*Assess sensory:* visceral sensitivity<br>*Manually* expand elastic balloon in rectum with air using continuous (1–2 mL/s) or intermittent (phasic or stepwise) distension protocols<br>*Sensory thresholds:* patient reports perceived sensations (first sensation, desire to defecate, urgency, maximum toleration/pain) and corresponding distending volume recorded | Abnormal visceral sensitivity:<br>• Rectal hyposensitivity<br>• Rectal hypersensitivity<br>Abnormal rectal stiffness/capacity:<br>• Rectal hypercompliance (lax)<br>• Rectal hypocompliance (stiff)<br>• Widely available, often included with HR-ARM<br>• Poorly standardized distension protocols<br>• if abnormal results should be followed by rectal barostat |
| Rectal barostat | *Assess motor and sensory*<br>*Computerized barostat* allows precise rate of distension to increase intra-observer reliability vs simple balloon<br>*Sensory thresholds* obtained similarly to simple balloon | • Not widely available<br>• Used in patients with abnormal rectal sensitivity or compliance seen on simple balloon distension or with high index of suspicion for abnormal compliance/capacity |

(continued on next page)

**Table 3**
*(continued)*

| Test | Description | Examples/Comments |
|---|---|---|
| Colonic transit | Sitz markers: 20–24 radio-opaque markers swallowed with abdominal radiograph taken on day 5; *colonic transit only*<br><br>Wireless motility capsule (WMC): records pH, temp., pressure; *regional (gastric, small bowel, colonic) and whole gut transit*<br><br>Scintigraphy: $^{111}$In capsule with pH sensitive release in terminal ileum, image at 24 and 48 h; regional and *whole gut transit*<br>• Measured as geometric center (GC), weighted average of isotope distribution throughout colon | Slow transit constipation values:<br>Sitz: >5 (20%) retained markers on day 5<br>WMC: colonic >59 h, whole gut >73 h<br>Scintigraphy: GC24 <1.47, GC48 <2.11<br>Delta GC48-GC24 <0.37<br>Transit alone cannot distinguish slow transit from rectal evacuation disorder; *requires adjunct anorectal test* |
| **Structural** | | |
| Endoanal ultrasound | Assess both external and *internal anal sphincters*<br>Lateral or prone positioning with rigid endoprobe<br>2-dimensional, multiplanar 3-dimensional image reconstruction | Various pathologies seen including sphincter atrophy, hypertrophy, or defects<br>Widely available but operator dependent<br>*Transperineal ultrasound also available for pelvic organ prolapse, urinary incontinence* |

| | | |
|---|---|---|
| Endoanal MRI | High-resolution imaging of external anal sphincter<br>Can also visualize structures pertinent to pelvic organ prolapse and fecal incontinence | Can differentiate between sphincter defects, scarring, and atrophy<br>Less available, less operator dependent |
| **Physiologic and structural** | | |
| Defecography | Barium defecography: *sitting* position, cheap, ionizing radiation<br>MRI defecography: *supine* position (unless open system used), costly, no ionizing radiation | Barium: poor interrater reliability, embarrassing for patients<br>MRI: excellent imaging of all pelvic floor compartments, but supine position often required (closed magnet at few centers) |
| Colonic manometry | Assess *resting,* and *stimulated* states<br>Assess *motor* and *sensory* components<br>Can assess *myopathy* or *neuropathy*<br>High-resolution multisensor solid state probe or conventional stationary water perfusion for 8 h | *Myopathy* (low-amplitude contractions)<br>*Neuropathy* (absence of response to stimulation with high-calorie meal, intraluminal bisacodyl, intravenous neostigmine) |

examination such as inadequate perineal descent, high anal sphincter tone at rest, puborectalis tenderness, and paradoxic contraction of the pelvic floor or anal sphincters during simulation of straining to evacuate the examining finger are highly suggestive of an evacuation disorder. The main findings that suggest a rectal evacuation disorder on anorectal manometry are high resting anal sphincter pressure, reduced anal sphincter relaxation, a high negative rectoanal pressure differential, and a prolonged rectal balloon expulsion time. The literature shows diverse normal values, most evident in the range of balloon expulsion times in the different articles, ranging from 60 seconds to 300 seconds. More recent data from our institution suggest that the upper limit of normal should be 30 seconds, based on the cohort of 449 patients in whom a cutoff of 22 seconds was associated with 77.8% sensitivity and 69.8% specificity, in contrast to a 60-second cutoff, which had a sensitivity of 29% and specificity of 93%.[11] Moreover, in a separate study of 163 healthy volunteers, the 90th percentile for balloon expulsion time in both male and female individuals was 24 seconds.[12]

Among the structural studies, endoanal ultrasound is rarely necessary in patients with chronic constipation unless there is concomitant incontinence of stool. On the other hand, MRI defecography is now the standard approach when a combined physiologic and structural assessment is required, because it provides excellent imaging of the pelvic floor as well as functional assessment of the defecatory process, including degree of perineal descent and opening of the rectoanal angle. In specialized centers, for patients who have refractory constipation that has not responded to second-line treatments or pelvic floor retraining for dyssynergia, colonic manometry is sometimes performed to identify colonic myopathies (typically diagnosed in children with refractory constipation), characterized by low-amplitude contractions in the absence of colonic dilatation, or neuropathic colonic inertia, which is typically associated with normal colonic compliance and failure of a colonic tonic and phasic response to a 1000-kilocalorie meal, as well as intravenous 1.0 mg neostigmine.[13,14] In the presence of enlarged colonic diameter, measurement of colonic compliance using a barostatically controlled balloon may be important to identify colonic megacolon when the measurements of colonic diameter do not provide a definitive anatomic diagnosis of chronic megacolon.[15]

## DIFFERENTIATING SUBTYPES OF PRIMARY CHRONIC IDIOPATHIC CONSTIPATION

Once the diagnosis of chronic idiopathic constipation is established, based on symptom criteria such as the Rome IV criteria[1] (**Table 4**), the next objective is to differentiate among normal transit constipation, rectal evacuation disorder, and slow transit constipation. **Fig. 1**A shows the proportion of respondents to a 2010 US population-based survey with regard to the overlap between irritable bowel syndrome with constipation (IBS-C) and chronic idiopathic constipation. Note that the reported proportions are 37.3% and 62.7%, respectively.[16] **Fig. 1**B shows the subtype stratification of normal transit constipation, rectal evacuation disorder, and slow transit constipation among 1411 patients evaluated over a 17-year period by a single gastroenterologist in a tertiary referral center based on clinical evaluation, anorectal manometry, balloon expulsion, and colonic transit measured by validated scintigraphy.[17]

The steps for achieving this differentiation are illustrated in **Table 4**, which also includes physical examination, vital clinical questions, and commonly performed clinical tests to achieve the diagnosis. In the diagnosis of normal transit constipation, it is important to perform a careful drug history and to exclude underlying conditions causing secondary constipation that would need to be addressed to achieve a satisfactory clinical outcome.

**Table 4**
**Differentiating subtypes of primary chronic idiopathic constipation**

Chronic Idiopathic Constipation (CIC) Rome IV Diagnostic Criteria
1. Must include ≥2 of following during ≥25% of defecations:
   - Straining
   - Lumpy/hard stools (Bristol Stool Form Scale [BSFS] 1–2)
   - Sensation of incomplete evacuation
   - Sensation of anorectal obstruction/blockage
   - Manual maneuvers to facilitate defecation
   - <3 spontaneous bowel movements/wk
2. Loose stools are rarely present without use of laxatives
3. Insufficient criteria for irritable bowel syndrome (abdominal pain and/or bloating not predominant symptoms)
   Duration: criteria fulfilled for last 3 mo with onset >6 mo before diagnosis

| Subtype | Normal Transit Constipation (NTC) | Rectal Evacuation Disorder (RED) | Slow Transit Constipation (STC) |
|---|---|---|---|
| Proposed diagnostic criteria[a] | • Satisfy Rome IV criteria for CIC<br>Rule out secondary causes[1]:<br>• Careful drug history:<br>  • Temporal associations<br>  • Diuretics<br>  • Over-the-counter medications<br>  • Recreational drugs<br>• Underlying conditions:<br>  • Metabolic<br>  • Neuropathy/Myopathy<br>  • Mechanical/pseudo-obstruction<br>  • Psychiatric<br>  • Diet/Exercise | Must meet *all* criteria[8,9]:<br>• Satisfy Rome IV criteria for CIC<br>• Dyssynergic pattern of defecation (types I-IV) on objective testing[b]<br>• Satisfy ≥1 of following:<br>  ○ Unable to expel 50 mL water-filled balloon within 1–2 min<br>  ○ Unable to expel ≥50% of barium during defecography<br>  ○ Slow colonic transit on validated testing | Must meet *all* criteria:<br>• Satisfy Rome IV criteria for CIC<br>• Slow colonic transit on validated test:<br>Sitz: >5 (20%) retained markers on day 5<br>Wireless motility capsule: colonic >59 h, whole gut >73 h<br>Scintigraphy: Geometric center (GC)24 <1.47, GC48 <2.11<br>Delta GC48-GC24 <0.37<br>Dyssynergic defecation may co-occur |
| Important clinical questions[c] | • Predominant BSFS type?<br>• Upper gastrointestinal symptoms?<br>• Systemic/neurologic symptoms?<br>• Abdominal pain/bloating predominant symptom?<br>• Is there a call to stool?<br>  ○ Postprandial?<br>  ○ Initiated by abdominal pain and/or rectal sensation? | • Abnormal digital rectal examination?<br>• Sexual abuse?<br>• Obstetric trauma? (multiple vaginal deliveries, vaginal tears)<br>• Sensation of incomplete evacuation/obstruction?<br>• Excessive straining?<br>• Digital maneuvers to facilitate defecation?<br>• Anal pain? | • Predominant BSFS type 1–2?<br>• Infrequent defecations?<br>• Over-the-counter medication history?<br>• Opiate use?<br>• Cannabinoid use?<br>*BSFS <3 more predictive of STC than decreased frequency[3]*<br>*Symptoms alone cannot differentiate between RED and STC[4]* |

(continued on next page)

| | Table 4 (continued) | | |
|---|---|---|---|
| **Subtype** | **Normal Transit Constipation (NTC)** | **Rectal Evacuation Disorder (RED)** | **Slow Transit Constipation (STC)** |
| Common testing | • Stool diary<br>• Investigations for alarm symptoms if present<br>• Complete blood count<br>• Thyroid cascade<br>• Fasting serum glucose<br>• Calcium[d]<br>• Colonoscopy:<br>  ○ nly if due for screening or alarm symptoms present | Physiologic:<br>• Balloon expulsion test<br>• Anorectal manometry<br>• Simple rectal balloon distension<br>• Pelvic floor electromyography<br>Physiologic and Structural:<br>• Defecography (barium, MRI)<br>Structural:<br>• Endoanal imaging (ultrasound, MRI) | • Appropriate testing to rule out RED<br>Physiologic:<br>• Sitz Marker study<br>• Wireless motility capsule<br>• Scintigraphy<br>Physiologic and structural:<br>• Rectal barostat<br>• Colonic manometry |

[a] Some criteria have been proposed by previous investigators but have not been formally established by consensus groups.
[b] Proposed diagnostic criteria by Rao and Patcharatrakul[8]: "Dyssynergic pattern of defecation (Types I-IV) is defined as a paradoxic increase in anal sphincter pressure or less than 20% relaxation of resting anal sphincter pressure, or inadequate propulsive forces observed on manometry, imaging, or electromyographic recordings."
[c] For RED: high sensitivity/low specificity: incomplete evacuation; high specificity/low sensitivity: sense of obstruction, digital maneuvers.[3]
[d] Fasting serum glucose, thyroid cascade, and calcium frequently tested but diagnostic utility and cost-effectiveness are questionable.[7]

Important clinical questions include the predominant stool consistency according to a standard scale such as the Bristol Stool Form Scale,[18] assessing possible systemic or neurologic disease, and determining whether the patient is experiencing a call to stool. In patients with suspected rectal evacuation disorder, the diagnosis rests on the identification of abnormal findings on the history including history of sexual abuse, obstetric trauma, excessive straining, sense of incomplete rectal evacuation, anal pain, and digitation of the anal canal or vagina to facilitate defecation. In addition, abnormalities on digital rectal examination described previously should be sought. In patients with suspected slow transit constipation, documentation of slow transit is required based on validated tests, of which the most commonly available is the radiopaque marker or Sitz markers test.

In specialized centers, other measurements of colonic transit include scintigraphy or wireless motility capsule. **Fig. 2** demonstrates regional transit profiles through the colon at 24 and 48 hours, illustrating the lower geometric center of radioisotopes in the colonic regions, particularly at 48 hours, as well as the prolonged $T_{1/2}$ ascending colon emptying time, indicating slow transit constipation, but not in patients with dyssynergic defecation. Because overall colonic transit is frequently retarded in patients with evacuation disorder, there is a clear advantage provided by measurement of regional colonic transit and, particularly, ascending colon emptying with scintigraphy to identify the proximal colonic emptying in slow transit constipation.[17] The degree of regional transit differentiation is clearly shown by the radiopaque marker transit measurement, but not by measurements obtained with the wireless motility capsule.

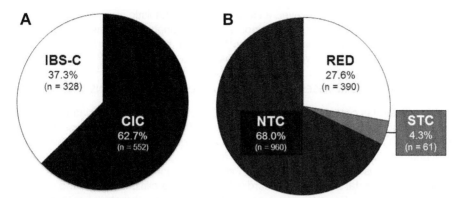

**Fig. 1.** (A) Respondents from 2010 US population-based survey meeting Rome III criteria for IBS-C versus chronic idiopathic constipation (CIC). (B) Constipation subtype stratification of 1411 patients using anorectal manometry, balloon expulsion, and colon transit scintigraphy between 1994 and 2011. NTC, normal transit constipation; RED, rectal evacuation disorder; STC, slow transit constipation. (*Adapted from* Heidelbaugh JJ, Stelwagon M, Miller SA, Shea EP, Chey WD. The spectrum of constipation-predominant irritable bowel syndrome and chronic idiopathic constipation: US survey assessing symptoms, care seeking, and disease burden. Am J Gastroenterol 2015;110:580-587; and *Data from* Nullens S, Nelsen T, Camilleri M, Burton D, Eckert D, Iturrino J, Vazquez-Roque M, Zinsmeister AR. Regional colon transit in patients with dys-synergic defaecation or slow transit in patients with constipation. Gut 2012;61:1132-1139.)

In patients with slow transit constipation, it is critically important to exclude exposure to medications that could retard colonic transit, particularly opioids. The potential effect of cannabinoid use in the development of slow transit or normal transit constipation is presently unclear because there have been no large studies to document the

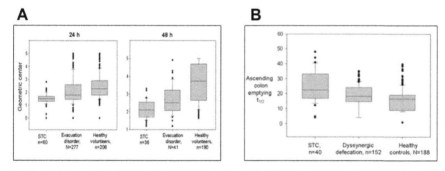

**Fig. 2.** (A) Colonic scintigraphy demonstrating distribution of geometric centers at 24 and 48 hours (median, interquartile range) in patients with slow transit constipation (STC) as compared with evacuation disorders and healthy volunteers. Note the large overlap of colonic transit in both STC and evacuation disorder groups. (B) Regional transit profile for stool predominantly in ascending colon for patients with STC as compared with those with dyssynergic defecation or healthy controls. (*From* Nullens S, Nelsen T, Camilleri M, Burton D, Eckert D, Iturrino J, Vazquez-Roque M, Zinsmeister AR. Regional colon transit in patients with dys-synergic defaecation or slow transit in patients with constipation. Gut 2012;61:1132-1139.)

effects of cannabinoids. However, a single-center mechanistic study with the nonselective cannabinoid agonist, dronabinol, showed dronabinol inhibited postprandial colonic tone and phasic pressure activity,[19] although it did not retard colonic transit in patients with irritable bowel syndrome associated with diarrhea.[20]

## COMMON PITFALLS IN ASSESSMENT OF REFRACTORY CHRONIC CONSTIPATION

**Table 5** illustrates common pitfalls in the assessment of chronic constipation that may contribute to the refractory symptoms. The first pitfall is incomplete assessment of a rectal evacuation disorder, either because of an inadequate digital rectal examination that had not assessed anorectal function at rest, during anal squeeze, and during bear down, or because of "normal" results on anorectal manometry, despite high pretest probability for rectal evacuation disorder based on the clinical history and a digital rectal examination. For example, inadequate effort during the straining to simulate the evacuation process may result in a low push pressure of less than 45 mm Hg. Another pitfall in the anorectal manometry results arises from the values obtained for rectoanal pressure gradient during bear down. The literature is replete with different normal values, based on inadequate control of sample sizes and lack of stratification based on age and gender. As mentioned previously, a balloon expulsion time of greater than 30 seconds should be considered in addressing a rectal evacuation disorder in the clinical consult. It is, therefore, important to interpret the anorectal manometry findings based on the totality of information obtained from the history, digital rectal examination, and an overall assessment of the evacuation function based on balloon expulsion time and manometric results.

A third common pitfall results from an incomplete drug history, and it is important to obtain a detailed history of over-the-counter medications, common prescription medications that cause constipation, such as antinausea medications, and recreational drug use. Finally, chronic constipation may be refractory because of failure to identify systemic, neurologic, or psychiatric diseases.

## SIGNIFICANT COLONIC DISEASES RESULTING IN SLOW TRANSIT CONSTIPATION

The most relevant colonic diseases that result in slow transit constipation reflect disturbances in the extrinsic or intrinsic neural control, or defects in the collagen and muscular layers of the colon. The most commonly encountered diseases of neural control that lead to refractory chronic constipation are Parkinson disease, multiple sclerosis, spinal cord injury, and, more rarely, peripheral and autonomic neuropathies, such as diabetes mellitus and amyloidosis. Such conditions are also aggravated by the medications used in the treatment of the neurologic manifestations. In the absence of such neurologic diseases, slow transit constipation and colonic inertia typically result from disturbances of enteric mechanisms including loss of interstitial cells of Cajal.[21] In the presence of dilatation of the colon or a marked increase in colonic compliance, chronic megacolon may be sporadic, syndromic or familial and may present in adolescence or adulthood.[15,22–24]

## CHOICE OF THERAPY FOR REFRACTORY CHRONIC CONSTIPATION

The choice of therapy is predicated by the correct classification of chronic constipation. Commonly used medications for chronic idiopathic constipation are summarized in **Table 6**.[25–27] In patients with rectal evacuation disorder, the gold standard for treatment is pelvic floor retraining with relaxation and biofeedback. Based on controlled clinical trials conducted predominantly in academic medical centers, symptoms and

**Table 5**
**Common pitfalls in assessment of refractory chronic constipation**

| Pitfall | Cause | Solution |
|---|---|---|
| Incomplete assessment for rectal evacuation disorder (RED) | A. Inadequate *digital rectal exam (DRE)* | A. *Perform* DRE and *look for pathology*:<br>3 phases: rest, anal squeeze, bear down<br>2 positions: lateral decubitus, squatting<br>*Visualize* and *palpate* at all 3 phases |
| | B. *"Normal"* results on anorectal manometry despite high pretest probability for RED | B. *Document pretest probability* for RED *before* testing<br>Most predictive of RED:<br>• Abnormal DRE<br>• low push rectal pressure <45 mm Hg<br>• Type IV dyssynergia<br>• positive rectoanal pressure gradient (normal) |
| | C. No testing for *structural* pathology despite high pretest probability | C. Obtain thorough *pelvic floor history*:<br>• *Obstetric* (vaginal deliveries, tears)<br>• *Sexual abuse* history<br>• Involuntarily reported symptoms:<br>  ○ Digital maneuvers<br>  ○ Sensation of obstruction<br>  ○ Sensation of incomplete evacuation<br>  ○ Fecal incontinence, urgency<br>  ○ Sensation of pelvic pressure/bulge<br>  ○ Anal pain<br>  ○ Impairment of sex life<br>• Urinary voiding dysfunction |
| Incomplete drug history | A. Over-the-counter medications not readily reported | A. Intentionally ask about common culprit medications:<br>• *Tylenol PM* (diphenhydramine)<br>• *Antiallergy* medications (cetirizine, fexofenadine)<br>• *Antacids* (Tums, Maalox, Gaviscon)<br>• Herbals (*peppermint oil*)[36,37] |
| | B. Common *prescription* medications with less-recognized effects on colonic motility | B. Intentionally ask about common culprit medications:<br>• 5HT3 antagonists (*ondansetron*)<br>• *Promethazine* |
| | C. Recreational substance use | C. Intentionally ask about *cannabinoids/opiates*:<br>• THC preparations (dronabinol)~ |

*(continued on next page)*

| Table 5 *(continued)* | | |
| --- | --- | --- |
| **Pitfall** | **Cause** | **Solution** |
| Inadequate assessment for systemic disease | A. Inadequate exploration of *extra-gastrointestinal symptoms* indicating systemic disease | A. Investigate important systems/examination findings<br>• *Skin* (sclerodactyly, laxity, easy bruising)<br>• *Neuro* (peripheral neuropathy, resting tremor)<br>• *Psychiatric* (body mass index, bulimia examination findings) |

anorectal parameters (eg, balloon expulsion time) improved to a greater extent after manometry-guided biofeedback therapy than after sham feedback and standard treatment, with approximately 70% of patients benefiting. The benefit was also sustained during long-term follow-up, although the proportion of patients dropped by approximately 10%.[28–30]

Biofeedback therapy significantly improves quality of life in patients with defecatory disorders, regardless of home or office setting. Home biofeedback is a cost-effective treatment option for defecatory disorders compared with office biofeedback, and it offers the potential of treating many more patients in the community.[31]

**Table 6** summarizes the different classes of medications used in the treatment of chronic idiopathic constipation, including the primary outcomes demonstrated with each medication, assessment of efficacy based on the number needed to treat, and adverse effects based on the number needed to harm, as well as the estimated cost of each of the medications in the United States. Although the different trials have not actually subselected patients with documented slow transit constipation in the assessment of efficacy of the treatment in patients with slow transit constipation among those with chronic idiopathic constipation, it is common in clinical practice to select a stimulant, over-the-counter agent (such as bisacodyl or a senna alkaloid), or a colonic prokinetic (such as the $5HT_4$ receptor agonist, prucalopride) for patients with slow transit constipation. For patients with normal transit constipation, osmotic or secretory agents are often preferred as first-line agents before considering stimulants or prokinetic agents. Elobixibat, an ileal bile acid transport inhibitor, is approved in Japan. Based on a network meta-analysis in which the relative efficacies of active medications were compared with the therapeutic benefits of placebo, the approved drugs for chronic idiopathic constipation showed similar efficacy for the primary endpoints, that is ≥3 complete spontaneous bowel movements (CSBMs)/wk and increase over baseline by ≥1 CSBMs/wk (which are used together as the combined endpoint in registration clinical trials for review and approval by the Food and Drug Administration). The most effective medication may be bisacodyl, based on the change from baseline in the number of spontaneous bowel movements per week and CSBMs/wk compared with other drugs.[4] However, it must be stressed that the relative efficacy was not based on head-to-head comparisons of the diverse medications.[4]

Infrequently, patients do not respond to all available medications or classes (fiber, osmotic, secretory, stimulant, or prokinetic) and may continue to experience constipation despite resolution of rectal evacuation disorder with biofeedback therapy and pharmacologic treatment. In such patients, further evaluation of colonic motor function with intraluminal colonic manometry and measurements of compliance and

**Table 6**
**Efficacy of common medications for CIC**

| Drug | Primary Outcome | Efficacy: NNT (95% CI) | Adverse Effects NNH (95% CI) | Cost/ mo |
|---|---|---|---|---|
| **Over the counter** | | | | |
| Soluble fiber (psyllium)[25] | Global symptoms | 2.6 | 5.6 | $16 |
| | Straining | 3.7 | *Abdominal pain* | |
| | Pain on defecation | 6.4 | | |
| | Increase in mean no. of stools/wk | 3.8 stools/wk after fiber vs. 2.9 stools at baseline | | |
| Laxatives[26] | ≥3 stools/wk, ≥3 CSBMs/wk or no need for rescue laxative use | 3 (2–4) | 3 (2–6) *Diarrhea* | |
| *Osmotic* | ≥3 stools/wk, ≥3 CSBMs/wk or need for regular laxative use | 3 (2–4) | | $11 |
| *Stimulant* | ≥3 CSBMs/wk | 3 (2–3.5) | | $3 |
| **Prescription** | | | | |
| *Intestinal secretagogues* | | | | |
| Linaclotide[27] | Increase in CSBM >1/wk and ≥3 CSBM/wk for at least 75% of weeks in a 12 wk trial | 72 μg 12 (6–29) 145 μg 10 (6–19) | 72 μg 9 (6–18) 145 μg 9 (6–13) *Diarrhea* | $423 |
| Lubiprostone[26] | ≥3–4 SBM/wk | 24 μg 4 (3–7) | 4 (3–7) *Total AEs* | $288 |
| Plecanatide[27] | Increase in CSBM >1/wk and ≥3 CSBM/wk for at least 75% of weeks and response in 3 of last 4 wk of trial | 3mg 11 (8–19) 6mg 12 (8–23) | 27 (11–89) 27 (13–72) *Diarrhea%* | $416 |
| *5HT4 agonists* | | | | |
| Prucalopride[26] | ≥3 CSBM/wk | 6 (5–9) | 10 (6–29) *Total AEs* | $428 |

*Abbreviations:* AE, adverse events; CI, confidence interval; CIC, chronic idiopathic constipation; CSBM, complete spontaneous bowel movements; NNH, number needed to harm; NNT, number needed to treat; RR, relative risk; SBM, spontaneous bowel movements.

tone[13–15] are recommended to definitively diagnose colonic inertia, as manifested by a lack of a colonic motor response to feeding, intravenous neostigmine,[14] or intraluminal bisacodyl.[32] After documenting colonic inertia and/or failure to respond to medical therapy, a small minority of patients could be considered for total colectomy with ileorectal anastomosis.[33]

## THE SPECIAL CIRCUMSTANCE OF DESCENDING PERINEUM SYNDROME AND EHLERS-DANLOS SYNDROME

Following multiple vaginal deliveries, especially those associated with forceps or vacuum-facilitated delivery, patients may present in the seventh or eighth decade with severe, refractory chronic constipation associated with descending perineum syndrome.[34] This is often associated with an anterior rectocele and, possibly, rectal mucosal or pelvic organ prolapse.[35] Such patients are often refractory to medical therapy and to pelvic floor retraining. Presentation with such a clinical picture in a young or nulliparous patient raises the clinical suspicion of Ehlers-Danlos syndrome or other connective tissue disorders. In such patients, the constipation may be refractory and may require surgical intervention, depending on the structural deficit identified, such as pelvic organ prolapse. It is imperative to manage these patients with a multidisciplinary team that includes physical medicine therapy, urogynecology, and colorectal surgery, in addition to gastroenterology. Sometimes it is necessary to treat the patient with an end-ileostomy to provide the best quality of life.

## SUMMARY

Refractory chronic constipation is typically responsive to therapy and is no longer refractory once a more detailed appraisal of the patient and a correct pathophysiological diagnosis are achieved. Optimal management requires a thorough clinical history, physical examination, measurements of defecatory as well as colonic motor functions, and management by a multidisciplinary team.

## REFERENCES

1. Lacy BE, Mearin F, Chang L, et al. Bowel disorders. Gastroenterology 2016. https://doi.org/10.1053/j.gastro.2016.02.031.
2. Saad RJ, Rao SS, Koch KL, et al. Do stool form and frequency correlate with whole-gut and colonic transit? Results from a multicenter study in constipated individuals and healthy controls. Am J Gastroenterol 2010;105:403–11.
3. Koch A, Voderholzer WA, Klauser AG, et al. Symptoms in chronic constipation. Dis Colon Rectum 1997;40:902–6.
4. Nelson AD, Camlleri M, Chirapongsathorn S, et al. Comparison of efficacy of pharmacological treatments for chronic idiopathic constipation: a systematic review and network meta-analysis. Gut 2017;66:1611–22.
5. Nelson AD, Mouchli MA, Valentin N, et al. Ehlers Danlos syndrome and gastrointestinal manifestations: a 20-year experience at Mayo Clinic. Neurogastroenterol Motil 2015;27:1657–66.
6. Voderholzer WA, Schatke W, Mühldorfer BE, et al. Clinical response to dietary fiber treatment of chronic constipation. Am J Gastroenterol 1997;92:95–8.
7. Muller-Lissner SA, Kamm MA, Scarpignato C, et al. Myths and misconceptions about chronic constipation. Am J Gastroenterol 2005;100:232–42.
8. Rao SS, Patcharatrakul T. Diagnosis and treatment of dyssynergic defecation. J Neurogastroenterol Motil 2016;22:423–35.

9. Rao SS, Rattanakovit K, Patcharatrakul T. Diagnosis and management of chronic constipation in adults. Nat Rev Gastroenterol Hepatol 2016;13:295–305.

10. Grossi U, Carrington EV, Bharucha AE, et al. Diagnostic accuracy study of anorectal manometry for diagnosis of dyssynergic defecation. Gut 2016;65:447–55.

11. Chedid V, Vijayvargiya P, Halawi H, et al. Audit of the diagnosis of rectal evacuation disorders in chronic constipation. Neurogastroenterol Motil 2019;31: e13510.

12. Oblizajek NR, Gandhi S, Sharma M, et al. Anorectal pressures measured with high-resolution manometry in healthy people: normal values and asymptomatic pelvic floor dysfunction. Neurogastroenterol Motil 2019;31:e13597.

13. Ravi K, Bharucha AE, Camilleri M, et al. Phenotypic variation of colonic motor functions in chronic constipation. Gastroenterology 2010;138:89–97.

14. Mouchli MA, Camilleri M, Lee T, et al. Evaluating the safety and the effects on colonic compliance of neostigmine during motility testing in patients with chronic constipation. Neurogastroenterol Motil 2016;28:871–8.

15. Wang XJ, Camilleri M. Chronic megacolon presenting in adolescents or adults: clinical manifestations, diagnosis, and genetic associations. Dig Dis Sci 2019. https://doi.org/10.1007/s10620-019-05605-7.

16. Heidelbaugh JJ, Stelwagon M, Miller SA, et al. The spectrum of constipation-predominant irritable bowel syndrome and chronic idiopathic constipation: US survey assessing symptoms, care seeking, and disease burden. Am J Gastroenterol 2015;110:580–7.

17. Nullens S, Nelsen T, Camilleri M, et al. Regional colon transit in patients with dyssynergic defaecation or slow transit in patients with constipation. Gut 2012;61: 1132–9.

18. Heaton KW, Radvan J, Cripps H, et al. Defecation frequency and timing, and stool form in the general population: a prospective study. Gut 1992;33:818–24.

19. Esfandyari T, Camilleri M, Busciglio I, et al. Effects of a cannabinoid receptor agonist on colonic motor and sensory functions in humans: a randomized, placebo-controlled study. Am J Physiol Gastrointest Liver Physiol 2007;293: G137–45.

20. Wong BS, Camilleri M, Eckert D, et al. Randomized pharmacodynamic and pharmacogenetic trial of dronabinol effects on colon transit in irritable bowel syndrome-diarrhea. Neurogastroenterol Motil 2012;24:358–e169.

21. He CL, Soffer EE, Ferris CD, et al. Loss of interstitial cells of cajal and inhibitory innervation in insulin-dependent diabetes. Gastroenterology 2001;121:427–34.

22. O'Dwyer RH, Acosta A, Camilleri M, et al. Clinical features and colonic motor disturbances in chronic megacolon in adults. Dig Dis Sci 2015;60:2398–407.

23. Gibbons D, Camilleri M, Nelson AD, et al. Characteristics of chronic megacolon among patients diagnosed with multiple endocrine neoplasia type 2B. United Eur Gastroenterol J 2016;4:449–54.

24. Camilleri M, Wieben E, Eckert D, et al. Familial chronic megacolon presenting in childhood or adulthood: seeking the presumed gene association. Neurogastroenterol Motil 2019;31:e13550.

25. Suares NC, Ford AC. Systematic review: the effects of fibre in the management of chronic idiopathic constipation. Aliment Pharmacol Ther 2011;33:895–901.

26. Ford AC, Suares NC. Effect of laxatives and pharmacological therapies in chronic idiopathic constipation: systematic review and meta-analysis. Gut 2011;60: 209–18.

27. Shah ED, Kim HM, Schoenfeld P. Efficacy and tolerability of guanylate cyclase-C agonists for irritable bowel syndrome with constipation and chronic idiopathic

constipation: a systematic review and meta-analysis. Am J Gastroenterol 2018; 113:329–38.

28. Chiarioni G, Whitehead WE, Pezza V, et al. Biofeedback is superior to laxatives for normal transit constipation due to pelvic floor dyssynergia. Gastroenterology 2006;130:657–64.

29. Heymen S, Scarlett Y, Jones K, et al. Randomized, controlled trial shows biofeedback to be superior to alternative treatments for patients with pelvic floor dyssynergia-type constipation. Dis Colon Rectum 2007;50:428–41.

30. Rao SS, Valestin J, Brown CK, et al. Long-term efficacy of biofeedback therapy for dyssynergic defecation: randomized controlled trial. Am J Gastroenterol 2010;105:890–6.

31. Rao SSC, Go JT, Valestin J, et al. Home biofeedback for the treatment of dyssynergic defecation: does it improve quality of life and is it cost-effective? Am J Gastroenterol 2019;114:938–44.

32. Preston DM, Lennard-Jones JE. Pelvic motility and response to intraluminal bisacodyl in slow-transit constipation. Dig Dis Sci 1985;30:289–94.

33. Singh S, Heady S, Coss-Adame E, et al. Clinical utility of colonic manometry in slow transit constipation. Neurogastroenterol Motil 2013;25:487–95.

34. Harewood GC, Coulie B, Camilleri M, et al. Descending perineum syndrome: audit of clinical and laboratory features and outcome of pelvic floor retraining. Am J Gastroenterol 1999;94:126–30.

35. Ellerkmann RM, Cundiff GW, Melick CF, et al. Correlation of symptoms with location and severity of pelvic organ prolapse. Am J Obstet Gynecol 2001;185: 1332–7 [discussion: 1337–8].

36. Amato A, Liotta R, Mule F. Effects of menthol on circular smooth muscle of human colon: analysis of the mechanism of action. Eur J Pharmacol 2014;740:295–301.

37. Grigoleit HG, Grigoleit P. Gastrointestinal clinical pharmacology of peppermint oil. Phytomedicine 2005;12:607–11.

Printed and bound by CPI Group (UK) Ltd, Croydon, CR0 4YY

03/10/2024

01040479-0008